Praise for *Supp*

"Attention must be paid to Mike Fillon's *Supplements Under Siege*. You ignore the information that this harbinger brings at your personal peril. Read, no, study this informative book now, or live by the legislation that will be enacted by your inaction."

—Louie Free, Host, Nationally syndicated
Louie Free Radio Show

"*Supplements Under Siege* is a timely and important book that anyone interested in preserving our freedom of health-care choices needs to read. Mike has definitely done his homework."

—Nicole Brechka
Editor in Chief, *GreatLife* magazine

"It's about time someone told the truth about the FDA."

—Norman Mark, Host, Nationally syndicated
radio show *Health Marks*

"Mike Fillon is a superb investigative reporter who has been able to discover and then connect many of the dots that may eventually lead to a full exposé and congressional investigation of what he boldly calls 'the conspiracy to take away your vitamins, minerals, and herbs.'

When Big Pharma demands that we surrender our most therapeutic supplements, an appropriate response might be 'Give up? Never!' Thanks to Mike Fillon, we have just begun to connect the dots."

—Clinton Ray Miller
Health Freedom Legislative Advocate

"Mike Fillon documents the concerted efforts of the drug industry, in conjunction with government agencies, to exert a double standard against dietary supplements, effectively limiting the choice of Americans to any color pill, as long as it's a drug. A must-read for anyone who values the freedom to choose the health care that's right for them."

—Robert Scott Bell, D.A.Hom.
Host, Nationally syndicated radio show
Jump-Start Your Health

Supplements Under Siege

INSIDE THE CONSPIRACY TO TAKE AWAY YOUR VITAMINS, MINERALS, AND HERBS

Mike Fillon

Here's To Health Freedom

Mike Fillon

WOODLAND PUBLISHING

For ordering information and bulk order discounts, contact:
Woodland Publishing, 448 East 800 North, Orem, UT 84097
Toll-free telephone: (800) 777-2665

Please visit our Web site: www.woodlandpublishing.com

Note: The information in this book is for educational purposes only and is not recommended as a means of diagnosing or treating an illness. All matters concerning physical and mental health should be supervised by a health practitioner knowledgeable in treating that particular condition. Neither the publisher nor author directly or indirectly dispenses medical advice, nor do they prescribe any remedies or assume any responsibility for those who choose to treat themselves.

Cover design: Joseph Bonyata
Cover art copright © Getty Images

A cataloging-in-publication record for this book is available from the Library of Congress.

ISBN-10: 1-58054-410-X
ISBN-13: 978-1-58054-410-8

Printed in the United States of America

06   07   08   09   10   1   2   3   4   5   6   7   8   9   10

For Evan

Contents

CONTENTS

Preface

"Oh, What a Tangled Web We Weave . . ."

You might think the title of this book is a bit over the top, but a few interesting things happened while I wrote it that only reinforced everything else included here. In fact, I crumpled up and threw away the original preface to the book after the Office of Complementary Medicine trumpeted a study they sponsored that appeared in the *New England Journal of Medicine* showing that echinacea, the second most popular selling herb, wasn't effective in preventing or treating the common cold. In other words, there was "no benefit" in taking echinacea.

If you read or viewed any of these news reports, you'd be perfectly justified in thinking you'd be wasting your money if you ever took the stuff again. But before you toss your echinacea, there are a couple of things you should know.

I reviewed seventeen of the dozens of articles appearing the next day about the study, and only one reported the actual dosages the subjects took (the *New York Times*). What's interesting is that both the abstract at the *NEJM* site—the full article requires a paid subscription—and the press release from the NIH's Office of Complementary Medicine did not reveal what dosage study participants took, so it's impossible for the average person to gauge the effectiveness of the herb versus what they might use themselves. Could it be they didn't want us to know?

Mark Blumenthal, founder and executive director of the nonprofit American Botanical Council (ABC) said in a released statement that it would have been optimal if this trial had tested the echinacea preparations at more frequent and/or higher doses. "Dosage is one of the most important aspects in assessing any therapeutic agent. Many clinicians who recommend echinacea for treatment of upper respiratory tract infections related to colds and flu normally utilize a frequency of use and/or a total daily dose that is higher than the one used in this trial."

Try this: if you take aspirin or ibuprofen for headaches try cutting one of the pills into thirds and take only one slice. Do you think it would be as effective? I doubt you'll ever see a study on the effectiveness of one-third of an aspirin tablet.

Since echinacea is an herb and therefore part of this book, I did a little digging. It turns out the lead investigator of the study, and the one quoted most often in news accounts is Ronald B. Turner, M.D., professor of pediatrics at the University of Virginia School of Medicine in Charlottesville, Virginia. While Dr. Turner's credentials are impressive, and he's considered an expert in the field, there's one aspect of his career he didn't disclose, and the press hasn't investigated. I think it could be a potentially serious conflict of interest.

At a roundtable discussion at the 2002 American Thoracic Society meeting about viral respiratory infections, Dr. Turner was compelled to reveal—these are ATS's words not mine—"A significant relationship with industry." It turns out Dr. Turner's "significant relationship" was with a company named ViroPharma that developed a drug named Pleconaril, a compound targeting the primary viral cause of the common cold.

This is an interesting drug. From 1997 to 2002 there were nearly a thousand news stories on Pleconaril in newspapers and on television. In an article in the *British Medical Journal,* reporters wore out their thesauri trying to come up with superlative terms for the drug such as "cure," "miracle," "wonder drug," "super drug" and "a medical first." It was described as "good news for physicians and their patients," "potentially huge," and as a treatment that "may drastically help relieve your misery." It was compared with the search for the Holy Grail and with humankind's landing on the moon. Most of the stories reported that the drug appeared to cause few side effects, none serious. In January 2000, the Associated Press wire service ran a story quoting one ViroPharma–funded investigator saying, "This *is* the cure for the common cold."

In December 2001, the *Los Angeles Times* ran a story entitled "The Cold Virus Meets Its Match." The article quoted Dr. Turner pontificating about Pleconaril and another drug under investigation, saying that "both of these drugs are very potent antiviral agents that work against a broad spectrum of different rhinoviruses." Wow! He should know, even though in that article Dr. Turner didn't admit he was involved in the clinical trials for Pleconaril.

A few months later the FDA issued a "not approvable" letter for an oral tablet formulation of Pleconaril for treatment of the common cold in adults. The FDA cited clinical data showing that the span of cold symptoms of subjects taking Pleconaril was reduced by only a day. As for those "few side effects, none serious," it seems the drug upset the menstrual cycle in many women and, to their dismay, a few women on birth control pills testing the drug became pregnant. Oops! I guess Dr. Turner missed that pesky little side effect. Oh, well, back to the drawing board.

In the same *BMJ* article, Dr. Turner blamed the media for the hype. He called the news coverage a disservice to the public, contributing to the public's science illiteracy. "People can't distinguish between valid results and charlatanism," he told the *BMJ*. "You pick up the paper one day and read that cholesterol causes heart attacks and you pick it up the next day and read that it doesn't. It becomes easy for people to feel that scientists don't know what they're doing."

OK, Dr. Turner. Thanks for clearing that up.

Three years after the oral formulation failed to receive approval, ViroPharma licensed rights to develop and commercialize intranasal Pleconaril in the United States and Canada from Sanofi-Synthelabo. Than late in 2004, ViroPharma entered into an option agreement to license ViroPharma's intranasal formulation of Pleconaril to Schering-Plough for the treatment of the common cold in the United States and Canada. The latest reports say it could be on the market in 2006.

So let's recap: an oral formulation of a drug fails, so the company develops an intranasal formulation. One of their researchers—

without revealing he has had ties to the company—then tests a low-dosage version of a popular herbal competitor against the drug being developed by the company he had or has "a significant relationship" with, and declares the herbal product doesn't work.

Neat trick—and his fingers never left his hand.

". . . when first we practice to deceive."

The other interesting event happened a few months earlier. In April, Nutraceutical Corporation successfully sued the FDA over its ephedra ban, and soon after ephedra-based products began appearing on the market. During the four months since they lost the case, the FDA hasn't uttered a peep about it. If they banned the herb because it was supposedly so dangerous, why didn't they file an appeal immediately?

Maybe they've been too busy lifting the thirteen-year ban on silicone gel–filled breast implants to worry about ephedra. Or maybe their time is occupied with reinstating Vioxx, even though there was suppression of evidence regarding its safety—between 88,000 and 139,000 people had heart attacks, of which 30–40 percent probably died—and the majority of the medical panel that approved it had ties to the pharmaceutical industry.

They couldn't turn to the RAND report, which they once touted, nor could they point to the white paper on the FDA Web site stating that ephedra isn't dangerous. Could it be they were caught pushing emotional appeals and shoddy evidence?

The FDA often says its hands are tied when it comes to regulating dietary supplements, which in addition to vitamins and minerals, includes herbs like ephedra and echinacea. That's hogwash. Numerous government agencies can recall or ban defective products whether it' a car that rolls over, flammable baby pajamas, or an herb that's dangerous. But, they need to have proof. With ephedra the FDA had none.

Supplements Under Siege? As you'll see, the title may not be over the top at all.

Introduction:
Why I Wrote This Book, and
Why I Wrote It Now

The ringing phone jarred me awake. Woodland Publishing had just released my latest book, *Real RDAs for Real People,* and I looked forward to a period of long walks and short naps as I recovered mentally. The phone call came during one of the latter.

On the other end of the line were Woodland's editor-in-chief and publisher. We exchanged a few perfunctory "atta' boys" and "good jobs" about the just-released book as I yawned myself awake. In the book, I described how the nutritional standards, principally developed by the U.S. Department of Agriculture, were heavily influenced by lobbying efforts of various food industries. I also reported how the standards were based on surveys of what people eat and had little scientific merit.

I also pointed out how the nutritional standards recommended minimum amounts to prevent diseases like beri-beri and scurvy, not the optimum quantities of nutrients our bodies need. The book required a lot of digging as well as the debunking of accepted truths. The book was the culmination of an agonizing journey, and it had also been an awakening, but nothing like I later experienced, as you'll see.

But I digress a bit.

After we exchanged pleasantries, the editors at Woodland asked me what I knew about ephedra. At the time of the conference call—February 2003—there was a great deal of media coverage about the dangers of the herb, the substance an estimated twelve to seventeen million people were taking annually to lose weight and stoke their athletic performance. Around the time of the phone call, blaring headlines reported that ephedra was in Baltimore Orioles pitcher Steve Bechler's locker when he died and that the substance was found in his stomach.

Keep in mind that I have been a health and medical writer for many years. I've written nearly two hundred articles for WebMD, the CBS HealthWatch Web site, and the original Dr. Koop site (named for the former U.S. Surgeon General). I had written a number of chapters for a *Reader's Digest* health book and covered and reported dozens of stories from a number of medical conferences for a Web site for medical doctors. I'd also been reporting on medical technological advances for *Popular Mechanics* magazine for more than fifteen years. While I've never been afraid to tackle controversial subjects, I could be best described as a truly mainstream health reporter.

This is my reality. Every day dozens of health reports and medical studies cross my desk. Plus, each day I scan newspaper headlines from across the country. I hadn't taken much interest in ephedra, probably because I never took it, and never planned to. I wrote one article about the herb a few years earlier for WebMD, but I wrote so many articles for them over a year or so, the details were lost in that region of the brain where so much of the data tucked into short-term memory goes and hides. I rake-combed my hair with my fingers, stifled another yawn, and answered, "From what I've read, ephedra is killing people."

They wondered that since it was in the news so much, and so many people were taking it, whether it might be an important topic for a short book. Frankly, I was lukewarm to the idea and I think it must have come across in my voice. They asked if I would look into it for a few days and let them know if I was interested.

So I thought, "What the heck?" I'd look at a few of the studies the press reports cited and if I could, build a case for consumers not to risk their health taking it. I figured it might be an easy gig. Another part of me wondered whether the topic would hold my interest since it appeared to be an open-and-shut case—ephedra was dangerous. "I'll let you know in a few days," I said.

Diving In

The next day I reviewed a few of the press reports from major newspapers and found they mostly quoted the FDA and not any meaningful medical studies. Then I stumbled upon the name Richard Kreider, Ph.D. I found out Dr. Kreider was and is professor and chair of the Exercise and Sport Nutrition Lab in the Center for Exercise, Nutrition and Preventive Health in the Department of Health, Human Performance and Recreation at Baylor University in Waco, Texas. What drew my interest was an eye-popping open letter Dr. Kreider and his colleagues wrote that appeared on the Baylor University Web site.

After I read the letter I muttered to myself, "This can't be right."

Kreider and his staff wrote that they didn't believe ephedra killed Steve Bechler. Their letter was chilling and went against everything I had read about Steve Bechler's death. I decided to see if Dr. Kreider might have had an alternative agenda. Perhaps he was a proponent of muscle-building supplements, including anabolic steroids or took money to promote an ephedra product. I simply didn't know. I discovered that Dr. Kreider was also president of the American Society of Exercise Physiologists, which in its bylaws forbids promoting products for money. I also checked some other written material attributed to Dr. Kreider. From all indications, he checked out as a reliable source.

I then discovered a 1997 transcript from a Congressional hearing during an earlier attempt by the FDA to ban ephedra. During the hearings, members of Congress criticized how the Food and Drug

Administration counted deaths attributed to ephedra, including a women who crashed her car into a pole. While it's true she had taken ephedra, her blood-alcohol level was far above the legal limit. The truth is, she was drunk and died from injuries sustained in the car crash.

During that same period, a General Accounting Office (GAO) report came out criticizing the manner in which the FDA's policy was developed, especially the adverse event reports (AERs) allegedly associated with ephedra. Members of Congress were appalled after reviewing the report. "I am concerned about the apparent lack of scientific data behind the FDA's actions," said House Science Committee Chairman F. James Sensenbrenner, Jr. (R-WI). "For the FDA—one of the most important regulatory agencies in government—to use such poor science for a dietary supplement raises warning flags for the other products the agency regulates."

A bell went off in my head. I rummaged around my office and dug up my notes from the ephedra story I wrote earlier for WebMD. While researching the piece, I spoke to a researcher who never questioned the effectiveness of ephedra for weight loss or to boost energy. Instead he harped on the lack of manufacturing standards some producers used. It suddenly came back to me. He claimed sometimes the amount of ephedra in the capsules exceeded what the label stated. I distinctly remembered him saying what was lacking was Good Manufacturing Practices, or GMPs.

With that information in mind I looked at the DSHEA law. It required the FDA to establish GMPs for dietary supplements. Nearly ten years later, the FDA still had not gotten around to it. As a result, many reputable dietary supplement manufacturers looked at the GMPs for food—and to add a margin of safety—exceeded them.

I found even more disturbing things during my initial research. Soon after Steve Bechler's death, one of his teammates made the following statement: "There's almost a witch hunt going on," said David Segui. "It hasn't been proven that ephedrine caused his death. There was probably some milk found in his system, too. Did that cause his death?" No, not milk, but there were reports he drank diet soft drinks containing aspartame, a controversial substance in its own right.

Have you ever had one of those cold-sweat moments when you discover a person you know was in actuality nothing at all like you thought, or something you firmly believed was an absolute truth was completely wrong? I did, and more than once as I researched the ephedra controversy.

I wondered, were the Department of Health and Human Services (HHS) and the FDA incompetent, lazy, or being purposely deceitful? Were they so inept that they found it impossible to sift through the facts? At best, could it be they were they being overly cautious and trying to "baby" us? I don't think so. Here's why.

As Dr. Kreider later wrote—in the introduction to the book I ended up writing (titled *Ephedra Fact & Fiction*):

> The debate over the safety and efficacy of ephedra is a classic example of how misinformation portrayed in the media and from various special interest groups can cause a political and legal firestorm about a dietary supplement. Although a significant body of scientific evidence indicates that use of synthetic ephedrine or herbal ephedra can safely promote weight loss when used as directed in overweight but otherwise healthy individuals, there have been unprecedented efforts made to see that ephedra is banned for sale in the U.S.

The untoward influence from the long, influential lobbying tentacles I discovered and wrote about in *Real RDAs for Real People* should have been a wake-up call. I guess I was just naïve enough to believe the outside pressure on our nutritional guidelines was an aberration, an isolated case. It now appeared to me it wasn't.

OK—Count Me In

I called Woodland back and agreed to write the book. They told me they were surprised. We settled on a contract, and I immediately dove back in.

I quickly learned things were worse than I thought. I uncovered misleading research on a few government Web sites from not just the

FDA, but also divisions of the National Institutes of Health (NIH). I also found reporters never questioning what the government agencies reported and often acted more like propaganda stenographers rather than journalists. I discovered numerous incidents of sloppy reporting, not just about ephedra, but about a number of other dietary supplements, including St. John's wort, kava, and vitamin E. I found and reported about staged government hearings, hidden evidence, misstatements (OK, lies), and other assorted shenanigans not the least bit representative of a country that historically prided itself on justice, freedom, and truth, or uncovering the lack thereof.

On more than one occasion I called my editor and pleaded, "Please tell me I'm not crazy. I just found such-and-such and no one is reporting it correctly. Am I being stubborn or just plain crazy?" One such incident had to do with St. John's wort, the popular herb used as a mental relaxant and, for some, an antidote for mild to moderate depression. I had been taking it for years and found it helped reduce stress and increased my concentration when deadlines loomed.

In this instance I was stunned when I read a headline appearing on a press release from the National Institute of Mental Health (NIMH): "Study Shows St. John's Wort Ineffective for Major Depression of Moderate Severity."

There are a few things of interest here. First, on the bottle of St. John's wort (SJW) I take, it says it is for "mood enhancement," not necessarily moderate depression. But here's the most interesting finding of the study that appeared in the April 10, 2002 issue of the *Journal of the American Medical Association* (*JAMA*). It found that neither SJW nor the prescription drug Zoloft (sertraline) were more effective than placebo in this particular trial. Media coverage fixed solely on SJW, erroneously reporting that, "St. John's wort doesn't work," yet they did not even mention Zoloft's ineffectiveness.

Here's something else. The whole time the safety of ephedra was being debated one common theme repeated over and over was how the Dietary Supplement Health and Education Act (DSHEA) passed in 1994 tied the FDA's hands when it came to removing dangerous dietary supplements from the market. But here's the truth. The FDA and the Federal Trade Commission (FTC)—and other government agencies—have always had the legal power to remove dangerous products from the market if scientific evidence shows the product is dangerous, and to act against companies who make false claims about their products. Whether they chose to do so is another matter. It seems as if they preferred complaining and hand-wringing rather than acting.

My editor's advice? "I believe you're fine, Mike. Keep going and just report what you find."

Hot Off the Press

When published, the book bore little resemblance to what I first envisioned. Also, my whole attitude and beliefs about the medical profession and our so-called government watchdogs were forever altered.

When the book came out it sold extremely well—at least for the few short months before ephedra was banned for sale in the U.S. So much for the FDA's "tied hands." And by the way, I've never seen the evidence they promised to release proving how dangerous ephedra was. In fact, I'm still waiting.

The announcement of the ban created hardly a ripple except for the die-hard ephedra devotees who ran to their health-food stores and stocked up.

Before the ban, I appeared on a number of radio talk shows to discuss the book. Radio host Robert Scott Bell had me on four times. (Once, he even tracked me down during a pharmaceutical press briefing I attended at a medical conference in Orlando.)

After one appearance on a station in upstate New York I received a terse e-mail from a doctor in the area. After a litany of insults he wrote, " . . . 167 deaths (from ephedra) were listed on the FDA Web site before they made it non-public, I find it hard to believe that you did any research before appearing on the show." He ended by calling me "just a shill for dishonest producers."

It was obvious he didn't know why the FDA stopped listing the number of deaths from ephedra on their Web site. As House Science

Committee Chairman F. James Sensenbrenner, Jr., stated above, Congress was so disgusted with their sloppy job the FDA had no choice.

Also, just before the ban, the FDA trumpeted the pending arrival of a special report from the RAND commission that would show how dangerous ephedra was. There was one tiny problem for the FDA: when the report came out it stated no such thing. Instead, the RAND commission revealed it could only find a handful of incidents where ephedra could be definitely linked to death or other sentinel events such as stroke. Did the FDA or its parent, HHS, report this? No. They just stopped discussing the RAND report.

And here's the kicker, and what I believe is the real reason for the ban: The RAND report stated ephedra was as effective as prescription diet drugs. We'll talk much more about this later.

As for the charge by the doctor that I was a shill, I believe shills are supposed to receive tons of cash in small unmarked bills in the dead of night, take luxurious cruises, and drive a fancy car. Here's the reality: I haven't even set foot in a rowboat in ages—much less taken a cruise—and I still drive the same old trusty van I've been tooling around in for years.

Now, in the interest of full disclosure, Woodland Publishing is a division of Nutraceutical Corporation, which, as its name implies, sells dietary supplements. As the DSHEA law states there has to be a wall between the two. Just as many big companies own other companies that may or may not be related—the conglomerates Lockheed Martin, IBM, and Johnson & Johnson come to mind—such is the case, at least in my experience, between Woodland and its parent, although those three companies are a heck of a lot larger. Here's a better example: Kraft Foods is part of the same company that owns Philip Morris, which manufactures and markets cigarettes, and yet people who know this—despite the companies distancing themselves under a new corporate umbrella known as the Altria Group—don't associate the dangers from smoking with macaroni and cheese.

The truth is, I wouldn't know anyone from Nutraceutical if I bumped into them on the street or if their names appeared on caller ID. And based on how I scrutinize their industry, the people at Woodland probably hope to keep it that way. After all, this is not a book to praise the dietary supplement industry. By and large the dietary supplement industry is a small and fragmented bunch that has been unable to corral the few bad apples that give it a collective black eye. Their trade associations have nowhere near the budget or lobbying footprint the pharmaceutical companies have in D.C.

There's something else you need to know. Despite the conclusions in the RAND report or other evidence I uncovered, I never argued that ephedra was safe. And this is the reason for this book—no one knows. It's as if it were more important for HHS, and its minions at the FDA and NIH, to flex their muscles and test the strength of the DSHEA law, which, in light of what they had been saying all along about how their hands were tied when dealing with DSHEA, would be comical if it weren't so sad and dangerous.

Some Vindication

Despite the nasty comments from the New York doctor, not everyone thought I was grinding someone else's ax. Gary Null is a well-known media celebrity, dietary consultant, and author. When I appeared on his radio show in October 2003 to discuss my books—time out to pat myself on the back—he called me "one of the most prolific researchers and writers on these topics in the United States for many years." And, at the end of the interview—man, my arm is getting tired—he said, "I find your work meticulously well researched and referenced and you have a long history of writing quality scientific reports."

So why was ephedra banned? The age-old reason—money. Was I able to find the smoking gun? Do I have a memo by a pharmaceutical executive or the ultra-powerful lobby group the Pharmaceutical Research and Manufacturers of America (PhRMA) stating, "Let's get rid of ephedra, and while we're at it, let's get rid of all dietary supplements." They don't operate that way. They've perfected the art of getting someone else to do their dirty work: politicians, front groups, strategic PR campaigns, and a media that no longer investigates what it's told if it doesn't deal with a celebrity or a damsel in distress.

I do have plenty of gun powder residue and enough wisps of smoke, though. As for the smoking gun? I believe it was tossed from a speeding car off a bridge into the Sea of Slander, Lake Innuendo, or the Bay of Subterfuge. Simply stated, pharmaceutical companies stood to lose tons of money selling diet pills as long as this low-cost pesky alternative remained on the market without a prescription. However, a witch-hunt and a smear campaign could take care of that and open the door to how the weak DSHEA law made it all possible.

If the safety of the public was the central reason for the ban, then why are antidepressants, linked to teenage suicides, and prescription pain relievers like Vioxx allowed to remain on the market after it was revealed how dangerous they were, and the evidence was covered up?

As a reminder, in November 2004, in front of the Senate Finance Committee, David Graham, M.D., the associate director for science and medicine at the FDA's own Office of Drug Safety testified that Vioxx was responsible for an estimated 38,000 excess heart attacks and sudden cardiac deaths. Graham also stated that this was a conservative estimate. He said that, "a more realistic and likely range of estimates for the number of excess cases in the U.S." was between 88,000 and 139,000. "Of these," he added, "30–40 percent probably died." Was this acceptable, as the drug manufacturers claim, by weighing "risk versus benefit?" Specifically, that this type of drugs eliminates the gastrointestinal problems from over-the-counter (OTC) pain relievers?

That too, it turns out, is not true. I'll explain all about the whole sordid tale later in the book. I'll also tell you troubling stories about cholesterol-reducing drugs, male potency pills, and a host of other troubling drug tales that, chances are, never appeared on the TV news or in your local newspaper.

Before you get the wrong idea, I do not hate the drug companies. Among their employees are top-notch workers and scientists. Many are devoted husbands and wives, sons and daughters. Among their ranks I'm sure are their fair share of field-trip chaperones, den mothers, and soccer coaches. Plus, the drug industry has produced some wonderful life-saving drugs. In one regard, they do what all companies are expected to do in a capitalist society, that is, they make money for their investors, just as the dietary supplement industry tries to do. If you are an investor, maybe with a 401(K) or other retirement account invested in mutual funds, that might mean you. No, my beef with the pharmaceutical industry stems from the the tactics they use, as you'll read later in this book.

Then there's another fundamental issue, which I'll talk to you about later. That is, what should our approach be towards sickness and health? To my way of thinking, sound nutrition and dietary supplements to ward off disease should be a fundamental concern for us all. But can't you see that could be a threat to an industry that needs you to be sick?

No Time to Quit

The ephedra ban didn't quench my interest in the whole dietary supplement issue. I continued to follow the story, and there have been some interesting developments since then.

Former U.S. Representative Billy Tauzin from Louisiana, who led the staged ephedra hearings by the House Subcommittee on Oversight and Investigations (which featured Steve Bechler's parents and a photo of the pitcher as props), is now the president of PhRMA. He earned it. Besides the ephedra charade, and before the left the House, he served as a key arm-twister in the new Medicare drug plan that forbids Medicare from negotiating drug discounts.

I saw another troubling trend continue. When there's a problem with a drug, reporters provide two sides of the story. If there's a question about a vitamin, mineral, or herb, you get one-sided spin.

Vitamin E is a perfect example. There have been over a thousand studies touting the benefits of vitamin E. And yet, when Edgar R. Miller, M.D., associate professor of medicine at Johns Hopkins University, presented findings at the American Heart Association's 2004 scientific meeting of his analysis of nineteen studies involving patients over age sixty who had preexisting conditions, such as cancer, heart disease, Alzheimer's disease, and kidney disease, the media jumped all over the story. Dr. Miller's research revealed that large dosages of vitamin E (400 IU or more) were linked to an increase in death, although no deaths were reported in association with levels of up to 150 IU.

My first reaction was to discontinue taking the 800 IUs I had been taking for years while I investigated. I quickly discovered flaws in the study. For one thing, it was a meta-analysis-type study, which allows researchers to pick and choose from the data. Also, the study did not take into account the poor health situation of the patients they studied, and the level of compliance of the subjects. In addition, over half of the study participants dropped out, and of the remaining participants it was not clear if the rules established in the study guidelines were followed.

Coincidence or Plot?

When I sent an e-mail to an editor of a popular health magazine I know asking what she thought about the study, she sent me the following reply: "There is some consensus that the vitamin E study was a planned 'negative' study—actually one among several others due out in the next few months—to create a 'soft landing' for Codex. Many people in the industry think that the Codex international guidelines are a back door being used by the pharmaceutical industry to control/regulate the natural products industry in the U.S."

During my many years of science, health, and medical writing, I have witnessed all sorts of shenanigans, shoddy interpretation, and manipulation when it comes to research. I've seen sound science shouted down by organizations with deep pockets, and sketchy findings overly publicized and underwritten by special interests. I sometimes find suspicious clinical studies hard to unravel, open to interpretation and requiring some down-and-dirty digging. But nothing prepared me for the subjects covered in this book.

Consider this: another recent "long-term study" reported that glucosamine was less effective than a placebo in relieving arthritis pain.

But a closer look at the published research reveals that the actual study period was only six months long, and all of the subjects had previously found glucosamine to be effective over a two-year period. (The researchers were counting those two years as part of the "long-term.") Nevertheless, this research was reported as a failure for glucosamine.

Now here's the key question: Is the timing of these and other deliberately negative studies a coincidence? Or, as my health editor wrote to me, is it part of a concerted effort to plant the seeds of doubt in the mind of the public? Could it be ephedra was the proverbial "toe in the water," and when the powers that be found the water's temperature just fine —meaning they got the ban they wanted with little fuss—that opened the spigot for further action against other dietary supplements?

That's why I wrote this book. That's what I set out to discover.

What Is Codex?

I may have dropped a term you're unfamiliar with—*Codex*. The United States is one of the 165 member countries of the Codex Alimentarius Commission, an international food standards program created by the Food and Agriculture Organization (FAO) and the World Health Organization (WHO). One of the purposes of the Codex commission is to "harmonize" international food trade. If passed here, many believe it could mean vitamins, minerals, and herbs will only be available at low dosages and by prescription—that is, those you can get at all. Needless to say, they'll cost a whole lot more.

Here are a few of the implications:

• WHO would get to classify all dietary supplements as drugs.
• The Codex commission would limit over-the-counter sales of dietary supplements while reclassifying others as pharmaceuticals, available only through a pharmacist.
• Under World Trade Organization (WTO) rules, Codex guidelines override the regulations of individual countries.

• Member countries (including the U.S.) that refuse to accept and enforce the WTO directives are subject to severe trade sanctions.

Just a few months ago, the Codex commission approved draft guidelines that will begin restricting the sale of dietary supplements as early as this summer. Can they get away with this? Do we risk waiting to see? And here's something else to ponder. The person who opened to door for U.S. participation in Codex recently resurfaced as a senior nutrition research scientist in the Office of Dietary Supplements (ODS) at NIH. ODS is supposed to be an objective research and information-disseminating arm of NIH regarding alternative medicine. At times, I've noticed them getting facts wrong either by an honest mistake or, perhaps deliberately. The Steve Bechler situation is one example.

There are also some reports that some of the dietary supplement associations have been infiltrated by executives from pharmaceutical companies.

Could this all be part of the Codex plot? As Jenny Thompson from the Health Sciences Institute writes, "Incredible, isn't it? Our freedom to make our own healthcare choices may simply be taken away by an international commission."

But at this point, the imposition of the Codex guidelines isn't necessarily a done deal. And although the situation is not promising, it's still not too late to help prevent it from happening."

Gary Null wrote about the Codex Alimentarius Commission in the September 1999 issue of *Penthouse* magazine:

In recent years, big medicine, the pharmaceutical establishment, and their allies in big government all joined forces to protect their own interests. These threatened groups engage in fear-mongering before Congress to get legislation that would sic state medical boards on alternative therapies, let dietitians control the dispensing of nutritional advice, and keep the public from having freedom of choice by turning as many nutrients as possible into prescription drugs. This is what the future will bring unless we take action.

He continues, "Not far into the twenty-first century you may be saying so-long to your St. John's wort, goodbye to your Ginkgo biloba. These and many other supplements may become things of the past, at least as reasonably priced over-the-counter items."

Paranoia? Perhaps. But as a friend once told me, "Just because you're paranoid doesn't mean people aren't out to get you."

I wish this book were unnecessary. I wish I didn't have to write about the FDA's inability to do its job. I wish I didn't have to report that some of my colleagues in journalism have continuously failed to do an even-handed job reporting on the dietary supplement industry.

This is a book exploring—and exploding, where appropriate—all the myths about DSHEA: "The FDA has no power over it," "Manufacturing standards don't exist," "There's nothing the FDA can do to curb product claims." I will also contrast the FDA's treatment of supplements with food and drugs. Lastly, I would talk about the future and what the industry and government—not just the FDA—need to do to maintain, or establish, a level playing field.

I'll be covering all these issues and more in the following chapters. As you read, it's important for you to keep asking yourself one question after I present evidence. That question is: "Who benefits?" Hopefully, when you finish you'll not only know the answer, but you'll know what to do about it.

PART I

"Oh, What a Tangled Web We Weave . . ."

1

Let's Talk About Freedom

In the movie *The Aviator,* Leonardo DiCaprio plays the enigmatic Howard Hughes, the head of Trans World Airways. It's the 1940s, and Hughes squares off against a hostile U.S. Senate committee led by Maine Senator Ralph Owen Brewster (played by Alan Alda), whom archrival Pan Am has plied with graft. Hughes is seeking transatlantic air routes, a market Pan Am holds in a virtual monopoly. By painting Hughes as a kook and an unscrupulous businessman, the senator attacks Hughes during a congressional hearing. But Hughes comes prepared, fights back, and TWA gains access to the North Atlantic air corridor.

While the story is indeed true, it is not too much of a stretch to say "only in the movies," especially if you apply the same scenario to dietary supplements. Instead of a senatorial hearing about transatlantic routes, the dietary supplement ephedra faced off with a U.S. House subcommittee hearing over the safety of ephedra and by extension every vitamin, mineral, and herb covered by the Dietary Supplement Act. Leading up to the hearings—and continuing ever since—the entire dietary supplement industry was slandered, just like Hughes, as being unscrupulous and yes, a little kooky. In place of the U.S. senator, the ephedra hearings were headed by a U.S. House member, who afterwards became president of PhRMA, the ultra-powerful lobby group for the pharmaceutical industry whose prescription diet drugs benefited greatly by the demise of ephedra—despite their own questionable record of safety and effectiveness. How did we get to this point?

No doubt the FDA has an awesome responsibility dealing with the health and safety of the American people. I'm not talking about nanny service, but ensuring things we eat and drink are safe so we don't have to worry about it.

Some people may argue against the role—and success—of government regulation and interference, but frankly, when it comes to product safety, I see little reason to skimp as long as it is effective. Frankly my bathtub isn't big enough to test drugs and the safety of food, and besides, it's been a long time since I took chemistry, and I'm kinda busy.

We need these objective government agencies, but they're supposed to be devoid of outside influences. We pay our taxes to ensure that.

Of Primrose and Black Currant Oil

In the early 1990s, Congress began investigating ways to battle health frauds including unsubstantiated nutritional and therapeutic health claims. During the same period, the FDA was considering tighter regulations for supplement labels.

In response, the health-food industry urged Congress to "preserve the consumer's freedom to choose dietary supplements" and warned retailers that the regulations under consideration would cripple their business. Consumers were told that unless they took action, the FDA would take away their right to buy vitamins. As a result, Congress received piles of letters from concerned citizens and, along with other evidence, voted overwhelmingly to pass the DSHEA act.

Here's how DSHEA came about according to Stephen N.

McNamara and A. Wes Siegner, Jr. These two are partners at the law firm Hyman, Phelps & McNamara, P.C., in Washington, D.C., and count among their clients both dietary supplement and pharmaceutical companies.

"DSHEA was enacted because FDA was viewed as distorting the law that existed before DSHEA to try to improperly deprive the public of safe and popular dietary supplement products," they wrote in an article appearing in the journal produced by the Food and Drug Law Institute. After abusing its powers regarding dietary supplements, the "FDA's authority needed to be better defined and controlled." Although Mr. Siegner is known as someone who has defended ephedra on occasion, the law firm assists the drug industry with respect to the regulation of foods, drugs, medical devices, cosmetics, and related products.

The attorneys say DSHEA was passed by unanimous consent because of abuse of power by the FDA. They provide two examples of FDA excesses described by a Senate committee. One was the FDA campaign to prevent the marketing of dietary supplements of black currant oil (from the same fruit used to make jam). The FDA argued the addition of black currant oil to a gelatin capsule caused the black currant oil to become a "food additive" as defined by FDCA, and that as a "food additive," the substance could not be marketed as a dietary supplement without first obtaining FDA issuance of an approving "food additive" regulation. Typically, the Senate noted, "the cost to a manufacturer to prepare a food additive petition can run to $2 million. FDA approval of a food additive petition typically takes from two to six years."

In case you're curious, black currant oil differs from other essential fatty acid oils because it contains both omega-6 gamma-linolenic acid and omega-3 alpha linolenic acid. It's believed to support the body's manufacture of hormone-like substances known as prostaglandins, which help regulate functions of the circulatory system.

After the Seventh Circuit Court ruled against the FDA, the U.S. Court of Appeals for the First Circuit ruled similarly, saying that the

"FDA's reading of the Act is nonsensical. . . . The proposition that placing a single-ingredient food product into an inert capsule as a convenient method of ingestion converts that food into a food additive perverts the statutory text, undermines legislative intent, and defenestrates common sense. We cannot accept such anfractuous reasoning."

A similar thing happened regarding the FDA's attempts to ban another dietary supplement: evening primrose oil. (In England, it is an approved treatment for breast pain and allergic dermatitis and eczema.) Although evening primrose oil was considered to be a safe and popular dietary supplement, the FDA claimed it, too, was an "unapproved food additive." These two rulings against the FDA helped pave the way for passage of DSHEA.

As an illustration of the agency's organized effort to undermine certain dietary supplements, evidence was presented before the House of Representatives and the Senate in 1993 that the FDA commissioner had awarded the Commissioner's Special Citation to more than FDA personnel, who at that time comprised the Evening Primrose Oil Litigation Team. Nevertheless, although two U.S. district courts and two three-judge U.S. courts of appeals had all unanimously rejected FDA's regulatory program, Congress concluded that unless it stepped in and passed DSHEA, the facts showed that the FDA would continue to try to prohibit the marketing of safe and proper dietary supplements. In the hearing on Dietary Supplements Before the House Committee on Appropriations, Subcommittee on Agriculture, Rural Development, Food and Drug Administration, and Related Agencies in October 1993, the committee wrote, "The committee is therefore concerned that the FDA will persist in such litigation, and thereby continue to subject small manufacturers to the choice of abandoning production and sale of lawful products, or accepting the significant financial burden of defending themselves against baseless lawsuits brought by the FDA."

McNamara and Siegner say it is important to remember this history, both because it helps to explain why, under current law, the FDA is not entrusted with blanket pre-approval authority over the marketing of all dietary supplement products, and because "it illustrates the risk of excessively restrictive regulation that might be presented if FDA were to be given such comprehensive authority in the future."

The Other Side of the Story

Of course, there are two sides to every story. In the case of the TWA–Pan Am squabble, TWA's critics contend the government went along with TWA because of racial prejudice against Pan Am President Juan Trippe because he was hispanic. And the awarding of TWA transatlantic routes fed by its network of domestic routes put Pan Am at a competitive disadvantage since Pan Am only had flight certificates for international travel.

Likewise, critics of DSHEA say the letter-writing campaign that prompted Congress to pass DSHEA was a public relations sham that successfully created a problem that didn't exist. According to a 1997 article appearing in *PR Watch*, which is published by the Center for Media and Democracy, in 1992 supplement makers called on the Rogers and Cowan PR firm to help launch the Nutritional Health Alliance, a grassroots PR campaign aimed at fighting what it called "the FDA's bias against preventive medicine and the dietary supplement industry."

Under the FDA's proposed rules for implementing its powers, supplements marketed simply as nutritional aids would be subject to the same rules as other food products, while substances marketed as disease cures or treatments would be held to the same "safety and efficacy" standard as drugs sold by the pharmaceutical industry.

According to *PR Watch*, one TV advertisement depicted mock FDA agents dressed in riot gear, who raided Mel Gibson's house and confiscated his vitamins. Gibson joined celebrities such as Whoopi Goldberg, Randy Travis, Sissy Spacek, Laura Dern, Mariel Hemingway, and Victoria Principal in making public service announcements claiming that the FDA was trying to block consumer access to vitamins.

Vitamin sellers, along with ten thousand health-food stores and their customers, supported the movement by targeted advertising and flyers calling on supporters to "act now to protect your right to use safe vitamins, minerals, herbs, and other dietary supplements of your choice." One brochure by the NHA urged consumers to "write to Congress today or kiss your supplements goodbye."

PR Watch says the goal of the campaign was to ensure passage of DSHEA, a bill sponsored by Utah Senator Orrin Hatch. Displays were set up at health-food stores with copies of letters to be sent to members of Congress. Some stores offered discounts to participants. Others provided free phone lines to call lawmakers. During a nation-wide "blackout day," stores refused to sell products that they claimed were threatened. NHA's director warned darkly of a "worldwide con-spiracy" led by the "Pharmaceutical-medical combine trying to make sure they are not being threatened worldwide by inexpensive, non-patented dietary supplements that will prevent the onset of chronic disease." In the space of twelve months, the campaign generated more than one hundred thousand letters to members of Congress, more than half of whom eventually agreed to cosponsor the legislation.

Bruce Silverglade, director of legal affairs for the Center for Science in the Public Interest, said the campaign was a "big lie":

> The consumers who wrote Congress had a financial inter-est in the matter or were duped into believing the FDA was using the new labeling law to ban their favorite vitamins. People should have the right to try any type of health care that they choose. But what we're talking about is whether the man-ufacturers have the right to hype supplements on the basis of unreliable scientific information or downright false claims.

Of course they can't. Maybe Mr. Silverglade should reconsider his position. No one was duped into writing. If people weren't already taking a vitamin, mineral, or herb and believed they were useful, they'd have no incentive to write. These were people who believed adamantly in the products. Did he think people would "stock up," increasing short-term sales? What would the point of that be? It would just lower demand while people used up their supply.

The end result was passage of DSHEA in 1994, which defined "dietary supplements" as a separate regulatory category. Some describe it as a subset of food since the industry depends on the safety standards established for nutrients encapsulated in the supplements.

DSHEA also created an NIH Office of Dietary Supplements and directed the president to appoint a Commission on Dietary Supplement Labels to recommend ways to implement the act. The commission's final recommendations were released on November 24, 1997.

A Quiet Conspiracy?

Unfortunately, many of the recommendations—such as Good Manufacturing Practices—were neglected and unfunded. It's an old trick known as "unfunded mandates." Members of Congress can vote for a popular bill, such as DSHEA, and then fail to fund it. It wasn't until just before the ephedra ban—ten years after DSHEA passed, that the FDA scrambled to issue a preliminary version of the GMPs. Two years later, they still haven't been finalized. As for the Office of Dietary Supplements, their efforts have been in direct conflict to their mission and in some cases, quite half-hearted, as I'll show later.

Anti-DSHEA criticism didn't end with the passage of the act. According to the Institute of Food Technologists' "IFT's Summary," published in the July 1999 issue of *Food Technology*, DSHEA broadened the definition of supplements to include ingredients not recognized as traditional nutrients, such as botanicals and hormones. "Prior to DSHEA, these ingredients could have been challenged by the FDA as unapproved food additives, exempt from additive regulations applicable to conventional foods," note summary authors Mary Ellen Camire, Ph.D., University of Maine, and Mark A. Kantor, Ph.D., University of Maryland.

Although supplement manufacturers should ensure that their products are safe and should be able to provide information to support any labeling claims, the FDA bears the burden of showing that a supplement is unsafe or mislabeled before it can restrict or ban the product's use, say Camire and Kantor, who note that:

> The passage of DSHEA has created an economic and regulatory environment favorable to the expanded marketing, sales, and distribution of dietary supplements. Opportunities for consumers to purchase supplements in a free market economy are vastly increased, but [false] expectations remain that government agencies provide [consumer] protection from unsafe or mislabeled products. One of the future challenges with respect to supplements will be to reconcile these apparently opposing forces.

As Always, the Truth Lies Somewhere In Between

Yes, there are some pretty far-out products being sold under the nutritional supplement umbrella, which DSHEA critics like to point to as representative of the unscrupulous dietary supplement industry.

I'm talking about the products claiming to grow crops of hair, make you lose incredible amounts of weight while you vegetate on your couch, build muscles on top of your muscles, and "enlarge" body parts on self-conscious men and women. There are even mainstream dietary supplements advertised making unrealistic promises via Saturday-morning infomercials. Ridiculous health claims for coral calcium come to mind. Fortunately, there are safeguards against these as the Saturday morning coral calcium hucksters learned. Their products are now banned.

Not only can the FDA put a stop to products like these, so can the FTC, the Interstate Commerce Commission, and many other government agencies both federal and local. If the products are sent via the mail, the U.S. Postal Service can charge the companies with mail fraud.

Free Enterprise Isn't Always So Free

"Effective propaganda must limit its points to a few and these points must be repeated until even the last member of the audience understands what is meant by them. . . . It must limit itself to a few themes and repeat them incessantly. Each change must never affect the content of propaganda, rather must always draw the same conclusions."
—Joseph Goebbels

The consumer advocacy group Public Citizen—founded by Ralph Nader—goes absolutely ballistic when talking about the pharmaceutical industry. For example, a Public Citizen report released on November 28, 2001 revealed how major U.S. drug companies and their lobby group, the Pharmaceutical Research and Manufacturers of America (PhRMA), have carried out a misleading campaign to scare policymakers and the public. PhRMA's central claim is that the industry needs extraordinary profits to fund expensive, risky, and innovative research and development (R&D) for new drugs. PhRMA's canned response goes something like this: If anything is done to moderate prices or profits, R&D will suffer, and, as PhRMA's president recently claimed, "it's going to harm millions of Americans who have life-threatening conditions." But this R&D scare tactic is patently untrue, says Public Citizen, and is built on myths, falsehoods, and misunderstandings, all of which are made possible by the drug industry's staunch refusal to open its R&D records to congressional investigators or other independent auditors.

Naturally, the exposés by Public Citizen and others immediately changed everything, right? Wrong. Not when you're dealing with an organization with much deeper pockets for marketing, self-promotion, and political contributions than its critics. Frankly, PhRMA has the resources to drown out any warning or plea Public Citizen and other consumer watchdog organizations try to make.

Marketing works, no question about it, and no one does it better or spends more on marketing than the pharmaceutical companies.

According to a study in the *New England Journal of Medicine,* in 2000 the drug companies spent $2.5 billion advertising drugs to consumers. This year, they are expected to spend over $3 billion to convince you their drugs are good for you. What they do spend might seem like a lot of PR, but the drug companies aren't worried. Americans are expected to spend over $500 billion on drugs this year—not including the extra $400 billion estimated for the Medicare drug benefit program.

Freedom of Speech

If you try to impose restrictions on what drug companies can say when they advertise, they trot out the old bromide that their freedom of speech is being stifled. One of our most cherished freedoms has sure been getting a workout lately. In June 2005 at their annual meeting in Las Vegas, the American Medical Association refused to back a ban on prescription drug ads, despite rising concerns about the dangers of certain heavily marketed painkillers and antidepressants, not to mentioned ads for heartburn and erectile dysfunction. As for the last, I'm still waiting to read a crawler across the bottom of the screen stating, "If you're not aroused by this ad you definitely need our little pill."

Besides the constant repetition of advertising messages convincing people that they need their drugs, advertising also serves as a "frame" for a more serious discussion. That is, wait until we're sick to treat what's ailing us, rather than prevention. Coupled with the questionable studies showing that certain vitamins, minerals, and herbs offer little benefit and great risk, and it should not come as a surprise that despite all of our economic might, the U.S. lags far behind most other industrialized nations in life expectancy and other measurements of health.

Then there's cost. Certainly, medical research has led to improvements in treatment. But, why is there no downward price pressure as a result? One of the reasons is that treating sickness is much more profitable than prevention. Another reason is public

Are We Overdosed?

John Abramson, M.D., wrote in his book *Overdosed America* that consumer demand for medications touted on TV leads to inappropriate treatment and dangerous drug interactions. Dr. Abramson said drug companies have infiltrated all legitimate sources of medical information, allowing them to produce "the knowledge that makes us believe we need their products." He estimated that 70–80 percent of medical journal articles are strongly influenced by commercialized drug interests, and research sponsored by pharmaceutical companies is five times more likely to show a given drug favorably.

policies that protect certain segments of the economy at the expense of others.

For years, the pharmaceutical industry has benefited from a double standard of government protectionism and free enterprise. On one hand, the federal government provides stringent intellectual property right protections and generous public subsidies for research, but on the other hand, has no say in regulating drug prices. As a result, the United States has been a leader in the development of new drugs, while faced with the highest drug prices in the world.

Until recently, there has been little public controversy over the pricing of drugs or the terms under which private firms obtain the rights to government-funded research. But as health-care costs have soared and policymakers attempt to deal with AIDS and the general crisis of health coverage and cost, the special treatment, power, and control the drug companies wield shows public interest and drug company interest collide more than intersect.

And what's happening to counteract it? Virtually nothing, even while the stakes are enormous. If the drug companies are to be believed, government attempts to control drug prices would cripple the industry's research and development efforts, slow the pace of innovation, and damage one of the nation's leading high-technology export industries.

Nowhere is there a greater need for more competition and the unleashing of free-market forces than in health care. So, does it make any sense to discourage and clamp down on an industry that promotes prevention, self-help, and healthy lifestyles when health-care costs are hyperinflating? Unfortunately the constant repetition and drum beat for drugs drowns out alternative messages. How often do you see an ad for a dietary supplement? Except for the occasional ad for One-a-Day vitamins and radio ads for a garlic formulation, virtually never. Instead we get press reports on the ephedra witch hunt and questionable studies about vitamin E, echinacea, and St. John's wort.

No doubt the pharmaceutical industry is fully exercising and exploiting its right to free speech. As a result, they're winning the war of message: treating sickness is more important—and profitable—even though common sense dictates that people would rather be healthy than sick. This is one of our most important freedoms, the freedom to make choices. But only when the influences on those choices are clear, fair, and above board.

2

No One Wants to Be Sick

If you or a family member takes at least one prescription drug, welcome to the club. It's a rather large club, and not very exclusive, mind you—gender, age, and race aren't barriers—and the dues are steep. Plus, the initiation is as daunting as any fraternity or sorority you can name. Often you have to be sick enough to warrant a prescription from a doctor—although you can demand entry to the club and your doctor more than likely will oblige you.

Americans spend about $200 billion per year on prescription drugs, but this does not include the drugs administered in hospitals, nursing homes, and doctors' offices.

A 2002 study by the Center on an Aging Society at Georgetown University estimates that more than 131 million people—66 percent of all adults in the United States—use prescription drugs. Specifically, the researchers found that the great majority of adults afflicted with at least one of five common chronic conditions—diabetes, heart disease, hypertension, arthritis, and cancer—use prescription drugs.

Too Cozy for Comfort

The relationship between drug companies and the FDA has changed significantly since the early 1990s. Much of the funding for new drug review now comes from the drug manufacturers, making the approval process faster and testing time shorter. Unbeknownst to most of us, the public increasingly plays a role in "testing" in the form of "post-marketing surveillance," and the resulting adverse drug reactions encountered are underreported. Marketing includes massive distribution of free samples to physicians, many of whom may not be familiar with precautions—and hence do not alert patients to warning signs and symptoms. Also, advertising of prescription medications has increased greatly in the last few years, which has significantly increased drug use and pressure on physicians to prescribe medications. I'll be talking about all these issues later in the book.

While the FDA clamors to ban herbs like ephedra—while lying about the risk—consider these facts:

• The fourth leading cause of death in the U.S. is properly pre-scribed and administered medication. When you add improperly prescribed medication, it becomes the third leading cause of death.

• There are over two million hospital admissions and 180,000 deaths each year in the U.S. due solely to adverse drug reactions

• When the FDA approves a medication for use by the general public, fewer than half of the serious drug reactions are known. The real clinical trial starts when doctors start writing prescriptions.

A Dose of Common Sense

Which seems more logical? Devoting most of our government's attention and resources to drugs for treating the symptoms of disease, or a strategy of sound nutrition and exercise supplemented by nutrients to boost health and prevent disease? Dr. Dean Ornish certainly thinks the latter approach is the wiser one. In 1999 and 2000, the University of California-San Francisco medical professor reported the results of his groundbreaking research linking diet and behavior with coronary diseases in the *Journal of the American Medical Association* (*JAMA*) and the *American Journal of Cardiology*.

One study showed that of forty-five people with partially clogged arteries, the twenty who made intensive diet and lifestyle changes had fewer blockages after five years. While ten patients dropped out, the fifteen patients who made smaller changes had more blockages after five years and nearly three times as many more heart attacks and other "cardiac events." The second study showed that more than three hundred people with severe heart disease were able to make the intensive changes that comprise Ornish's program and improve their health as a result.

The idea that heart disease was reversible was thought impossible until Dr. Ornish conducted his first study more than two decades ago. Until then, most people viewed heart disease as primarily the amount of blockage, or stenosis, in the arteries. Since it was known that the blockages take decades to build up, the idea that they could change in a short time was radical. So how could so much blockage clear in so little time? Besides improved metabolism, Dr. Ornish and his research team found decreasing triglyceride levels in the blood and increasing the HDL cholesterol (good cholesterol) levels made it harder for fats to collect inside artery walls.

In his studies, Ornish and his research team found that blood flow to the heart, angina and chest pain, and the ability of the heart to pump blood improved after only one month. In later studies, they saw 90 percent reductions in the frequency of chest pain within weeks. No drugs required.

This is probably a good place to look at the top-selling pharmaceutical drugs in the U.S.

Top-Selling Drugs in the United States—2003

Here are the top selling drugs in the United States in 2003—their annual sales, what they treat, and their manufacturer.
(Source: IMS Health)
1. Lipitor, $6.8 billion, cholesterol, Pfizer, Inc.
2. Zocor, $4.4 billion, cholesterol, Merck & Co.

3. Prevacid, $4.0 billion, heartburn, TAP Pharmaceutical Products, Inc.

4. Procrit, $3.3 billion, anemia, Johnson & Johnson

5. Zyprexa, $3.2 billion, mental illness, Eli Lilly & Co.

6. Epogen, $3.1 billion, anemia, Amgen, Inc.

7. Nexium, $3.1 billion, heartburn, Merck & Co.

8. Zoloft, $2.9 billion, depression, Pfizer, Inc.

9. Celebrex, $2.6 billion, arthritis, Pfizer, Inc.

10. Neurontin, $2.4 billion, epilepsy, Pfizer, Inc.

11. Advair Diskus, $2.3 billion, asthma, GlaxoSmithKline PLC

12. Plavix, $2.2 billion, blood clots, Bristol-Myers Squibb Co.

13. Norvasc, $2.2 billion, high blood pressure, Pfizer, Inc.

14. Effexor XR, $2.1 billion, depression, Wyeth

15. Pravachol, $2.0 billion, cholesterol, Bristol-Myers Squibb Co.

16. Risperdal, $2.0 billion, mental illness, Johnson & Johnson

17. OxyContin, $1.9 billion, pain, Perdue Pharma

18. Fosamax, $1.8 billion, osteoporosis, Merck & Co.

19. Protonix, $1.8 billion, gastrointestinal reflux disease, Wyeth

20. Vioxx, $1.8 billion, arthritis, Merck & Co.

That's quite a list, don't you think? Let's take a closer look at some of these top sellers.

Unclogging Arteries

It's worth noting that the number-one and number-two—as well as the number-fifteen—best-selling drugs help lower cholesterol. I guess it's possible to argue that lowering our "bad" LDL cholesterol prevents disease, most notably heart disease and stroke. But what if I were to tell you that lowering bad cholesterol doesn't prevent heart disease and strokes, but rather can cause other serious health problems, including muscle weakness, impotence, and liver disease? With the number of ads promoting these wonder drugs known as statins, a reasonable response by you could be, "you better have a boat-load of evidence, buddy. I'm paying top dollar every month for my Lipitor."

That would be a reasonable request. And I will present most of the evidence in a later chapter. For now, let's look at the Lipitor Web site.

Here, on the first page where it says at the top, "Drug for Reducing Cholesterol and Reducing Risk of Heart Attacks," near the bottom is this caveat: "It has not been shown to prevent heart disease or heart attacks."

Should I repeat that?

"[Lipitor] has not been shown to prevent heart disease or heart attacks."

So which message is correct—the one at the top of the page or the one at the bottom?

Not long ago, most doctors thought of heart attacks as primarily a clogged plumbing problem. Over the years, fatty deposits would slowly build up on the insides of major coronary arteries until they grew so big that they cut off the supply of blood to a vital part of the heart. A complex molecule called LDL, the so-called bad cholesterol, provided the material for these deposits causing the blockage. It made sense to think that people with high LDL levels were at greater risk of developing heart disease. One problem is that half of all heart attacks occur in people with normal cholesterol levels. Not only that, as imaging techniques improved, doctors found, much to their surprise, that the most dangerous plaques weren't necessarily all that large. Something that hadn't yet been identified was causing those deposits to burst, triggering massive clots that cut off the coronary blood supply.

In the 1990s, Dr. Paul M. Ridker, director of the Center for Cardiovascular Disease Prevention at Brigham and Women's Hospital in Boston, believed some sort of inflammatory reaction was responsible for the bursting plaques, and he set about trying to prove it. He and others found that blood levels of a molecule called C-reactive protein (CRP) are just as important as cholesterol readings when measuring cardiovascular risk.

By 1997, Ridker and his colleagues at Brigham and Women's proved healthy middle-aged men with the highest CRP levels were three times as likely to suffer a heart attack in the next six years as were those with the lowest CRP levels.

Despite the huge amount of prescriptions being written for statin drugs to lower bad cholesterol levels, heart disease, stroke, and related diseases continue to be the biggest killers in the U.S. Through extensive research, Dr. Richard M. Fleming, a cardiologist and founder of the Fleming Heart and Health Institute in Omaha, Nebraska, discovered the immune system was the crucial piece missing from the diagnosis and treatment equation. He saw that when key elements in the blood became elevated they triggered a dangerous inflammatory chain reaction. These elements, ranging from bacteria to triglycerides, when combined with a high-protein diet and sedentary lifestyle, cause arterial inflammation, a damaging, debilitating, and sometimes deadly condition, leading not only to heart disease, high blood pressure, and stroke, but also diabetes and cancer.

Just so you know, Dr. Fleming has had his own measure of controversy. Information Fleming obtained from the New York City medical examiner's office on diet guru Robert Atkins showed he was obese when he died in April 2003 from the complications of a fall. The examiner's report suggested Atkins had a history of congestive heart failure and high blood pressure, which his widow and supporters have denied. Fleming's book, titled *Stop Inflammation Now!*, is critical of high-protein diets like the one made famous by Atkins.

A critic of Fleming accused him of having a "profit motive" by sharing the report with the Physicians Committee for Responsible Medicine. That group has received more than $1 million from People for the Ethical Treatment of Animals (PETA) and the animal-rights movement. But that's besides the point.

In his research, Dr. Fleming shows that anti-inflammatory strategies can slow the chronic and degenerative diseases of aging—even aging itself. The antioxidant vitamins E and C, modifying lifestyle factors, food and nutritional supplements, and nutraceuticals can be useful in reducing the risks of inflammatory disorders.

Elation, Then Reality

Recently, two studies looked at the CRP issue in different groups of patients and came to the exact same conclusions. Both studies, including one directed by Dr. Ridker whom I mentioned above, appeared in the January 6, 2005 issue of the *New England Journal of Medicine* (*NEJM*).

CRP is a marker of inflammation, and it works in tandem with LDL cholesterol—the bad kind—to increase the risk of cardiovascular problems, said Dr. Ridker. While LDL cholesterol forms the fatty plaques that accumulate in arteries to block blood flow, "inflammation is causing those plaques to rupture and cause heart attack and stroke."

Both *NEJM* studies dealt with people who had coronary conditions and were treated with statins, drugs marketed because they reduce LDL cholesterol levels. The Boston study included 3,745 patients with acute coronary syndromes who were given statins. As expected, the incidence of heart attack and death from heart disease was related to LDL cholesterol levels and the rate of adverse events was roughly 50 percent lower in persons with LDL levels less than 70 milligrams per deciliter of blood. That's all well and good. We know clogged arteries restrict blood flow, and statins reduce LDL levels, but then why don't the reduced amounts result in fewer heart attacks?

The other *NEJM* study—known as the Cleveland study—included 502 patients with coronary disease who were given statins and whose arteries were assessed by ultrasound for eighteen months. Again, lower cholesterol levels meant slower progression of arterial blockage, but "the decrease in CRP levels was independently and significantly correlated with the rate of progression," the study said.

Physicians still don't know for sure how inflammation might cause a plaque to burst. But they have a theory. As the level of LDL cholesterol increases in the blood, they speculate, some of it seeps into the lining of the coronary arteries and gets stuck there. Macrophages—a type of white blood cell that functions as a patrol cell and engulfs and kills foreign infectious invaders—are alerted to the presence of something that doesn't belong, come in, and try to clean out the cholesterol. If cytokines, which facilitate communication among immune system cells and between immune system cells and the rest of the body, signals begin elevating the inflammatory process instead of reducing it, the plaque becomes unstable.

Dr. Ridker says this discovery does not replace cholesterol as a risk factor, since cholesterol deposits, high blood pressure, smoking—all contribute to the development of underlying plaques. What inflammation seems to contribute is the propensity of those plaques to rupture and cause a heart attack. Don't get too excited just yet. There's more.

When the CRP story broke in the media, Dr. Ridker predicted that the findings would likely encourage widespread use of the CRP test, and this in turn will greatly expand the market for statins. John Abramson, M.D., author of *Overdosed America* and a clinical instructor at Harvard Medical School said hold on, one gosh-darn minute. For one thing, he noted that both studies were funded by companies that make statin drugs, and the lead authors of each study, like most cardiovascular research physicians, have strong financial ties to the cardiac drug industry. Greater scrutiny of the studies was needed, especially if it would lead to a greater use of statins by people for whom the drugs may cause harm.

Abramson noted that the participants in both studies had severe heart disease. And the CRP test has yet to be proven useful to people in the early stages of heart disease or to healthy people who are at risk for developing heart disease.

High CRP levels may merely be an indicator that a person is at higher risk for another heart attack or stroke. He also noted the high percentage of the study participants who smoked. He said since 36 percent of the subjects were smokers—if the goal is really to reduce heart disease, then it doesn't make sense to focus attention exclusively on CRP without addressing smoking cessation and other lifestyle modifications like exercise that are at least as effective as statin therapy. After careful review of this study, Dr. Abramson said that he remains unconvinced that the researchers proved that reduced CRP levels account for the reduced incidence of heart attack and stroke.

This doesn't mean CRP levels aren't a possible contributing factor to heart disease, but could it be the conclusions reached in the two studies seemed more in tune with building a new market for statin drugs than careful analysis would suggest?

So, are we tackling the wrong problem? Maybe the focus should be more on something else, maybe triglycerides? Yet, the common answer in today's world is to write statin prescriptions. One thing we can bet the farm on is, as syndicated radio personality Robert Scott Bell often says, heart disease isn't caused by a "statin-deficiency." There's obviously something else going on here. More in a later chapter.

WARNING! This News Might Raise Your Blood Pressure

Number 13 on the best-selling list is Norvasc, prescribed for high blood pressure, a leading contributor to cardiovascular disease (CVD.) Norvasc is a type of drug known as a calcium-channel blocker (CCB). These slow the rate calcium passes into the heart muscle and into the vessel walls. Since calcium is important in muscle contraction, blocking calcium transport relaxes artery muscles and dilates coronary arteries and other arteries of the body. The relaxed vessels let blood flow more easily through them, thereby lowering blood pressure.

Common side effects from CCBs include feeling tired, flushing, swelling of the abdomen, ankles, or feet, and heartburn. Doesn't sound too bad does it? If you look at risk versus benefit, a little ankle swelling might be worth it, right? Well, there's more.

As far back as 1997, calcium channel blockers and certain kinds of diuretics were associated with brain damage and memory loss, according to a report in the *Journal of the American Geriatrics Society.* These results come from an analysis of participants with high blood pressure in the Cardiovascular Health Study (CHS), the largest study ever of the natural progression of heart disease and stroke in the elderly. The study, sponsored by the National Heart, Lung and Blood Institute and begun in 1989, involves 5,888 residents of Forsyth County, North Carolina; Sacramento County, California; Washington County, Maryland; and Pittsburgh, Pennsylvania.

Curt D. Furberg, M.D., Ph.D., professor and chairman of the Department of Public Health Sciences at the Wake Forest University School of Medicine, and, at the time, national chairman of the CHS Steering Committee, called the results "a surprise finding." He said there was no reason to suspect that drugs that reduce high blood pressure would have such an adverse effect on the brain.

The researchers looked at the 1,268 CHS participants who were being treated for high blood pressure by their personal physicians, but who had never had a stroke or reported a transient ischemic attack (a ministroke).

But that's not all. As a result of a recent study, B. Zane Horowitz, M.D., medical director, Oregon Poison Center, professor, Department of Emergency Medicine at Oregon Health Sciences University, stated calcium channel blocker overdose is rapidly emerging as the most lethal prescription drug ingestion. For one thing, he found that overdoses by short-acting agents are characterized by rapid progression to cardiac arrest. Overdose by extended-relief formulations result in delayed onset of arrhythmias, shock, sudden cardiac collapse, and bowel ischemia.

Here are the numbers tallied by the American Association of Poison Control Centers (AAPCC):

• In 1996, the AAPCC reported 58 fatalities and 225 major outcomes.

• In 1997, the AAPCC reported 44 fatalities and 232 major outcomes.

• In 1998, the AAPCC reported 61 fatalities and 277 major outcomes.

• In 1999, the AAPCC reported 61 fatalities and 243 major outcomes.

• In 2000, the AAPCC reported 44 fatalities and 317 major outcomes.

• In 2001, the AAPCC reported 60 fatalities and 286 major outcomes.

• In 2002, the AAPCC reported 68 fatalities and 365 major outcomes.

Horowitz disclosed no conflicting financial interest in competing drugs.

But even when used correctly the drugs may not be as effective as advertised. Pfizer, the maker of Norvasc, presented a study at a cardiology conference in Orlando in March 2005, and attempted to show that patients taking Norvasc were less likely to die than those on another regimen of hypertension medications. In addition, Pfizer demonstrated that the Norvasc treatment appeared to raise good cholesterol levels. Still, the study failed in its initial goal of proving that Norvasc lowered the rate of heart attacks or fatal coronary heart disease compared with the other hypertension treatment.

There were other questionable conclusions. The study, which followed almost twenty thousand patients with high blood pressure from 1998 until 2004, showed that patients taking Norvasc had a 15 percent lower death rate from all causes than those taking beta blockers, a different type of blood pressure drug. While deaths from heart attacks and other cardiovascular problems alone were 25 percent lower in patients taking Norvasc, the drug failed to show a statistically significant reduction in deaths from fatal coronary heart disease, the initial goal of the trial.

Here's some more bad news about channel blockers. Diuretics—which have been around for half a century, and have proven in multiple studies to prevent the complications of high blood pressure and are much cheaper—work better than other drugs at lowering high blood pressure and reducing the risk of heart disease, so they should be a first-line treatment for hypertension, new research suggests.

In a study reported in the April 6, 2005 issue of *JAMA*, researchers found that diuretics are at least as effective as other drugs in preventing coronary heart disease, that they are more effective in preventing heart failure, and they are more effective than beta blockers and ACE inhibitors in preventing stroke. For this study, 33,357 participants, about 35 percent of whom were African-Americans, were randomly assigned to receive either a calcium channel blocker, an ACE inhibitor, or a thiazide-type diuretic.

Participants taking calcium channel blockers had a 37 percent higher risk of heart failure compared to those taking diuretics. Diuretics were more effective in preventing cardiovascular disease (especially heart failure) than ACE inhibitors, among all participants. That reduction in high blood pressure and prevention of stroke was even more pronounced in African-Americans, the researchers note. But, as pointed out in the *Journal of the American Geriatrics Society* study I mentioned above, certain kinds of diuretics were associated with brain damage and memory loss.

There's a better way to fight high blood pressure. Lifestyle changes that can lower blood pressure combine sound dietary principles, weight loss, exercise, reduced sodium intake, increased potassium intake, and moderate alcohol use.

I Can't Believe I Ate the *Whole* Thing

The third and seventh best selling drugs are prescribed to relieve heartburn and acid indigestion. Drugs such as Prevacid, Nexium, and Prilosec—not to mention those friendly little cylinders of Tums and Rolaids—are among the most profitable on the market, with annual sales approaching $20 billion. You'd think we were a nation besieged by ulcers, heartburn, and acid reflux. Wait a minute—we are. But probably not because of excess stomach acid. Let's take a closer look.

The lining of our stomachs contains millions of special cells that produce acid via "acid or proton pumps." It is the job of these pumps to produce the acid to help digest food. There are actually three different ways that the acid-producing cells in the stomach are stimulated to secrete acid. One is with histamine. Another is through gastrin, which is a hormone in the body that stimulates acid secretion. The third is with acetylcholine, which, again, stimulates acid secretion. For people with gastroesophogeal reflux disease (GERD), the "pumped" acid backs up into the esophagus where it doesn't belong. PPIs disable the cell-level pumps that move acid into the stomach.

We have been told for years that heartburn is the result of too much stomach acid. However, what we're never told is that hydrochloric acid made by the stomach lining promotes health and prevents a wide range of ills:

• It helps digest food and process it for the absorption of nutrients in the small intestine. This is probably its best-known function. Acid produced in the stomach has to break down all the protein, fat, and carbohydrates we eat. There is a popular notion that too much acid causes our gastric ills, when in fact the opposite may be true: when we produce too little acid to sufficiently digest our food, we get very uncomfortable.

• It keeps us well nourished. As it breaks down dinner, stomach acid releases vital nutrients, such as vitamin B12, folic acid, calcium, iron, and zinc from the food we eat. Deficiencies of these nutrients can cause or worsen myriad ailments, such as anemia, diarrhea, osteoporosis, and brittle nails.

• It kills infectious bacteria. Food poisoning from listeria, salmonella, and *E. coli* is not as common as it might be because, on ingestion, bacteria are quickly plunged into a cauldron of hydrochloric acid in the stomach—from which they rarely escape alive.

In light of all this, do we *really* want to "turn off" the pumps? When there are lower levels of stomach acid, foods sit in the stomach much longer than normal. This extra waiting time means stomach acids have a longer time to back up into the esophagus, causing heartburn.

We should also ask why there's too much acid in the stomach. Tom Cowan, M.D., believes one answer could be that the person is eating too much food, which "tells" the body to secrete acid. Since protein foods are what cause the stomach cells to produce acid, the therapy is simple—stop eating so much protein. Dr. Cowan, who is a holistic doctor in private practice in San Francisco, says as a result, the stimulus to produce acid will be lessened, less acid will be produced, and eventually the symptoms will abate.

Dr. Cowan says another theory states that stomach acid helps the stomach and pancreatic enzymes maintain a balance, so without stomach acid the whole digestive system is thrown off.

Stomach acid is beneficial in other ways. As I've already said, stomach acid kills the microorganisms ingested with food. Stomach acid thus protects us from infections, both acute and chronic, in our GI tract.

On the flipside, according to an article recently published in *Alternative & Complementary Therapies,* by Leo Galland, M.D., people with low stomach acid or who chronically take antacids actually increase their risk of intestinal infections because the acid in the stomach helps to kill off bacteria in contaminated food and water. Unfortunately, the drugs reduce the acidity of the stomach and allow those bacteria to survive and enter the intestines, where they can cause trouble, not only acute food poisoning, but also by disrupting the normal and healthy flora, which can contribute to chronic health conditions. It's not surprising that a factor often overlooked regarding food poisoning is whether the patient is taking antacid medications.

Not making enough stomach acid puts you at increased risk for gastritis (an inflammation of the stomach lining usually resulting from infection) and stomach cancer. Research conducted by Dr. Juanita Merchant at the University of Michigan offers a recent example. Her investigations on bacteria living in the stomach suggest that low acidity allows for an overgrowth of unfriendly species, which can lead to a pre-cancerous condition known as atrophic gastritis. This type of gastritis usually develops in people infected with *Helicobacter pylori,* a type of bacteria that can cause ulcers, but may not be directly responsible for the gastritis. Half of the U.S. population aged sixty and over is infected with *H. pylori,* compared with only 20 percent of those under forty. In addition, *H. pylori* was found to thrive in slightly acidic stomachs, therefore exonerating excess stomach acid as the direct cause of ulcers.

It's important to know that decreased production of stomach acid (a condition known as hypochlorhydria) can be caused by alcohol abuse, gastritis, and certain drugs. Prolonged use, or overuse, of common pain relievers, such as aspirin or ibuprofen and other similar remedies, can cause gastritis, which can kill acid-producing cells that line the stomach. Again, this can lead to the overgrowth of unfriendly bacteria.

Contrary to what pharmaceutical companies say, heartburn *is not* caused by too much acid in the stomach. Research shows that for every decade, adults lose about 13 percent of their ability to produce stomach acid. Ironically, a lack of stomach acid promotes indigestion.

Even now the medical community is starting to question the chronic use of acid-blocking drugs. For example, in a study published in the *Journal of Drug Safety,* rats that were given acid-blocking drugs throughout their lifetime developed tumors in their stomach. So think twice before you decide to "turn off the pumps."

Food, Glorious Food

We are a society that consumes a diet too high in calories, too low in fiber, low in vitamins and minerals, and deficient in phytochemicals. No wonder obesity has become a major health problem. These deleterious, health-limiting dietary characteristics could be corrected with a simple, inexpensive plant-based diet. Researchers have targeted a handful of specific foods containing phytonutrients (disease-fighting plant-based chemicals), vitamins, minerals, and healthful fatty acids. These nutrients act as powerful antioxidants to fight heart disease, cancer, the aging process, and as anti-inflammatories to reduce inflammation that can lead to heart disease, eye disease, and cancer, and as immunity boosters to help ward off infections of all kinds.

Oxidation happens to all living cells in nature, including those in our bodies. That's what makes a sliced apple turn color and other substances become rancid—including cholesterol in our arteries. While the body metabolizes oxygen very efficiently, one or two percent of cells will get damaged in the process and turn into free radicals. Free radicals are missing a critical electron, which sends them on a rampage to pair with another molecule. These free radicals often injure the cell and damage the DNA, paving the way for diseases.

External toxins, including cigarette smoke, air pollution, and other environmental contaminants, are free-radical generators. Food and water also harbor free radicals in the form of pesticides and other toxins. Drinking excessive amounts of alcohol also triggers substantial free radical production.

Free radicals don't just damage one molecule but trigger a damaging chain reaction. For example, when a free radical oxidizes a fatty acid, it changes that fatty acid into a free radical, which then damages another fatty acid. This can happen rapidly.

These external attacks can overwhelm the body's natural free-radical defense system. In time, and with repeated free-radical attacks that the body cannot stop, and the damage can lead to a host of chronic diseases, including cancer, heart disease, Alzheimer's disease, and Parkinson's disease.

To combat the ravages of oxidation and protect our health, we need to consume the thousands of antioxidants found in foods such as fruits, vegetables, whole grains, nuts, and legumes. This makes sense. As I explained in my previous book, the *Good Digestion Guide,* as much as 90 percent of all illnesses begin in the digestive tract—a sort of a "garbage in, garbage out" analogy.

Flavonoids are the biggest class of antioxidants. Researchers have identified some five thousand flavonoids in various foods. Polyphenols are a smaller class of antioxidants, which scientists often refer to as phenols. Phytonutrient and phytochemical are terms that researchers use to describe nutrients and chemicals in plants. Though not considered essential nutrients, they provide important protection against toxins, cancer, and other common illnesses. Carotenes in yellow fruits and vegetables, lycopene in tomatoes, allicin in garlic and onion, curcumin in turmeric, phytoestrogens in soybeans, gingerol in ginger, quercetin and limonene in citrus fruits—these are just a few more examples of phytochemicals that may protect against allergies, heart disorders, arthritis, and other degenerative diseases.

While it is virtually impossible to get all the antioxidants we need from food, and to fortify our need for antioxidants—especially from the added stress from environmental factors including nutrient-depleted soils—many people take antioxidant supplements such as vitamins C and E. Vitamin C can stop the chain reaction before it starts by capturing the free radical and neutralizing it. Vitamin E acts as a "chain-breaking" antioxidant. Notice that we don't take pharmaceutical drugs to prevent the diseases. We only take those after the body has been damaged from any number of diseases. However, taking vitamins and other supplements is never a substitute for a good balanced diet. Thus the word "supplement."

No doubt, sound nutrition, combined with a healthy lifestyle, is the basic necessity for lasting good health. Even in this modern contaminated world, good nutrition is attainable, as is a healthy lifestyle. But both require a serious personal commitment. What has received little publicity or research until now is the way in which prescription drugs disturb the body's ability to absorb nutrients. So, when you use prescription drugs, not only are you increasing the load of possibly toxic chemicals in your body from which these drugs are made, you might be starving it of essential nutrients that could exacerbate the problem. This lengthens the period of recovery.

When Food Is Not Enough

Taking daily supplements of fish or soy oil may improve cardiac function and protect against heart attacks in the short term. Study results published in the April 2005 issue of *Chest*, the journal of the American College of Chest Physicians, are the first to show that soy oil increases heart rate variability (HRV), a measure of cardiac autonomic function. "Our findings contradict the current belief in the medical community that increasing the intake of omega-3 fatty acids produces only long-term cardiac benefits," said the study's lead author, Fernando Holguin, M.D., Emory University School of Medicine. "In fact, our study group showed improvements in heart function in as little as two weeks."

Vitamins are also taking on a new role in health care—to help manage or treat disease. It's best to replace medicines with vitamins under your doctor's supervision.

Foods for Health

The Mayo Clinic has identified ten must-have foods that provide energy for your body to function and also ward off illness.

1. Whole grains: Whole grains may lower the risk of cardiovascular disease, type 2 diabetes, and cancer.

2. Fish: Salmon and tuna that are rich in omega-3 fatty acids help protect against heart disease.

3. Walnuts and almonds: Nutrient dense and cholesterol free, nuts may help reduce the risk of heart attacks.

4. Plant stanols and sterols: These natural substances from plants in margarine-like spreads such as Benecol and Take Control can decrease LDL cholesterol up to 14 percent.

5. Soy: Found in tofu and other products, soy helps lower cholesterol and the risk of cardiovascular disease.

6. Fat-free dairy products: While not suitable for everyone, skim milk and fat-free cottage cheese, yogurt, and cheese may help prevent stroke, colon cancer, and obesity.

7. Berries: Rich in antioxidants, blueberries, raspberries, and strawberries may lower cancer and cardiovascular disease risk.

8. Broccoli and cauliflower: These cruciferous vegetables, along with cabbage, Brussels sprouts, bok choy, and kale, are packed with phytochemicals that may help reduce the risk of colorectal and other cancers. They also contain fiber, have no cholesterol, and are naturally low in fat and calories.

9. Tomatoes: Contain nutrients that include vitamins C and B-complex as well as iron and potassium and the antioxidant lycopene. In numerous studies, lycopene has been shown to help lower the risk of heart attack and prostate cancer.

10. Green tea: Rich with phytochemicals known as flavonoids, green tea has been shown to help lower the risk of some cancers and heart disease.

Here are some examples from the March 2005 issue of the *Mayo Clinic Health Letter*:

• B vitamins to manage cardiovascular health: When your body breaks down protein, a by-product is homocysteine. High homocysteine in the blood is linked to heart disease and stroke. A number of factors are thought to influence increased homocysteine, including a lack of certain B vitamins.

• Niacin (vitamin B-3) to improve "good" cholesterol: Taken at prescribed levels, niacin can potentially boost high-density lipoprotein (HDL), the "good" cholesterol by 15 percent to 30 percent—or occasionally up to 50 percent.

• Riboflavin (vitamin B-2) to help prevent migraines: Very preliminary evidence has found that high doses of riboflavin might help prevent migraines for some people.

Eat This and Lower Your Blood Pressure

A high-fiber diet can not only lower your blood pressure, but also can improve healthy blood pressure levels, according to new research from Tulane University that examined data from twenty-five clinical trials representing 1,477 adult study participants. It works like a magic pill—only better because it's not. The study participants who ate 7.2 to 18.9 grams of fiber a day in the form of fruits, vegetables, and cereal experienced a reduction in both systolic and diastolic blood pressure. "All the data pointed to one strong conclusion: Adding fiber to a person's diet has a healthy effect on their blood pressure," said study leader Seamus Whelton in a news release announcing the study results. "Analyzing a large number of studies lends strength to the conclusions of clinical trials that involved too few participants to show an effect of dietary fiber on blood pressure." The study was published in the *Journal of Hypertension*.

The bottom-line: The researchers recommend that all of us—no matter our blood pressure—add fruits and vegetables to our diets in order to increase dietary fiber intake. People can also get dietary fiber from cereal, whole-wheat bread and pasta, and in pill form.

Exercise Lowers Cardiovascular Risk Factors

Aerobic exercise and stress-management training can reduce levels of depression and emotional distress, as well as improve markers of cardiovascular risk in patients with heart disease, according to a study in the April 6, 2005 issue of *JAMA*.

Psychosocial factors are now recognized as playing a significant and independent role in the development of ischemic heart disease (IHD) and its complications. Consequently, efforts to alter psycho-social risk factors, particularly in the setting of cardiac rehabilitation, have received increased attention. However, it's uncertain whether the effects of behavioral interventions to reduce adverse cardiac events have been effective.

James A. Blumenthal, Ph.D., of Duke University Medical Center, and colleagues compared the impact of two behavioral intervention programs, aerobic exercise and stress management training, with routine medical care on psychosocial functioning and cardiovascular risk. The randomized controlled trial included 134 patients (ninety-two male and forty-two female, aged forty to eighty-four years) with stable IHD and exercise-induced myocardial ischemia (decreased blood supply to the heart muscle). The trial was conducted from January 1999 to February 2003.

Participants received either routine medical care (usual care), usual care plus supervised aerobic exercise training for thirty-five minutes three times per week for sixteen weeks, or usual care plus weekly 1.5-hour stress management training for sixteen weeks.

The researchers found that patients in the exercise and stress management training groups exhibited lower average depression scores and reduced distress scores compared with patients receiving usual care only. Exercise and stress management training were also associated with favorable improvements in certain cardiovascular risk markers, compared with usual care patients.

"Results of this randomized controlled trial demonstrate that behavioral treatments provide added benefits to routine medical management in patients with stable IHD," the authors wrote.

We're Number One!

No doubt, exercise and a healthy diet go a long way in warding off all major diseases, and in many cases, they can even supplant the need for prescription drugs. But too many of us resist changing habits, and many doctors don't even bother suggesting it. No doubt there is a growing reliance on drugs as the first option.

That's why more than 130 million Americans swallow, inject, inhale, infuse, spray, and pat on prescribed medication every month, according to the U.S. Centers for Disease Control and Prevention. In fact, Americans buy much more medicine per person than residents of any other country in the world. We also spend almost as much on drugs as we do to fuel our cars.

The national appetite for drugs has sharpened over the past decade, driving up the number of prescriptions by two-thirds to 3.5 billion yearly, according to the pharmaceutical consulting company IMS Health. And that doesn't even count the over-the-counter nonprescription drugs we dump into our shopping carts.

Lately, safety questions have beset some depression and anti-inflammatory drugs, pushing pain relievers Vioxx and—more recently—Bextra from the market. Well, look at the above list again. Since there's so much controversy surrounding both anti-inflammatory drugs (Numbers 9 and 20,) along with other pain relievers, and anti-depressants and mental health drugs (Numbers 5, 8 and 16), I've devoted entire chapters to both.

Death by Medication

For a sizable minority of Americans, the consequences are dire. Well over 125,000 people die from drug reactions and mistakes each year, landmark medical studies of the 1990s suggest. It bears repeating: pharmaceutical drugs are the fourth leading cause of death—after heart disease, cancer, and stroke—in the United States today.

Foods for Health

"Garlic Is Top-Selling Herb; Herb Combinations See Increase"
Mark Blumenthal

The sales of herbal dietary supplements continued their downward slide in mainstream retail stores in 2004. For the 52-week period ending January 2, 2005, sales of all herbal supplements sold in food (grocery), drug, and mass market (FDM) stores decreased by 7.4 percent to a total of $257,514,900 according to sales data compiled by Information Resources Inc. (IRI) of Chicago.

The biggest increase was in the "multi-herb" category, referring to combination herb products, where sales rose 29.1 percent to $52,049,290. The sales for the top-selling 20 single herbs as well as for combination herbal formulas and total herb sales are shown in Table 1.

Table 1: Top-Selling Herbal Dietary Supplements in 2004*
1. Garlic
Prevents or reverses plaque buildup in arteries.
2. Echinacea
Prevents and treats the common cold, flu, and upper respiratory tract infections and strengthens the immune system.
3. Saw Palmetto
Treats enlarged prostate symptoms.
4. Ginkgo
Improves circulation and mental function.
5. Soy
Reduces the risk of coronary heart disease, aids in weight loss, promotes healthy bones, prevents cancer, and alleviates menopausal symptoms.
6. Cranberry
Helps to prevent urinary tract infections caused by *E. coli* bacteria.
7. Ginseng*
Siberian ginseng and schizandra. Asian ginseng (Chinese and Korean) increase energy and endurance.

8. Black Cohosh

Treats the physical and emotional symptoms of menopause.

9. St. John's wort

Used to treat mild to moderate depression, insomnia, injuries involving nerve trauma and bedwetting in children.

10. Milk thistle

Improves liver function, protects against liver damage, and enhances regeneration of damaged liver cells.

11. Evening primrose oil

Counteracts deficiency of essential fatty acids, which may be responsible for conditions/diseases, including cardiovascular ailments, menstrual irregularities, inflammation, and hyperactivity in children.

12. Valerian

Relieves anxiety and nervous irritability. Also used as a sedative and sleep aid. Non-habit-forming.

13. Green tea

Used as an antioxidant for prevention of heart disease, ulcers, cancer, and plaque formation.

14. Bilberry

Increases microcirculation by stimulating new capillary formation, strengthening capillary walls, and increasing overall health of the circulatory system.

15. Grape seed

Reduces risk of heart attack and stroke by preventing plaque development. Other blood vessel disorders such as diabetes, leg cramps, varicose veins, arm and leg numbness or tingling. Also used for macular degeneration and cataracts.

16. Horny goat weed

Increases libido in men and women, and improves erectile function in men.

17. Yohimbe**

Used by males to relieve impotence or achieve an erection.

18. Horse Chestnut

Treats the discomforts of varicose veins and other leg vein problems and reduces hemorrhoids.

19. Eleuthero (Siberian ginseng)
Invigorates and fortifies the body during fatigue or weakness, increases work and concentration and aids in patient rehabilitation.
20. Ginger
Treats nausea, motion sickness, and vomiting and can help to increase appetite.

SOURCES: Information Resources, Inc., and the American Botanical Council.
NOTE: Sales data from IRI represent only a minor segment of the total herbal dietary supplement market (estimated to be just under 7 percent of the $4.2 billion market). Sales data do not include sales from Wal-Mart stores, or sales from other market channels: health and natural food stores, mail order, MLM companies, health professionals, warehouse buying clubs, and convenience stores. Data do not include herbal tea sales.
*Includes Asian ginseng (*Panax ginseng*) and American ginseng (*P. quinquefolius*)
**Yohimbine is also sold as a prescription drug. It is on the FDA's supplement ingredients of concern warning list and is under investigation by the FDA.

But don't we need our drugs? Don't they save us from almost certain death? Some do, like some antibiotics and AIDS medicines. However, too many Americans have demanded antibiotics for viral diseases they can't possibly cure—often for minor infections—which has allowed bacterial strains to develop resistance.

Other drugs, like cholesterol-cutting statins, while possibly unclogging arteries, don't reduce the number of heart attacks and don't address what clogged the arteries in the first place—while exposing users to possible side effects like liver and muscle damage. The right balance of risk and benefit is still harder to strike for a raft of heavily promoted drugs that treat common, persistent, daily life conditions: anti-inflammatories, antacids, and pills for allergies, depression, social phobias, menstrual emotional discomfort, waning sexual powers, and excitable children. As Marcia Angell, M.D., former editor of the *New England Journal of Medicine* and author of *The Truth About the Drug Companies*, says, "We are taking way too many drugs for dubious or exaggerated ailments."

"What the drug companies are doing now is promoting drugs for long-term use to essentially healthy people. Why? Because it's the biggest market," Angell said.

Drug makers, doctors, and patients have all been quick to medicate some conditions that were once accepted simply as part of the human condition. Americans instinctively trust science and medical technology, say public health experts, and they expect drugs to smooth over even the routine bumps of life.

The United States buys 18 percent more pharmaceuticals per person annually—even adjusting for higher prices—than second-ranking France, according to the Organization for Economic Co-operation and Development, while lagging well behind other industrial nations in important measures of health, like life span and rates of heart disease and cancer. With so many medications at hand, mounting numbers of patients abuse them. About 4 percent of the nation's adults and teenagers misuse prescription drugs annually, suggests a 2001 report by the National Institute on Drug Abuse.

In a recent report, the U.S. Centers for Disease Control and Prevention voiced concern about the huge off-label growth of antidepressants. They are being used to treat often loosely defined syndromes of compulsion, panic, anxiety, and premenstrual discomfort.

Good thing we have a federal agency to monitor all these things and act as our advocate, right?

Right? We do, don't we?

3

The Regulators

In June 2001, Milton Cole, a seventy-one-year-old man in generally good health, went to his cardiologist complaining of chest pains. After undergoing a series of cardiac tests that turned up nothing, the doctor gave his patient a prescription and some free samples of Prozac, an antidepressant drug. Thirteen days after that visit, Cole's wife found him hanging from a beam in a back room of their shop. Even though Prozac isn't approved for treating chest pain, technically, the doctor—unaware that experts had debated for years whether Prozac caused suicide—did nothing wrong in the eyes of the Food and Drug Administration.

As you probably are aware, the FDA impacts the lives of every American every day, and as in the case of Mr. Cole, some more than others. The FDA regulates over $1 trillion worth of products, which is about one of every four dollars spent annually by American consumers. As impressive as this sounds, the FDA's reach is greater—and more controversial—than people realize; again, Mr. Cole, whom I'll talk about later. In the meantime, consider the following scenario.

You enter the waiting room at your doctor's office, and sign in at the reception desk. You scan the crowded room and spot an empty seat next to a middle-aged woman flipping through *Better Homes & Gardens*. As you plop into the chair you notice her magazine is opened to an ad for the acid reflux drug Prilosec OTC. She flips again and there's a picture of former quarterback great John Elway in an ad for Prevacid, then one for the allergy medicine Allegra-D.

You nervously pick up *Money* magazine and as you begin your own flipping, you notice an ad with the headline, "Mommy, where do pharmaceuticals come from?" The ad, sponsored by GlaxoSmithKline begins, "Surveys show most Americans credit the government for most of the drug research and development done today. But, in fact, pharmaceutical companies developed 91 percent of today's top-selling medicines on their own. According to the National Institutes of Health, only 9 percent of medicines were developed with government help and none by government alone." You hear your name called and you follow the nurse to a smaller waiting room where she hands you a striped crinkly paper gown.

It's about forty-five minutes later, and you've undergone a battery of tests and a bunch of poking and prodding. After sitting for some time on the examination table, the nurse pops in. Forcing a smile, she says after you remove the paper gown you should meet with the doctor in his office.

On the way, you pass a well-groomed young man and woman hovering over a large spread of food. The doctor's staff surround the table, picking at the cold cuts, cheeses, and an assortment of cookies and fruit. You have a chance to look around the doctor's office before he comes in. You see his degrees and stacks of files, printouts, and large manila envelopes labeled "radiology." There's also a tray full of medical journals including the *Journal of the American Medical Association* and the *New England Journal of Medicine*.

The doctor sits down behind his desk. He looks grim. He tells you both your blood pressure and cholesterol count are too high, and if you don't lose weight you're a prime candidate for diabetes. For these he scribbles out two prescriptions. He then says that your heartburn complaints are due to gastroesophageal reflux disease, known as GERD, which also could be caused by the extra pounds you're carrying. He recommends you take Prilosec. You're mildly disappointed, remembering that's not the heartburn remedy John Elway recommends.

He starts to write a prescription for it and stops. He tells you it's unnecessary since Prilosec is now available over the counter. Almost as an afterthought he slides two vacuum-sealed plastic packets toward you. "In the meantime, why don't you take these?"

When you tell him you've had some chest pains he tells you your heart is fine, "so far." He rummages through his desk drawer and hands you samples of Prozac. Noticing your surprise, he says, "I know it's an antidepressant but it treats pain, also." You're relieved he hasn't suggested you exercise more. There's simply no time.

On the way out, you notice nametags on the well-heeled young man and woman by the food spread. You realize they're sales reps for a major pharmaceutical company.

At the drugstore, the pharmacist tells you they have a generic equivalent for only one of your prescriptions. You cringe, knowing your health plan requires a higher co-pay for brand-name medications.

As you wait for the prescriptions to be filled, you wander through the rows of aisles. You grab the Prilosec. The next few rows contain a wide variety and assortment of vitamins, minerals, herbs, and other supplements, including ginseng, garlic, coenzyme Q10 (coQ10)—whatever that might be—vitamin E, a B-complex vitamin, trimethylglycine (which you can't even pronounce), and licorice root. You chuckle to yourself when you see bottles of fish oil, green tea extract, and grape seed extract. "What a waste of money," you think to yourself. You eat plenty—maybe too much—but you're sure you get all the nutrients you need. Why eat grapes or fish in a pill? Probably just expensive urine, you figure.

You look at the label of a popular brand of multivitamins and see that it contains over 500 percent more of a vitamin than is "recommended." You put it back, fearing an overdose.

You then notice displays for diet pills. One catches your eye—it has a picture of a man with washboard abs. You check the ingredients to make sure it doesn't contain ephedra, since you've read it kills people. Then you remember it's already been banned. An ingredient you don't recognize, synephrine, is listed. The label describes it as an

What Is the HHS?

Overseeing the network of federal government agencies that promote, monitor, and ensure the health of all Americans by providing essential human services is the U.S. Department of Health and Human Services (HHS). With a $581 billion budget in the 2005 fiscal year, HHS controls over three hundred programs administered by agencies with defined roles. These include:

- Administration for Children and Families (ACF)
- Administration on Aging (AoA)
- Agency for Healthcare Research and Quality (AHRQ)
- Agency for Toxic Substances and Disease Registry (ATSDR)
- Centers for Disease Control and Prevention (CDC)
- Centers for Medicare and Medicaid Services (CMS)
- Health Resources and Services Administration (HRSA)
- Indian Health Service (IHS)
- Program Support Center (PSC)
- Substance Abuse and Mental Health Services Administration (SAMHSA)
- Food and Drug Administration (FDA): Assures food and drug safety.
- National Institutes of Health: Conducts health and social science research.

Also under HHS are the Office for Civil Rights, the Office of Public Health and Emergency Preparedness, and the Center for Faith-Based and Community Initiatives. The Social Security Administration was formerly under HHS but became an independent agency in 1995.

There's another government agency that deals with food outside of HHS. The U.S. Department of Agriculture (USDA) is responsible for the safety of meat, poultry, and egg products and researches a

> variety of related fields including human nutrition (such as nutritional standards like the Food Pyramid) and new crop technologies. If you suspect there might be conflicts between HHS—especially the FDA and the USDA—with agencies operating at cross purposes you'd be right.

"effective and safe ephedra substitute." You shrug and put it in your basket, not really knowing whether or not its ingredients are effective—or safe, for that matter.

You remember your daughter asked you to pick up something for her congestion so you go to the cough and colds section and absently drop a bottle of Sudafed into your basket.

Pretty soon, you've drifted over to the food section. You brighten when you see a box of artificial sweetener near the low-fat potato chips. You figure you can reduce calories by using aspartame instead of sugar.

Your prescription is still not ready, so you sit in the waiting area and watch the overhead TV. During a break there are three drug commercials: one for an allergy medicine, another for acid reflux disease, and one for impotence. You blush, and head back to the prescription counter. The pharmacist rummages through dozens of white bags with forms stapled to the front. She soon hands you two bags. As you head for the register, you pass the shelves of pain relievers. Remembering that you're out of Tylenol, you grab a bottle.

What does this little scenario have to do with the FDA? More importantly, what does it have to do with you? As you'll see, plenty.

"In the Beginning": How the FDA Got Its Start

The FDA is one of our nation's oldest consumer protection agencies. Its nine thousand employees monitor the manufacture, importation, transport, storage, and sale of about $1 trillion worth of products each year, costing taxpayers about $3 per person.

First and foremost, the FDA is a public health agency, charged with protecting American consumers by enforcing the Federal Food,

Drug, and Cosmetic Act (FD&C Act) and several related public health laws. To do this, the FDA has some 1,100 investigators and inspectors in district and local offices in 157 cities across the country, covering nearly 95,000 FDA-regulated businesses.

The FDA originated in the late 1930s after the Massengil company marketed an antibiotic product called Elixir Sulfanilamide without prior toxicity testing of its solvent. The solvent—diethylene glycol (which is used today as automotive antifreeze)—caused the death of 107 people, mostly children. The Elixir Sulfanilamide tragedy prompted the passage of the FD&C Act in 1938 and eventually led to the establishment of the FDA.

Today the FD&C Act authorizes the FDA to regulate drugs, medical devices, foods, and cosmetics under different standards. For decades, the FDA regulated dietary supplements as foods, in most circumstances to ensure that they were safe and wholesome, and that their labeling was truthful and not misleading. An important facet of ensuring safety was the FDA's power to judge the safety of all new ingredients, including those used in dietary supplements, granted to it by the 1958 Food Additive Amendments to the FD&C Act.

Other FDA Tasks

Another major FDA mission is to protect the safety and wholesomeness of food. The agency's scientists test samples to see if any substances, such as pesticide residues, are present in unacceptable amounts. If contaminants are identified, the FDA takes corrective action. The FDA also sets labeling standards to help consumers know what is in the foods they buy. Another FDA responsibility is to make sure medicated feeds and other drugs given to animals raised for food do not threaten the health of consumers.

The FDA is also responsible for the safety of the nation's blood supply. The agency's investigators routinely examine blood bank operations, from record-keeping to testing for contaminants. The FDA also ensures the purity and effectiveness of biologicals (medical preparations made from living organisms and their products), such as insulin and vaccines.

Medical devices are classified and regulated according to their degree of risk to the public. Devices that are life-supporting, life-sustaining or implanted, such as pacemakers, must receive agency approval before they can be marketed. After a drug or device is approved for marketing, the agency collects and analyzes tens of thousands of reports each year to monitor for any unexpected adverse reactions.

Cosmetic safety also comes under the the FDA's jurisdiction. The agency can remove unsafe cosmetics from the marketplace. The dyes, preservatives, and other additives used in drugs, foods, and cosmetics must pass FDA scrutiny, and the agency must review and approve these chemicals before they can be used.

Unlike most drugs and devices, foods (and dietary supplements) do not require pre-market approval because of their inherent safety and history of use. Rather, the law requires that manufacturers of dietary supplements, prior to marketing, submit data to the FDA for any new dietary ingredient that is not already present in the food supply.

If a company is found to be violating any of the laws that the FDA enforces, the agency can "persuade" the firm to voluntarily correct the problem or to recall a faulty product from the market. A recall is generally the fastest and most effective way to protect the public from an unsafe product.

When a company can't (or won't) voluntarily correct a public health problem with one of its products, the FDA can bring to bear legal sanctions. The agency can go to court to force a company to stop selling a product and to have items already produced seized and destroyed. When warranted, criminal penalties—including prison sentences—are sought against manufacturers and distributors.

About three thousand products a year are found to be unfit for consumers and are withdrawn from the marketplace, either by voluntary recall or by court-ordered seizure. In addition, about thirty thousand import shipments a year are detained at ports of entry because the goods appear to be unacceptable.

The Brouhaha Involving Vitamins, Minerals, and Herbs

For decades the FDA tried to regulate the sale and use of vitamins, herbs, and other dietary supplements. By law, the FDA ruled that any ingested product intended by its manufacturer to prevent or treat a disease is a drug. Products—other than food—that are intended to affect the structure or function of the body are also considered drugs. Throughout the 1950s and 1960s, the FDA brought hundreds of court actions against nutritional supplement manufacturers for making health-related claims for their products. Under threat of law, food manufacturers were even prevented from labeling the fat, cholesterol, or other nutritional content of their food. (Note: Such labeling was later allowed, and with the Nutrition Labeling and Education Act of 1990, nutrition labeling became mandatory.)

The FDA actively prosecuted vitamin retailers that sold vitamins and other supplements in conjunction with books or pamphlets that extolled their use. It was illegal for a health food store to sell vitamins and books touting the virtues of vitamins.

The FDA justified such practices, which many considered to be a violation of the First Amendment, under the theory that literature sold near a product was thereby converted into a product label, and if health claims were made in the literature, then the product had to be regulated as a drug (and thus had to go through FDA clinical trials before being sold).

In 1973, the FDA published regulations expanding its control over supplements by declaring that any dietary supplement that it considered to lack nutritional usefulness was a drug and was thus under the FDA's control. The regulations took effect in 1975. For instance, high-potency vitamins, defined by the FDA as vitamins sold in dosages as little as twice the federal recommended daily allowance (RDA), were automatically considered drugs.

As a result, high-potency vitamins were effectively made illegal by this ruling because they could not be sold without FDA approval, and the FDA would not approve supplements that it considered to be "unnecessary." Vitamin manufacturers and consumers fought back, and in response Congress passed the Proxmire Vitamin Mineral Amendment of 1976, which stated that the FDA could not classify a mineral or vitamin as a drug "solely because it exceeds the level of potency the FDA determines is nutritionally rational or useful."

Under the protection of the Proxmire Amendment, the dietary and nutritional supplement industry expanded. Undaunted, the FDA stepped up enforcement again in the early 1990s after thirty-eight deaths were attributed to L-tryptophan, an amino acid widely used for treating depression and building muscle mass. (Note: The Centers for Disease Control and Prevention later exonerated L-tryptophan in the deaths, which were caused by a contaminant and not L-tryptophan. However, the FDA did not lift its ban on over-the-counter sales of L-tryptophan.)

In 1985, the FDA lost a bitter turf battle with the Federal Trade Commission and the National Institutes of Health. Under recommendation from the National Cancer Institute, a division of the NIH, the FTC permitted Kellogg's to claim that a high-fiber diet reduced the probability of certain types of cancer. The FDA wanted to sue Kellogg's, but the FTC argued that the ads presented "important public health recommendations in an accurate, useful, and substantiated way." Under pressure, the FDA backed down, and as a result it was established that food products could advertise a "substantiated" health claim without going through the FDA drug-approval process. Later, in 1993, the FDA announced that it planned to regulate as drugs all amino acids, herbs, and other supplements including fibers and fish oils. The FDA immediately found itself under a furious attack from millions of consumers and the supplement industry in general.

Enter DSHEA

In response to the rising controversy between the FDA and its regulation of the supplement industry—and no doubt, at least partially in response to the outpouring of letters and phone calls from health-conscious consumers, retailers, and manufacturers— the Dietary Supplement Health and Education Act (DSHEA) was passed by Congress unanimously in 1994. With passage of DSHEA, Congress amended the FD&C Act to include several provisions that apply only to dietary supplements and ingredients of dietary supplements. As a result, this new law created a new regulatory framework for the safety and labeling of dietary supplements.

Signed by President Clinton on October 25, 1994, DSHEA acknowledges that millions of consumers believe dietary supplements may help augment daily diets and provide health benefits. Congress' intent in enacting DSHEA was to meet the concerns of consumers and manufacturers and to help ensure that safe and appropriately labeled products remain available for those who want to use them.

In the findings associated with DSHEA, Congress stated that there may be a positive relationship between sound dietary practice and good health, and that, although further scientific research is needed, there may be a connection between dietary supplement use, reduced health-care expenses, and disease prevention.

So, what allowances do DSHEA codes make for supplement manufacturers and distributors? Under DSHEA, nutritional supplements can make substantiated "statements of nutritional support" that do not thereby invoke FDA control. Supplements, however, cannot make claims regarding disease without becoming regulated as drugs. The distinction between statements of nutritional support and claims regarding disease is vague. Manufacturers of St. John's wort, for example, may claim that St. John's wort "promotes healthy emotional balance and well-being," but they cannot say St. John's wort "is useful in the treatment of depression." The difference is of most interest to lawyers—not consumers—when you consider how many people take St. John's wort for mild cases of depression (more on this later).

Under DSHEA, a supplement company is responsible for determining that the product it manufactures or distributes is safe and that any representations or claims made about it are not false or misleading and are supported by adequate evidence. This means that dietary supplements do not need approval from the FDA before they are marketed. Except in the case of a new dietary ingredient, where pre-market review for safety data and other information is required, a manufacturer does not have to provide the FDA with the evidence it relies on to substantiate safety or effectiveness before or after it begins to market its products. The rationale is that like food, these ingredients have already passed muster for safety.

The FDA Modernization Act of 1997

By the late 1990s, numerous academic studies and government reports had indicted the FDA for dragging its feet regarding the approval of drugs and the monitoring of them afterwards. Pressure for reform finally began to be felt by members of Congress, a portion of which had recently promised deregulation in their "Contract with America." In 1996, the House wrote an FDA reform bill that would have significantly threatened some of the FDA's central powers, but the FDA and its supporters in the Clinton administration defeated it. Facing a veto, Congress abandoned the bill and the following year passed a watered-down bill, the FDA Modernization Act of 1997.

Much of the Modernization Act merely put in writing what was already FDA practice. For one thing, it authorizes the FDA to appoint panels of scientific experts to assist the agency in evaluating new drugs, a practice the FDA has followed for decades. Similarly, it codified the rule that only one adequate and well-controlled clinical study in addition to confirmatory evidence could be the basis of approval for a new drug. The most important provisions of this act were the reauthorization of user fees for another five years. As you'll see later in this chapter, these user fees are very controversial.

The FDA's Powers

Despite what you've been led to believe, a dietary supplement that is adulterated or misbranded or bears an unauthorized drug claim can be seized, condemned, and destroyed. A perfect illustration of this ability occurred recently when the Federal Trade Commission and FDA charged the marketers of a dietary supplement called Coral Calcium Supreme with making false and unsubstantiated claims about the product's health benefits, especially during their oft-seen infomercials on cable television. In a complaint filed in federal district court, the agencies allege that Kevin Trudeau, Robert Barefoot, Shop America (USA), LLC, and Deonna Enterprises, Inc., violated the FTC act by claiming, falsely and without substantiation, that Coral Calcium Supreme can treat or cure cancer and other diseases such as multiple sclerosis and heart disease.

DSHEA codes include other safety requirements regarding the introduction of new dietary ingredients. The law clarified that dietary supplement ingredients marketed prior to October 15, 1994 do not require pre-market approval. However, manufacturers marketing a new dietary supplement ingredient after this date must submit safety information on the new dietary ingredient to the FDA.

The FDA can remove products from the market for the following reasons:

• *The Product Poses a Significant and Unreasonable Risk:* The FDA does not have to prove that a product actually harmed anyone, but simply that it presents a "significant or unreasonable risk" of illness or injury.

• *The Product Contains Poisonous or Deleterious Substances:* The FDA does not have to prove that a product has a substance that will injure, but simply that it may render injury under the recommended or suggested conditions indicated on a product's label.

• *The Product Is Unfit for Food:* The FDA has authority to stop the marketing of any dietary supplement that the agency believes is not fit for human consumption.

• *The Product Makes Drug Claims:* If a dietary supplement's label indicates that the product can diagnose, cure, mitigate, treat, or prevent a disease, then it is clearly being represented as a "drug" and is no longer considered a dietary supplement. Responsible manufacturers have labels, warnings, and directions for use of their products and are careful not to represent their products as drugs. As in the coral calcium case I mentioned above, the FTC and FDA charge that these and other claims go far beyond existing scientific evidence regarding the recognized health benefits of calcium. This action, by the way, is part of a series of initiatives the FTC and FDA are taking against the purveyors of products with unsubstantiated health and medical claims.

• *The Product Lacks Truthful and Informative Labeling:* By law, all dietary supplement products must contain extensive informative labeling, including detailed information about the nutrients in the product, such as name and quantity of all ingredients in the product and the name and place of business of the company. (By the way, most legitimate companies in the dietary supplement industry support the enforcement of this provision.)

A couple of years ago, the Secretary of Health and Human Services announced enforcement efforts to remove products that were marketed to minors and for illicit purposes. No one objected. The supplement industry says it has consistently urged the FDA to use its enforcement powers to remove such products from the marketplace. Plus, DSHEA already gave the secretary the authority to remove any dietary supplement or supplement ingredient that poses an "imminent hazard."

This bears repeating: DSHEA already gives the Secretary of HHS the authority to remove any dietary supplement or supplement ingredient that poses an "imminent hazard."

The procedure is rather straightforward. If the HHS Secretary makes this decision, the government must conduct an administrative review of the case and the product cannot be sold to the public. Of course, it's expected the secretary will have solid evidence when he does remove a product.

Familiar Words

Dietary supplements that make nutritional claims must carry the following two disclaimers, which are probably familiar to most of us:

- "This statement has not been evaluated by the Food and Drug Administration."
- "This product is not intended to diagnose, treat, cure, or prevent any disease."

Though subject to certain conditions, such as the information presented is not false or misleading and not biased in favor of a particular manufacturer or brand, DSHEA also restricts the FDA's ability to ban the dissemination of information on dietary supplements. Health food retailers, for example, can now market books, magazines, and scientific literature describing the uses of dietary supplements (though there are very specific regulations as to where the literature can be shown in relation to the supplements and food shelves). As a result, in recent years consumers have had much more information—for better or worse, some may argue—pertaining to the health benefits of vitamins and other supplements.

Different Standards

Prescription drugs need to undergo various steps before they are approved for use (for more on this, see chapter 5, So You Want to Be a Human Guinea Pig?). The industry boldly claims the cost of developing a new prescription drug is probably over $800 million. The consumer watchdog group Public Citizen scoffs at this estimate. Suspecting the pharmaceutical industry is either not being truthful or they have really lousy accountants, they believe the true figure is more than likely at least 75 percent lower, in large part because much of the research is conducted under government grants.

One thing is for sure—drug companies aren't too fond of untested dietary supplements that compete against their drugs. Especially when you consider that supplements can bypass the costly FDA approval process by simply carrying a statement saying the product hasn't been evaluated by the FDA. The argument would almost be laughable if not for the death of Mr. Cole and other scams perpetrated on the public.

Back to Our Scenario

As you can see, the FDA wields enormous clout over what we eat, drink, and take as "medicine." And, they also have the power to look the other way.

Because of this power, there are plenty of outside factors trying to muscle in and influence their regulatory authority and decisions. Remember the scenario we set up at the beginning of the chapter? Let's go back and examine other ways in which our well-being is often compromised.

Let's start in the waiting room. Our patient saw the John Elway ad for Prevacid and was disappointed his doctor recommended Prilosec instead. Let's be honest. Whether we want to admit it or not—even to ourselves—we are influenced by celebrity endorsements. Is Prevacid a superior medicine because it (supposedly) works for John Elway? Would it be as effective for weekend warriors or those who live with weekend warriors like you? Who knows?

Then there was this little beauty of an ad. To repeat:

"Mommy, where do pharmaceuticals come from?" The ad, sponsored by GlaxoSmithKline states, "Surveys show most Americans credit the government for most of the drug research and development done today. But, in fact, pharmaceutical companies developed 91 percent of today's top-selling medicines on their own. According to the National Institutes of Health, only 9 percent of medicines were developed with government help and none by government alone."

Let me be as frank as possible—that's bunk, pure bunk, as you will clearly see later in this book.

On the way to the doctor's office, we passed a young man and woman hovering over a food table. We later learn that they're pharmaceutical sales representatives. There are currently approximately eighty thousand pharmaceutical sales people in the United States, which is slightly more than one for each ten physicians. The cost of face-to-face promotion (or detailing) in 2000 was approximately $4.8 billion, or $6,400 for each practicing physician in the United States. It's quite obvious that these reps are exerting significant influence over physicians.

According to industry estimates, drug companies spent $15.7 billion dollars on promotion in 2000. Over $7 billion worth of free samples were distributed that year. According to a study from the Department of Medicine at the University of Washington, pharmaceutical companies often use drug samples as a marketing strategy. Based on interviews with 131 doctors, they found the availability of drug samples led physicians to dispense and subsequently prescribe drugs that differ from their preferred drug choice. While physicians most often report using drug samples to avoid cost to the patient, they would dispense a drug sample that differed from their preferred drug choice.

What does this mean? While your physician undoubtedly had to go through a grueling medical school curriculum after college, many pharmaceutical sales reps have only a bachelor's degree and/or marketing background. This wouldn't much matter except when you consider the major pull that pharmaceutical sales reps have over what ends up in your medicine cabinet.

On the Other Hand

Not everyone agrees with the notion that pharmaceutical reps have too much power and influence. One recent study suggests that doctors are more wary of pharmaceutical companies' aggressive market-

More About the University of Washington Study

Here are a few more details about the study from the University of Washington. The researchers asked physicians to self-report their prescribing patterns for three clinical scenarios, including their preferred drug choice, whether they would use a drug sample and subsequently prescribe the sampled medication, and the importance of factors involved in the decision to dispense a drug sample. A total of 131 of 154 physicians (85 percent) responded. When presented with an insured woman with an uncomplicated lower urinary tract infection, 22 respondents (17 percent) reported that they would dispense a drug sample; 21 of these sample users (95 percent) stated that they would dispense a drug sample that differed from their preferred drug choice. For an uninsured man with hypertension, 35 respondents (27 percent) reported that they would dispense a drug sample; 32 of 35 sample users (91 percent) indicated that they would dispense a drug sample instead of their preferred drug choice. For an uninsured woman with depression, 108 respondents (82 percent) reported that they would dispense a drug sample; 53 of 108 sample users (49 percent) indicated that avoiding cost to the patient was the most consistent motivator for dispensing a drug sample for all three scenarios.

ing than generally believed and don't easily yield to pressure to switch prescriptions. In a study presented at a conference of the Institute for Operations Research and the Management Sciences at the Robert H. Smith School of Business at the University of Maryland in June 2003, Natalie Mizik of Columbia University and Robert Jacobson of the University of Washington write, "Are physicians easy marks? To the contrary, our results show that physicians are 'tough sells' in that sales force activity has modest to very small influence on prescribing behavior."

The authors, noting accusations that pharmaceutical sales representatives (PSRs) compromise physician integrity, obtained access to a database that allowed them to assess the impact that interactions with sales reps have on the number of new prescriptions issued by physicians.

The study sample involved three different drugs and 74,075 American physicians. The database contained information for twenty-four months on the number of new prescriptions issued for a drug by a given physician, the number of detailing sales calls the physician received that month for the drug, and the number of free drug samples that the rep left with a physician. The data was provided on condition of anonymity.

The drugs differ: they come from different therapeutic areas, they have been on the market from less than one year to eleven years, and they have achieved different levels of commercial success—their annual sales range from under $500 million to over $1 billion. In total, the data represent over four million interactions between physicians and pharmaceutical sales representatives.

For each of the drugs in the study, the authors used statistical modeling and operations research methods to assess the effect of changes in the amount of detailing and sampling on the number of additional new prescriptions the physician issued over the subsequent six-month period for the drug.

They found that pharmaceutical companies had to invest heavily to produce even a small increase in prescriptions. For the three drugs studied—drug 1 is prescribed by psychologists and psychiatrists, drugs 2 and 3 are prescribed by primary care physicians—the results indicate that it would take an additional 0.64, 3.11, and 6.54 visits by pharmaceutical sales reps, respectively, to induce one additional new prescription and 6.44, 25.39, and 73.05 additional free drug samples to induce one new prescription.

The authors say that the most important reason why sales reps are having limited influence is that they are not the only source of information for physicians. Doctors consult scientific papers, advice from colleagues, and their own experience when developing prescribing practices. "Indeed, most physicians view these influences as far more important than that of PSRs," write the authors. "Many physicians view skeptically or hold negative attitudes toward PSRs. They recognize that information presented is biased toward the promoted drug and is unlikely to be objective."

Benefit of Drug Samples

A related study by a second set of researchers at the same conference suggests that distributing drug samples is less a method to sway physicians than a way of contrasting medications and helping manufacturers maintain market share.

In "Prescription Drug Promotion: The Role and Value of Physicians' Samples Under Competition," Kissan Joseph of the University of Kansas and Murali K. Mantrala of ZS Associates in Evanston, Illinois, used a mathematical model to analyze drug samples' impact on patients, physicians, and pharmaceutical manufacturers. They conclude that supplying samples plays a positive role in making the choice between medications.

"While critics often argue that this practice adversely affects patient welfare," they write, "we contend that samples provide a benefit by facilitating the match between drugs and patients' underlying disease state by reducing the cost of comparing drugs."

If patients are incorrectly matched to a drug, the researchers observe, they lose money and suffer the lack of physical relief from their ailment. Providing free samples helps reduce out-of-pocket cost to patients and alleviates some of the non-financial costs as well.

Surprisingly, they suggest that pharmaceutical companies are often the losers in the samples war, incurring great expense by distributing free samples purely as a defensive marketing tactic to maintain market share. Still, while this might sound logical, I believe that we should expect doctors and health-care professionals to make their medical decisions based on science, not marketing.

Hypothetical Health Risks

While we're on the subject of prescriptions, it's important to note a few other things in the scenario at the pharmacy. Remember all the prescription bags on the pharmacist's table? Granted, doctors in the U.S. write three billion prescriptions each year, yet according to the Institute of Medicine, prescription errors due to misreading physician's handwriting kill up to seven thousand Americans annually. In addition, overmedication and adverse reactions to prescription drugs also cause unnecessary deaths. In 1994, these accounted for 106,000 deaths, according to the *Journal of the American Medical Association*. In fact, more people are killed by adverse reactions to prescription drugs than by pulmonary disease or accidents. To top it off, it's now estimated that an average of 137,000 people die each year just as a result of taking prescription medication where no mistakes or abuse is involved. Today, prescription drug deaths are surpassed only by heart disease, cancer, and stroke. The elderly, whose bodies often can't tolerate the dosages and combinations of pills doctors prescribe for them, are particularly susceptible.

We also have to consider that while many drug interactions may not kill people, they do seriously injure them. Studies estimate that two million Americans are hospitalized annually from drug side effects. True, some dangerous drug side effects are simply a consequence of taking medicine, such as when chemotherapy treatments leave a patient vulnerable to infection.

There's another aspect of this problem. New drugs are tested on only a few hundred to a few thousand patients before they're sold to millions, meaning rare side effects that didn't show up in clinical studies can wind up hurting hundreds of people. In essence, the real clinical trial begins when the drug is prescribed to you and yours.

Part of the FDA's job is to track side effects of medications after they're approved for sale so that health officials can take action if unexpected problems arise, and to develop strategies for preventing drug-related injuries. But the FDA learned of just 9,961 medication-related deaths and 33,541 hospitalizations in 1997, said a 1998 report from the Health and Human Services inspector general.

Why? The problem lies in the voluntary nature of the injury reporting system, the report said. In simple terms, the FDA can require drug manufacturers to report only the injuries they learn about that involve their drugs. The FDA does not have the authority to require doctors and hospitals to report injuries, either to the government or to the drug companies themselves. But unless the FDA finds proactive ways to uncover patterns of injuries, it can't take the next step of helping to prevent them, the inspector general concluded.

Here's a perfect illustration: At the first World Congress on Lung Health and Respiratory Diseases in Florence, Italy, where fifteen thousand specialists from eighty-four countries met in September 2002, researchers noted that hundreds of medicines are routinely prescribed against a variety of disorders, including high blood pressure, allergies, rheumatism, certain cancers, or even common nonrespiratory inflammations that can cause all kinds of lung diseases. These diseases can develop within a very short time or after several years. They are mostly unpredictable and some are irreversible, resulting in permanent damage. Yet the information provided with the packaging rarely warns patients that the medicine could potentially cause a lung disorder, and there still aren't many doctors who even know to give the matter due thought when they prescribe a treatment.

Bet you never heard about this, right? It's somewhat ironic when you read in the press a negative article on supplements—they always talk about the lack of government regulation, which must mean that the safety of these products is highly questionable. Yet by comparison, nutritional supplements void of government regulation seem to be far safer than highly regulated and enormously profitable prescription drugs. And what do our fearless leaders in Washington want to do? Set up a new procedure for reporting adverse events tallied by manufacturers.

This self-reporting system for adverse events doesn't work for the pharmaceutical industry, so why do they want to make the same mistake twice with dietary supplements? I'll tell you more about this foolish proposal later in the book.

Meanwhile, consider this: remember our patient looking over the wide selection of assorted vitamins? While there have been over five hundred studies published in the medical literature about the dangers of homocysteine, our patient had never heard about it—not even from his doctor. While our patient of course knew about cholesterol (although he could never keep straight whether HDL was the good one or the bad one), elevations in homocysteine can lead to arteriosclerosis of the blood vessels in the heart and brain and is up to five times more deadly than elevated cholesterol. It is widely accepted that vitamins B6, B12, folic acid, and trimethylglycine promote healthy homocysteine levels.

As for the patient's heartburn, licorice increases the production of protective mucus in the stomach and may reduce acid secretion, making it a useful treatment for inflammatory stomach conditions. It contains vitamin E, B-complex vitamins, biotin, niacin, pantothenic acid, lecithin, manganese and other trace elements. One warning for our patient, though—it shouldn't be used by people with hypertension.

As for Prilosec, the drug the doctor started to prescribe and stopped since it is now available over the counter, the fact is that insurance companies are unlikely to pay for a drug that's available over the counter. "The insurance companies might abandon their patients who need this drug. That could be very problematic to many patients who can't afford it," says Dr. Peter J. Baiocco, associate chief of the gastroenterology section at Lenox Hill Hospital in New York City. Doctors already have to provide extra information to insurance companies when they want to prescribe Prilosec to a patient for more than a couple of months, said Baiocco.

Gastroenterologists say some patients do have to take Prilosec each day—typically one pill—to treat chronic heartburn. If insurance companies don't pay, that could add up to more than $300 a year, much more than proven herbal remedies. After all, there's a lot of advertising to pay for.

If It's on TV, It Must Be True

Let's face it. We are a culture depending on—and convinced of—the "healthy" practice of taking drugs. As our friend found out while waiting for his prescriptions, television commercial breaks are in no shortage of ads pushing pharmaceutical drugs. And these ads all have the same basic message: "Feel bad? Take our drug and feel good." Is that why the media always touts new unproven drugs, and rarely mentions prescription drug deaths or alternative therapies for health? Don't want to tick off our advertisers, now, do we?

In 2000, pharmaceutical companies spent $2.5 billion on mass media ads for prescription drugs. Admittedly, this is a small portion of the $101.6 billion spent on advertising of mainstream consumer products in the United States. But consider the following:

• PepsiCo spent $125 million advertising Pepsi Cola—less than the $160 million Merck spent advertising Vioxx to consumers.

• Vioxx also beat out Budweiser's beer ad campaign of $146 million and was close to the most heavily advertised car—GM's Saturn—with ad spending of $169 million in 2000.

• Each of the top seven most heavily advertised prescription drugs beat Nike's ad budget of $78.2 million for its shoes.

• More was spent on advertising in each of the top fifteen individual drugs than Campbell's $58 million for its soups.

While we're on this topic, how many ads have you seen for fruits and vegetables? (Not counting the rubbery pellets found in soups and frozen foods.) One, two, none?

The bottom line? Drugs are as much or more a pedestrian part of our existence as is our lunchtime soup or the shoes we wear. And what about the foods crucial to our health and well-being—vegetables, fruits, whole grains, etc.? As they say in New York, "fuhgetaboutit."

Increasing Spending on Prescription Drugs

Spending on prescription drugs escalated more than 12 percent per year in five of the eight years between 1993 and 2000. Spending on retail prescription drugs increased 18.8 percent from 1999 to 2000 and it's anticipated that the increase will continue to be between 15 and 20 percent annually for the foreseeable future.

A 2002 study by the Center on an Aging Society at Georgetown University estimates that more than 131 million people—66 percent of all adults in the United States—use prescription drugs. Specifically, the researchers found that the great majority of adults who have one of five common chronic conditions—diabetes, heart disease, hypertension, arthritis, and cancer—use prescription drugs.

The dramatic rise in spending on prescription drugs can be attributed to a few related factors. In 1992 there were roughly 1.9 billion prescriptions dispensed in the United States, and in 2000 there were 2.9 billion. Americans are demanding, and physicians are prescribing, a higher volume of medicines each year. The rising volume of prescriptions is driven by three factors:

- An increase in the general U.S. population and the aging of the population.
- An increase in the number of people being prescribed drug therapy.
- An increase in the number of prescriptions per person.

The average number of prescriptions per person in the United States increased from 7.3 in 1992 to 10.4 in 2000. Along with this increase in demand, there has been a shift toward the use of more expensive medications. It's more than a coincidence that many of the most expensive medications happen to be those medications that are most heavily advertised.

About half of the increase in retail drug spending between 1999 and 2000 occurred among just eight drug classes—antihypertensives, antilipemics, COX-2 inhibitors, antidepressants, proton pump inhibitors, antidiabetics, antiepileptics, and pain relievers. Major drugs in these classes are extensively advertised both to prescribing physicians and directly to consumers. Interestingly, the ten drugs with the heaviest direct-to-consumer advertising accounted for 34 percent of the total increase in spending. Those drugs will probably sound familiar. They include:

- Vioxx and Celebrex (COX-2 inhibitors, for pain)
- Claritin and Allegra (for allergies)
- Paxil (for depression)
- Prilosec and Prevacid (for GERD)
- Zocor and Pravachol (for hyperlipidemia, cholesterol)
- Viagra (for erectile dysfunction)

Based upon the dramatic increases in spending for heavily advertised drugs, it is evident that the consumer advertising campaigns are working very well. Of course some of these are now under a cloud because it's been discovered:

- They don't work as well as advertised.
- They aren't as safe as reported from clinical studies.
- Side effects warp the FDA's "risk versus benefit" ratio.

How many ads for dietary supplements like multivitamins have you ever seen on TV? (Infomercials for coral calcium on cable TV don't count!) There are a handful (like Centrum), but very few in comparison to prescription drugs.

If you remember our patient selected a weight-loss product containing the ephedra substitute synephrine. The fact is, there's much less evidence about synephrine's health benefits and safety than there is about ephedra, which has been heavily studied. In fact, no one really knows if there are risks with ingesting synephrine or not. But hey, the important thing is that it's not that dangerous herb ephedra, right?

Here's some irony for you. Remember when the shopper put a bottle of Sudafed into the basket? Its sole active ingredient is pseudoephedrine, a key ingredient in the illegal stimulant methamphetamine. When the FDA banned ephedra, it allowed cold and bronchial remedies containing the substance to remain on the market. Why? Take a wild guess. The problem is, law enforcement officials soon discovered people producing meth from pseudoephedrine, often cooked up in clandestine labs in kitchens, trailers, and sheds. Meth is a highly addictive, synthetically produced central nervous system stimulant with effects similar to cocaine, and is the most prevalent synthetic drug manufactured in the United States (because it is so easily produced in makeshift labs). According to the U.S. Department of Justice, in 2002 meth labs caused 194 fires, 117 explosions, and 22 deaths.

To combat the meth labs, many states have proposed that Sudafed and similar cold and sinus remedies only be sold from behind the pharmacy counter. In Georgia, a bill requires pseudoephedrine products to be sold in blister packaging, and retailers are prohibited from selling more than three packages at once. Why didn't they ban it outright since meth is so dangerous? Dream on. It will never happen and not because officials want to preserve the free enterprise system and entrepreneurial spirit of the meth makers. Once again, think of the FDA's risk versus benefit formula. To their way of thinking, I suppose, combating post-nasal drip far outweighs the plague meth labs bring on communities. Now, if people started using the substance for weight loss, the FDA would probably take a more serious look.

Food Fights

As I mentioned earlier, the FDA also has control over approving new foods and ingredients. Do you remember how the patient in our scenario passed by the low-fat potato chips in the food section of the pharmacy? Let's examine the case of the fat substitute olestra. When first announced, many people were excited about olestra because of the possibility it could assist people in eating diets lower in saturated and overall fat—and thereby prevent obesity and heart disease.

But there were some problems. Simply put, olestra causes gastrointestinal disturbances (which are sometimes severe), including diarrhea, fecal urgency, and more frequent and looser bowel movements. (Some reports also described olestra's cause of "underwear staining" associated with "anal leakage.") The Center for Science in the Public Interest (CSPI) reports that a variety of gastrointestinal symptoms occurred in subjects who consumed on a daily basis the amount of olestra that would be found in less than one ounce of potato chips (about sixteen chips), as well as higher doses.

Data is lacking on the health effects of olestra on potentially vulnerable segments of the population. Key tests were unacceptably brief. According to the CSPI, "Only poor studies have examined the effect of olestra on gastrointestinal disturbances in children, while no studies at all have focused on gastrointestinal problems and nutrient loss in healthy people over forty-four years of age and people with poor nutritional status."

After much fanfare when introduced, olestra-laced products were largely rejected by consumers. Having lost the public relations war, Frito-Lay did what so many companies do. They don't remove the product from the market, they simply change the name. So, if you're at the grocery store you may want to check the label of Lay's Light, Ruffles Light, Doritos Light and Tostitos Light chips formally known as WOW! Chips. And, I suggest you check the packages before hosting your next barbecue or Super Bowl party.

Sweet Stuff

You might recall that our imaginary patient bought the sugar substitute aspartame—commonly known by the brand names Nutra-Sweet and Equal—to reduce his intake of sugar calories. Good thought, but probably the wrong solution. In 1996, Ralph G. Walton, M.D., chairman of the Center for Behavioral Medicine, Northeastern Ohio Universities College of Medicine, conducted a survey of peer-reviewed medical literature about the safety of aspartame using various research databases. Dr. Walton analyzed 164 studies that he believed were related to human safety questions. Of those studies, seventy-four had aspartame industry–related sponsorship and ninety were funded without any industry money.

Of the seventy-four aspartame industry–sponsored studies, all seventy-four (100 percent) claimed that no problems were found with aspartame. Of the ninety non-industry-sponsored studies, eighty-three (92 percent) identified one or more problems with aspartame. Of the seven studies that did not find a problem, six were conducted by the FDA. Given that a number of FDA officials went to work for the aspartame industry immediately following approval (including the former FDA commissioner), many consider these studies to be equivalent to industry-sponsored research.

Now let's contrast the story of aspartame with that of another sweetener, commonly called stevia. If you go to your local health food store, you will probably find a stevia product (scientific name *Stevia rebaudiana*) on the shelves. Originating in various parts of Asia and South America, stevia is commonly used throughout the rest of the world. Why? Well, it's easy to grow, it's cheap, and most of all, it's up to three hundred times sweeter than table sugar. To top it off, stevia has no calories.

Unlike most of us, the FDA most definitely has heard of stevia. In 1991, the FDA blocked the importation of stevia leaves and extracts. In 1995, they issued a revision that allowed stevia leaves or stevioside extracts to be imported if explicitly labeled as a dietary supplement or for use as an ingredient of a dietary supplement. However, it is not allowed to be imported or used as a commercial sweetener or flavoring agent. You usually have to go to a health food store to find it. Though commonplace in countries throughout the world, here it is labeled as a "supplement," and can't be called an "additive" or "food." Since the mid-1980s, the FDA has labeled stevia an "unsafe food additive" and has gone to extensive lengths to keep it off the U.S. market—including initiating a search-and-seizure campaign and full-fledged "import alert."

Is stevia dangerous? To judge from the extensive measures the FDA has employed to keep stevia away from the public, one might think so. The truth is, no ill effects have ever been found. However, the FDA has remained so adamant on the subject that even though stevia can now be legally marketed as a dietary supplement under legislation enacted in 1994, any mention of its possible use as a sweetener or tea is still strictly prohibited. To top things off, since stevia has been designated as "unsafe"—almost certainly to benefit the politically powerful sweetener industry—the agency has insisted on stonewalling any and all evidence to the contrary.

As Rob McCaleb, president and founder of the Herb Research Foundation, has said, "Sweetness is big money." In other words, the powers that be don't want to see a product that is cheap and easy to grow on the market competing with their own products. (More on sweeteners later.)

Finally, there's one other point in our scenario that requires mentioning—the vitamin with "500 percent more of the nutrient than recommended." We can't blame the FDA for this one. Instead this is the handiwork of the U.S. Department of Agriculture, although some would argue this area—the determination of nutritional standards—should fall under the FDA. Simply put, the 500 percent figure is the amount above the minimum daily requirement and has nothing to due with toxicity. Many experts argue that these "minimum daily requirements" (which were once called RDAs and are now called DRIs) are woefully inadequate. Therefore, we have need of higher intake of various nutrients. Either way, it's very unlikely that you'll suffer drastic side effects from taking a multivitamin. (For more information on this topic, see Woodland Publishing's *Real RDAs for Real People*.)

Wait, I almost forgot! There's one more thing—the Prozac samples the doctor gave our patient.

The Off-Label-Use Scam

Well, this may come as a surprise, but drug companies have a scam they'd rather not talk about. It's called "off-label use." Drug companies only have to test drugs for a particular malady while medical doctors are free to prescribe anything they want for any condition, whether it has been tested for that condition or not. You can bet there are a lot of side conversations between drug sales reps and doctors about off-label uses. You don't have to take my word for it. In a 2003 Knight Ridder study, off-label sales of the top-selling drugs hit $12.9 billion in the preceding year, producing nearly a quarter of those drugs' retail sales. I doubt doctors across the country all had the same off-label prescribing ideas occur to them via telepathy.

But are doctors and patients in a position to gauge the safety or effectiveness of off-label treatments? Aren't clinical trials one of the bulwarks and prime defenses in favor of prescription drugs and against dietary supplements?

Here's a reality check: Even in the busiest of practices, doctors see too few patients to assess any drug's range of side effects. They also have no way of knowing whether the drugs are working, if it's a placebo effect, or whether the patients simply got better on their own. Typically they base their prescribing decisions on secondhand anecdotes, small published studies or their own experiences or lapel-pulling asides by drug reps. Off-label prescribing often goes on for years before a clinical trial investigates a drug's efficacy or safety, if a clinical trial is conducted at all.

Frankly, there are too many sad stories about doctors who were convinced that an off-label therapy was safe and effective, and turned out to be wrong, in some cases disastrously so. In the 1990s, there was Fen-Phen, an unapproved cocktail of two prescription appetite suppressants that was widely prescribed until 1997, when the Mayo Clinic noticed that some Fen-Phen patients were suffering from a rare heart-valve disease.

The same thing happened more recently, with the widespread off-label prescribing of hormone replacements. Though they were approved for treating specific menopause symptoms, such as hot flash-es, doctors put millions of women on the drugs for life. They believed hormones would prevent heart disease, breast cancer, and Alzheimer's disease, uses the FDA hadn't approved. They even started women on the drugs years after they had gone through menopause.

A massive government-run study, the Women's Health Initiative, found that hormone replacement therapy actually increases a woman's risk of getting these diseases. Many doctors don't believe the findings, theorizing that the study's outcome would have been different if the participants had started hormone therapy earlier and had taken it longer.

Sylvia Wassertheil-Smoller, Ph.D., professor in the Department of Epidemiology and Population Health at Albert Einstein College of Medicine in the Bronx, New York, says the findings of WHI about hormone therapy in general, and stroke in particular, are very important to women because before these results were available it was thought that estrogen protects the brain. But, WHI found that both estrogen alone—for women who have had a hysterectomy—and estrogen plus progestin—for women who have an intact uterus—pose increased risks of stroke as well as dementia.

"The implications are that hormones should not be used to prevent cardiovascular disease or protect the brain," says Dr. Smoller, adding that the FDA indications are for menopausal symptoms at the lowest dose and duration to achieve relief. "The point is that menopause is not a disease, so it is not is if hormones are used to treat a disease—rather they were thought to prevent disease. While they do prevent osteoporosis fractures and colorectal cancer, they do not prevent heart disease and stroke or Alzheimer's, and so the risks outweigh the benefits." Because of these surprising findings, the estrogen plus progestin arm of the WHI study ended earlier than scheduled in July 2002, solely due to the potential dangers to the participants' health.

No, Not Us

Despite decades of off-label prescribing, drug makers universally deny that they push these uses at doctors. "We don't track what you're calling prescribing for unapproved uses," Doug Petkus, a spokesman for Wyeth, which makes an antidepressant as well as hormone replacement therapy, told the Knight Ridder investigators. "We don't recommend that our products be used off-label." I guess then the only explanation is a collective coast-to-coast brain-freeze by doctors, or it could be they well remember when Warner-Lambert pleaded guilty a couple of years ago and paid more than $430 million to resolve criminal charges and civil liabilities in connection with its

Parke-Davis division's illegal and fraudulent promotion of unapproved uses for the drug Neurontin (gabapentin). The drug was approved by the Food and Drug Administration in December 1993 solely for use with other drugs to control seizures in people with epilepsy. The company promoted Neurontin for the treatment of a number of other disorders, including attention-deficit disorder, migraine, bipolar disorder, drug and alcohol withdrawal, seizures, and restless leg syndrome.

Which brings us to back to Mr. Cole, whom I mentioned at the beginning of this chapter. Even though Prozac isn't approved by the Food and Drug Administration for treating chest pain, the doctor, unaware that experts had debated for years whether Prozac caused suicide, technically did nothing wrong.

The day Mr. Cole came in for his checkup and complained of chest pains, according to Knight Ridder, his doctor had a drug closet stocked with dozens of medicines that cardiologists commonly prescribe, as well as some that general practitioners and other specialists use. "I chose Prozac probably because I had samples of it," he said in an interview. "I thought it was a pretty harmless thing to do."

Until then, the FDA has approved Prozac to treat depression, panic, obsessive-compulsive disorder, and an eating disorder, none of which conditions afflicted Mr. Cole. Besides his pain, which you should notice was not one of the conditions approved for Prozac, Cole was described as upbeat and active.

The sad truth is, doctors have prescribed antidepressants off-label for years to manage chronic pain. The Knight Ridder analysis found that during the 1990s, 40 percent of Prozac prescriptions were written by non-psychiatrists and in 2000 alone, a *half-million* Prozac prescriptions were issued for off-label uses.

His doctor, knowing how popular the drug was, but not aware of any serious side effects, including the risk of suicide, went ahead and recommended the antidepressant. It didn't help Cole's chest pain, in fact, soon after he began taking it he complained of feeling jittery, his fingers tingled, and he became easily aggravated. Days later, he committed suicide.

His wife blamed Eli Lilly for not warning that Prozac can cause suicidal behavior, and her lawyer accused Lilly of over-promoting Prozac to non-psychiatrists. At the time, Lilly said they had settled "some lawsuits" for economic reasons, but wouldn't comment on specifics. There were no reports that the FDA reprimanded or fined Eli Lilly. How could they? Lilly has long contended that depression causes suicide, not Prozac. And, as with Wyeth's statement above, Lilly spokeswoman Tarra Ryker said Lilly "does not condone or encourage off-label use of any of our medications, including Prozac."

So what's the FDA's stand on off-label drugs? Here's a 1998 brief it produced entitled "Guidance for Institutional Review Boards and Clinical Investigators" entitled "'Off-Label' Use of Marketed Drugs, Biologics and Medical Devices." Here' s what it says:

> Good medical practice and the best interests of the patient require that physicians use legally available drugs, biologics and devices according to their best knowledge and judgement. If physicians use a product for an indication not in the approved labeling, they have the responsibility to be well informed about the product, to base its use on firm scientific rationale and on sound medical evidence, and to maintain records of the product's use and effects. Use of a marketed product in this manner when the intent is the "practice of medicine" does not require the submission of an Investigational New Drug Application (IND), Investigational Device Exemption (IDE) or review by an Institutional Review Board (IRB).

What? No clinical study? No report of adverse events?

Well, if that's OK with the FDA and HHS, it's OK with me, I guess. After all, they are our public safety watchdogs. Obviously, Mr. Cole's good mood was an act, and the pain caused him to be depressed enough to kill himself. And, his suicide coinciding with taking Prozac was merely a coincidence, right?

It's obvious that the pharmaceutical companies learned from Parke-Davis's expensive lesson. Be careful what you say, but still say it.

Maybe the problem is that not enough people are watching the FDA.

4

Does the FDA Need Its
Own Warning Label?

On October 8, 2003, the FDA sent out a letter warning of deaths and serious adverse events from accidental overdose of a liquid morphine sulfate product named Roxanol. "In most of these cases," the FDA wrote, ". . . morphine oral solutions ordered in milligrams (mg) were mistakenly interchanged for milliliters (mL) of the product, resulting in 20-fold overdoses." You read that right. A potentially lethal drug was being administered at twenty times the properly prescribed dosages. The FDA letter followed a letter from the maker of the drug, Elan Pharmaceuticals, called "Dear Healthcare Professional," released two days earlier.

There are a couple of things here I hope you noticed. "Deaths," of course, and "20-fold overdoses" should grab your attention. A 20-fold error is a huge error, an error that caused deaths.

You heard about this on television, right? "Serious adverse events and deaths resulting from accidental overdose of high concentration morphine sulfate . . ." You didn't? Neither did I. That's right—the FDA didn't send the letter to the media to warn the public of a potential life-threatening situation for anyone taking Roxanol. Instead they sent it to the same people Elan had, "Healthcare Professionals." Again not to the media, which could have warned patients and their loved ones to be on the alert.

This was Elan's second warning letter following one they sent the previous June, four months earlier. It's important to note that our government watchdog agency, the FDA, said nothing in June, when the problem first cropped up. Rather, they waited four months before uttering a peep. Did you notice—and doesn't it seem odd—that Elan sent their first letter about the problem the previous June, but the FDA's first mention of it took four months, and their response was their own "Dear Healthcare Professional" letter? There is no indication that doctor's offices, clinics, or hospitals were called or visited and the public made aware. I mean, what happens if "Dear Healthcare Professional" didn't see the letter, or overlooked it, or it was misfiled, or the person who received it quit their job?

To Elan's discredit, according to their own listing of press releases in 2003, neither time did they report it to the media or offer evidence that they did more than send the letters.

Just so you know the danger here. Morphine is an opioid analgesic extracted from Asian poppy plants and is used to relieve moderate to severe pain. (It works by affecting the way the body senses pain.) This is powerful stuff. Heroin is processed from morphine. Yes, heroin. The Drug Abuse Warning Network, which is part of the government's Substance Abuse and Mental Health Services Administration (SAMHSA), lists heroin/morphine among the four most frequently mentioned drugs reported in drug-related death cases in 2002, and reports that nationwide, heroin emergencies increased 35 percent between 1995 and 2003.

Can you imagine if someone inadvertently received a dose twenty times what's prescribed? I hope you or a loved one wasn't affected. Sadly, most of you probably read it here first.

An obvious question should be, "why did this mistake happen?" Did a bunch of doctors or nurses go on a collective spell of stupidity? Were the bottles mislabeled or was the packaging insert incorrect? None of the Elan or FDA letters tell us. From what I gathered from the scant evidence, there was some confusion between milligrams and milliliters as well as teaspoons and tablespoons. Why? Who knows—no one was, nor is, currently discussing it.

And here's another puzzling thing. One of Elan's explanations states the following:

". . . For example, a prescribed dose of 5 mg was mistakenly administered as 5 mL (100 mg) of the morphine sulfate concentrated solution."

The U.S. National Library of Medicine states that a usual prescribed adult dose of Roxanol varies from 10 to 30 milligrams every four hours or as directed by a physician. Could it be they are deliberately understating the problem? In other words, a 10 milliliter (200 milligram) dose instead of a 10 milligram dose, or worse, 30 milliliters (600 milligrams) instead of 30 milligrams—an extra 570 milligrams?

I checked Elan's Web site for all press releases issued in 2003. There are many product-related announcements, but nothing about this problem. Strange, but soon after the second letter went out, I notice Elan *did* issue the following press release: "Elan to Sell Four Pain Products for $100 Million" (22 October 2003).

Surprise! Roxanol was one of the products Elan sold. Another surprise, I guess, there was no mention about the morphine deaths—not in the press release, nor any other press releases issued that year, not in Elan's annual report, nor in the SEC filings and annual report from the purchaser, aaiPharma Inc. It wasn't just Elan clamming up. The FDA never mentioned the problem again.

My theory is if the press got hold of this story it would have been a PR nightmare, and heaven forbid, might have affected the stock value and sale price. But that shouldn't have influenced the FDA alerting the public of potential danger, right? As it stands people died, we know that, and to this day the survivors may be wondering why.

Mistakes happen, but cover-ups and complacency are inexcusable for an agency that is supposed to be the guardian of our food and drug supply. I think the public had a right to know.

Ironically, early in 2004, the *National Pharmacy Compliance News*—which is not a periodical you'd find on too many coffee tables—reported the death of a ninety-one-year-old man being treated for a mild heart attack, who was mistakenly given a 100-milligram dose of Roxanol instead of 5 milligrams as prescribed. The error may have contributed to the patient's death the following day. Ironic, because the same issue of the publication mentioned the FDA's final rule for banning the sale of ephedra supplements because of concerns over adverse reactions.

It's time for me to ask—Is the FDA still part of our Public Health Service network or is it a drug-sales-promoting adjunct to the pharmaceutical industry?

Gut-Wrenching News

Consider the case of the popular heartburn drug Propulsid, which now, fortunately, is off the market. In March 1998, after dozens of patients died and over one hundred patients suffered serious heart problems after taking the drug, the FDA told the company they were considering banning it for use by children, who seemed to be at greater risk for serious complications. Instead, the government and the company negotiated new warnings for the drug's label. Two years later, as reports of heart problems and deaths mounted, Johnson & Johnson continued defending the safety of Propulsid until a government hearing threatened to draw attention to the drug's mostly hidden record of trouble. Only then did they withdraw it from the market, even though sales continued to top $1 billion, meaning the company reaped an additional $2 billion in sales while the drug was under a cloud. A survey that year found that about 20 percent of infants in neonatal intensive care units were being given the drug.

That evidence, pieced together from corporate and government documents obtained by the *New York Times,* provided an in-depth view of a pharmaceutical company trying to save a lucrative drug in the face of growing proof of harmful side effects. Among the documents included proof of lawsuits against Johnson & Johnson showing the company did not conduct safety studies urged by federal regulators and their own consultants that may have headed off the disastrous results of taking Propulsid. Even more revealing is that "our" watchdog agency, the FDA, did not disclose company research that cast doubt on Propulsid's effectiveness against digestive disorders it was being used to treat, since the studies are considered "trade secrets." Despite these public warnings about Propulsid, much of the conversation between the company and regulators remained private as the drug thrived.

According to the documents obtained by the *Times*, government regulators did start to press Johnson & Johnson executives when evidence mounted that Propulsid could interfere with the heart's electrical system. But shades of the Roxanol story above, physicians and the public were never made aware of the full depth of the agency's concerns.

Last year, Johnson & Johnson agreed to pay up to $90 million to settle lawsuits that eventually involved claims that three hundred people died and as many as sixteen thousand were injured from taking Propulsid. Unfortunately, this news didn't generate the headlines we saw when Steve Bechler the baseball player died while using an ephedra product.

Here's something that could help shed some light on the cozy relationship that's evolved between the FDA and the pharmaceutical companies. A couple of years ago I covered a medical conference in Tampa, Florida, that featured up-to-date research into pharmacological issues. The keynote speaker was a top official from the FDA who gushed from the podium about how thrilled he was to be there with his "partners," the pharmaceutical companies. By the way, after I reported accurately about a certain drug that was being over-prescribed to children at the time, I received an irate phone call from the association that sponsored the conference. In no uncertain terms I was told I would not be welcomed back, since I was an ungracious guest.

Fortunately, my editor—who vets my copy very closely and checks the abstracts from the studies I report on—continues to post this story. Maybe we saved some youngsters' lives.

Again I ask—why would the FDA allow them to get away with this? Why do you think?

Controversy and Conflicts of Interest

The Propulsid fiasco wasn't an isolated instance for Johnson & Johnson. In October 2000, the pharmaceutical company sent a team of executives to a Holiday Inn ballroom in Silver Spring, Maryland, for a specific purpose—to persuade the FDA's panel of independent experts that an expensive antibiotic, Levaquin, should be the first drug approved to treat penicillin-resistant pneumonia. For Johnson & Johnson executives, the FDA's Anti-Infective Drug Advisory Committee included some people it knew quite well. According to *USA Today*, at least two of the experts were paid consultants to the drug company and had worked on the very same medicine they were being asked to evaluate for approval in an important new market.

The expert panel's "consumer representative," whose assignment is to defend consumers' interests, had the most extensive financial relationship with Johnson & Johnson. Keith Rodvold, a pharmacy professor at the University of Illinois-Chicago, served on a company anti-infective drug advisory board, according to Johnson & Johnson spokesman Marc Monseau. Rodvold advised the company on how to design and analyze the clinical trials that got the drug approved. In 1999, he designed a study to measure how Levaquin is absorbed in the lungs. The company also used him regularly as a consultant on a variety of issues.

When approached by *USA Today*, Rodvold declined to discuss his relationship with Johnson & Johnson and his work on Levaquin. Likewise, Johnson & Johnson would not say how much Rodvold had been paid during the five years of consulting with the company.

The case of Levaquin shows how deeply money and influence from the pharmaceutical industry can penetrate the drug-approval process. The fact is, FDA advisory committees consist almost entirely of pharmaceutical industry consultants and researchers. Even consumers' and patients' representatives on the committees—the people who are supposed to look out for you and me—often receive drug company money.

The law requires the FDA to screen all committee members for financial conflicts. It states members have conflicts when committee action could have the "direct and predictable effect" of causing the member a financial gain or loss. The only way around it is for the agency to issue a waiver, usually on the grounds that the experts' value outweighs the seriousness of the conflict. The FDA grants these waivers routinely.

In the period analyzed by *USA Today*, the FDA granted 803 conflict-of-interest waivers. In seventy-one other instances, members had financial conflicts that were voluntarily disclosed but did not require a waiver. In the 746 other member appearances on the committees, there was no conflict of interest.

Dallying for Dollars

While the FDA is required to disclose the existence of financial conflicts, it has kept details under wraps since 1992, making it nearly impossible to uncover the amount of money or the drug company involved. Since then, the FDA stopped making public the details of financial conflicts after controversies about whether the financial interests of committee members had unduly influenced decisions on breast implants, Prozac, and a drug to treat Alzheimer's disease. The FDA said it stopped releasing details on conflicts because of concerns about violating the privacy rights of committee members—not because of the controversies.

In its research, *USA Today* found at least one committee member had a financial stake in the topic under review at 146 of 159 FDA advisory committee meetings held from January 1, 1998, through June 30, 2000. At eighty-eight of those meetings, at least half the advisory committee members had financial interests in the topic being evaluated; at 92 percent of the meetings, at least one member had a financial conflict of interest; at the 102 meetings dealing with the fate of a specific drug, 33 percent of the experts had a financial conflict. As you would expect, more often than not the FDA followed the committees' advice.

The experts hired to advise the FDA assist in deciding which medicines should be approved for sale, what the warning labels should say, and how studies of drugs should be designed. It might seem unnecessary for the FDA to seek outside advice. After all, the agency employs its own full complement of scientific specialists. But the FDA says outside experts add a wide spectrum of judgment, outlook, and state-of-the-art experience to drug issues confronting the FDA. "We seek scientists with a broad range of expertise and different backgrounds," said John Treacy, director of the advisors and consultants staff in the FDA's Center for Drug Evaluation and Research (CDER).

The FDA believes expert advisers add to the agency's understanding, so that final agency decisions will more likely reflect a balanced evaluation. While committee recommendations are not binding, the agency considers them carefully when deciding drug issues.

The FDA said most members of its drug advisory committees are physicians whose specialties involve the drugs under the purview of their committee. Others include registered nurses, statisticians, epidemiologists, and pharmacologists (who study drug effects in the body). Consumer-nominated members serve on all committees. As voting members, they must possess scientific expertise to participate fully in deliberations. They must have worked with consumer groups so they can assess the impact of decisions on consumers.

This does not jive with what *USA Today* found. The paper discovered that more than half of the experts hired to advise the government on the safety and effectiveness of medicine have financial relationships with the pharmaceutical companies that had a financial stake in the decisions. In other words, very often the people playing critical roles in making decisions affecting the health and well-being of millions of Americans and influencing billions of dollars in drugs sales are people who benefit financially.

After the *USA Today* story broke, FDA senior associate commissioner Linda Suydam, who was in charge of waiving conflict-of-interest restrictions, defended the FDA's practices. "The best experts for the FDA are often the best experts to consult with industry," she said. While that may be true, isn't it also true that the public has a right to know?

"The industry has more influence on the process than people realize," said Larry Sasich, a pharmacist who works for Public Citizen's

Health Research Group, a consumer advocacy organization founded by Ralph Nader. "It is outrageous that the pharmaceutical industry's influence is so great that even some consumer representatives are on drug companies' payrolls."

Another Big "Uh-Oh!"

An obvious question is why the FDA bends over backwards to appease the drug industry. Here's one piece to the puzzle. Because of the increased expense due to reforms and other costs, the FDA, Congress and the pharmaceutical industry negotiated the Prescription Drug User Fee Act of 1992. In essence, these user fees "forced" (or allowed, depending on your take) drug companies to pay a portion of the FDA's cost to review marketing applications for drugs.

Since user fees were first authorized more than ten years ago, the FDA has taken in over $160 million from the pharmaceutical industry. User fees also have provided Congress with a good reason to continue to underfund the FDA. As a result, the agency often cannot carry out many of the public protection duties assigned to it.

Since the inception of the user fees, the FDA's staff devoted exclusively to new drug and biologics pre-approval has doubled—financed in part by the user fees—while staff for all other oversight activities has shrunk by 15 percent. As a result, there aren't enough inspectors to regularly visit drug manufacturing plants in the U.S. and abroad to make sure good manufacturing standards are maintained, nor are there enough to regularly inspect the safety of the thousands of food products that come under FDA authority. Before the introduction of user fees, the FDA was free to allocate its resources as its scientists felt necessary. Now, a smaller discretionary budget means some important items do not receive funding.

Pain Pills Panned

Here's a more recent example. In November 2004, drug maker Merck & Co. withdrew the popular anti-inflammatory drug Vioxx from the market after a study showed patients taking the drug had twice the risk of heart attack compared to those taking a placebo. Vioxx became the first prescription drug to be pulled from pharmacy shelves for safety concerns in three years. Later it was revealed that ten of the thirty-two FDA drug advisers whose total votes favored not only Vioxx but also other COX-2 drugs Celebrex and Bextra had financial ties to the industry.

According to public records and disclosures in medical journals, the ten advisors had recently consulted with the drugs' makers. It turns out that Vioxx was significantly more dangerous than the over-the-counter remedy Aleve (naproxen), provides no better relief, and cost almost twenty times as much. Also, its trumpeted advantage, that it did not cause the gastrointestinal distress of aspirin or ibuprofen, turned out to simply not be true. Even worse, although this all came to light in 2004, Merck and the FDA knew this three years earlier.

As I've asked before, who benefits? I'll be covering this story and others about pain relievers in a later chapter.

For now, the Vioxx imbroglio raises questions about the FDA's review process and the foot dragging by the FDA and Merck to remove the drug from the market. At the time, an FDA spokeswoman said the agency has been pressured from all sides—medicine, industry, and consumers—to approve new drugs more quickly or slowly depending on the demand or risk. Demand or risk? What demand? Response to "demand" generated by multi-million-dollar advertising budgets that trumpeted the drug while downplaying the risks?

It turns out this wasn't an isolated case. At Wake Forest University in North Carolina, a professor who researched clinical trials for three decades discovered that more than half of all FDA-approved drugs caused a new side effect after their approval and after they entered the marketplace. It appears that once drugs are approved there is little effort on the part of the FDA to monitor their safety.

It's been suggested that longer clinical trials are the answer, since the increased risk of heart attacks and strokes among Vioxx users didn't happen until after eighteen months of usage. If that's the solution, who would pay for the trials, the drug companies? They'll balk at the added expense, claiming it's not just a hardship, but would slow down the introduction of "important" drugs. How about as a first step we and the FDA demand a bit more honesty?

Another Blood-Boiling Discovery

But it's not just the COX-2 inhibitors that have raised eyebrows recently. In May 2005, Tufts University researchers in Boston reported more people suffered serious side effects from the cholesterol drug Crestor than from other drugs, and recommended that millions of people use it only as a last resort, contradicting findings by the FDA. Specifically, researchers found Crestor induced markedly more cases of rhabdomyolysis—a serious muscle disorder—and kidney problems than rivals Zocor, Pravachol, or Lipitor. In fact, patients taking Crestor suffered six times the number of side effects than those using Lipitor. It turns out the FDA had received a relatively high number of anecdotal reports of side effects from the drug through its adverse event reporting system, or AER. A year earlier, FDA whistle-blower David Graham said the drug's safety merited further scrutiny.

The FDA and AstraZeneca, the maker of Crestor, played down the AER rates as deceptively high because of negative publicity around an earlier statin drug named Baycol. On March 14, 2005, the FDA rejected calls by a consumer group, Public Citizen, to ban Crestor.

On his well-respected Web site, Dr. Joseph Mercola, a doctor of osteopathy (D.O.) wondered how the Food and Drug Administration could possibly have made the decision that Crestor did not increase the risk of muscle damage any more than other cholesterol-lowering drugs, when they reviewed the same data that not one, but two, different research groups used to determine otherwise. "It is clear evidence of the influence of further FDA conflict of interest," writes Dr. Mercola. "The nearly $1 billion that Crestor sales amount to each year provides plenty of potential to influence purchasing. Not only would you be better off with Crestor off the market, but statins of any kind, whether or not they are safer than Crestor, are rarely needed to control high blood cholesterol anyway."

As I discussed in an earlier chapter, statin drugs such as Crestor aren't the miracle drugs we've been led to believe they are. You don't have to take my word for it. Many are starting to say statins may be the most dangerous class of drugs ever developed. More studies now show they may actually precipitate the onset of the disease they are supposed to prevent. For one thing, they reduce levels of coenzyme Q10, which protects the heart muscle and its function.

According to Ron Rosedale, M.D.—and a number of other doctors and medical studies that have been systematically drowned out—cholesterol is not the major culprit in heart disease or any disease for that matter. Dr. Rosedale says our focus and worries about cholesterol as a major cause of heart disease run counter to fifteen years of research and detract from real causes such as the damage that sugars such as glucose and fructose inflict on tissues, including the lining of arteries, resulting in inflammation and plaque buildup.

In other words, reducing your level of LDL (bad) cholesterol has less to do with your risk of heart attacks, heart disease, or stroke than we've all been led to believe.

That bears repeating, don't you think?

Reducing your level of LDL (bad) cholesterol has less to do with your risk of heart attacks, heart disease, or stroke than we've all been led to believe.

The truth is, cholesterol is not the evil, heart-threatening substance that's been pounded into us with constant repetition. Abut 80 percent of it is produced by our livers to assist in the manufacture of hormones and vitamins. It breaks down carbohydrates and proteins, helps form a protective coating around nerves, and builds cell walls and produces bile—a digestive juice secreted by the liver and stored in the gallbladder that aids in the digestion of fats. When free radicals nab electrons from your cholesterol it creates unhealthy oxidized cholesterol.

Crestor was the first of the cholesterol-lowering drug class known as statins introduced since Baycol was withdrawn from the market in 2001 because of the muscle problem rhabdomyolysis. But this isn't the only question mark about statin drugs. While you may not be familiar with the term "statin," the drugs in this class are all too familiar since they're advertised constantly. Do the names Lipitor, Zocor, Mevacor, Vytorin, and Pravachol ring any bells? I'm sure they do since their ads run constantly. Did you ever notice the creeping text along the bottom when their ads run? Well, maybe you never noticed or you don't have a TV. In either case I'll tell you what it says, and this is taken right from one of AstraZeneca's Web sites: "Crestor has not been shown to prevent heart disease or heart attacks."

I mentioned Pfizer's Lipitor in chapter 2, but it bears repeating. On the same page where at the top it says, "Drug for Reducing Cholesterol and Reducing Risk of Heart Attacks," near the bottom is this caveat: "It has not been shown to prevent heart disease or heart attacks."

Zocor? Well, Merck doesn't offer that disclaimer, but instead states: "The Heart Protection Study proved that people who suffer from heart disease or diabetes could benefit from treatment with Zocor." Is this true?

Let's take a look at this study that was conducted at Oxford University in the U.K. in 2002. This study received widespread press coverage when researchers claimed "massive benefits" from lowering cholesterol. But as Uffe Ravnskov, M.D., Ph.D., points out in his book *The Cholesterol Myths: Exposing the Fallacy that Saturated Fat and Cholesterol Cause Heart Disease,* the benefits weren't quite "massive." According to Dr. Ravnskov, an independent researcher born in Copenhagen, Denmark, and head of The International Network of Cholesterol Skeptics (THINCS), those who took Zocor (simvastatin) had an 87.1 percent survival rate after five years compared to an 85.4 percent survival rate for the controls—and these results were independent of the amount of cholesterol lowering. The authors of the Heart Protection Study never published cumulative mortality data, even though they received many requests to do so.

Say what? With at least twelve million Americans taking cholesterol-lowering drugs, mostly statins, and experts' recommendations that another 23 million should be taking them, it's reasonable to ask, what the heck am I taking this expensive drug for? And why does an article I read in *USA Today* in August 2002 state, "Most evidence on statins is positive: a clear reduction in strokes and heart attacks," when the drug's manufacturers can't even claim that?

Side effects include muscle weakness, liver problems, and loss of sex drive (no sweat—we have erectile dysfunction medicines to take care of that!). But some researchers say side effects should be considered by patients at lower risk of heart disease.

Of course we only hear how great the drugs are and how successful they were in clinical trials. If you delve deep into the major studies you'll find it's just not so. (At the end of this chapter I'll list a summary of the most often quoted studies.)

The Wrong Focus

A Boston University research team recently concluded that not having *enough* dietary cholesterol can cause a measurable deficit in mental functioning. According to Reuters Health, the team used data from nearly two thousand men and women who originally participated in the world-renowned (yet largely inaccurate) Framingham Heart Study to calculate the relationship between total cholesterol and cognitive performance.

Their findings: when the lowest cholesterol group was compared with the highest cholesterol group (those with blood levels of 240–380), the low-lipid subjects were as much as 80 percent more likely to perform poorly on tests of similarities, word fluency, attention, and concentration.

According to Public Citizen, the evidence for treatment, especially with cholesterol-lowering drugs, is much weaker for people who have not yet had cardiovascular disease known as primary prevention. This is especially so for those people who do not have more than one of the following risk factors: hypertension, diabetes, smoking, obesity, or a close family history of premature heart attacks or strokes.

Even more telling about the way the FDA works, Crestor became the sixth cholesterol-lowering statin drug in the U.S. Why would you need to take Crestor when there are more effective statins, in terms of reducing cardiovascular events, on the market? What the drug companies know is it's good business, what with the PR machine cranked up, and a compliant distribution channel known as the U.S. medical community willing to prescribe them rather than stressing improved diet, more exercise, and an overall healthy lifestyle.

Even when the FDA tries to do the right thing it often flubs it. Take the case of Lipitor, the best-selling drug in the country, with annual sales of about $7 billion. In the early 1990s, the drug's developers—the Parke-Davis research division of Warner Lambert—sent a team of researchers and executives to Rockville, Maryland, to persuade the FDA to give the drug priority status, meaning they could get it on the market quickly. To its credit, the FDA declined, saying the drug was not significantly different from the four other statins on the market at the time.

Undeterred, the company's research discovered a small group of children—there were no more than ten of them in the U.S.—with a rare genetic defect that prevented them from clearing cholesterol from their bodies. Parke-Davis took out its eraser and changed its application with a new protocol to conduct clinical trials with this underserved market of individuals. The fact that they were children? All the better.

Of course the FDA kicked them out of the office and told them "Don't waste our time and the taxpayers' money," right? In your dreams. The FDA said "Oh, OK," granted them a priority review, and Lipitor soon hit the market. The rest, as they say, is history, even though the priority review meant some other drug—possibly truly unique—was pushed back into the pipeline.

Let's face it. The drug companies are clever. Beatrice Golomb, M.D., Ph.D., assistant professor of medicine, University of California at San Diego, has stated that people typically take statins for life, yet the statin trials lasted no more than five years. She also pointed out that no study that has released gender-specific information has shown a survival benefit for statin use in women, yet the drugs are routinely prescribed for them. (Dr. Golomb is also the principal investigator of the University of California San Diego Statin Study.)

"What matters is not just whether the person has a heart attack or not," she continued, "What matters is the overall complications and overall mortality, yet in most cases, the drug companies have not released the non-cardiac data." Dr. Golomb explained that the few statin trials that have done so, either showed the benefits and harms of the drug were even or there was "a trend toward harm"—that is, more women died in the statin group than in the placebo group, but this was not statistically significant.

All government-funded trials, Dr. Golomb continued, are obligated to make their serious adverse events data available to the public. This includes hospitalizations, prolonged hospitalizations, and deaths from all causes. "But the reality is that all the major statin trials are funded by drug companies, and there is no obligation to release this critical information," Dr. Golomb said, adding that she wrote each drug company that has failed to release its data and was turned down. "They [the drug companies] claim it's irrelevant."

The Choice of a New Generation

In chapter 2, I talk about C-reactive protein (CRP). In the 1990s, researchers found that blood levels of the CRP molecule are just as important as cholesterol readings when measuring cardiovascular risk but what that actually means no one really knows. But here's another culprit that looks like it may contribute to elevated risk of heart troubles. This one may seem like it's out of left field since it's consumed by most of us every day, but it's not.

You may have noticed something Dr. Rosedale said earlier in this chapter. I'll repeat the crux of it: "Cholesterol as a major cause of heart disease runs counter to fifteen years of research and detracts from real causes such as the damage that sugars such as glucose and fructose inflict on tissues, including the lining of arteries, causing inflammation and plaque as a result."

Did you see it? Fructose, also known as high-fructose corn sweeteners (HFCS), have been used as a sweetener since the 1970s and are often cited as a major contributors to the rapid increase in obesity. HFCS, which is made from cornstarch, is now used to sweeten soft drinks, fruit juices, baked goods, canned fruits, dairy products, and other products. Food and beverage manufacturers began switching from table sugar or sucrose to corn syrup when they discovered that HFCS was both cheaper and much sweeter—nearly twenty times sweeter than table sugar. Researchers say consumption of high-fructose corn sweeteners increased more than 1,000 percent between 1970 and 1990, far exceeding changes in intake of any other food or food group.

Research shows that fructose has the ability to significantly raise triglyceride levels, which may increase the risk of heart disease. Researchers from the University of Minnesota note that, "About 9 percent of average dietary energy intake in the United States comes from fructose." In 1966, sucrose made up 86 percent of sweeteners. Today, 55 percent of sweeteners used are made from corn. And while the average American ate no high-fructose corn syrup in 1966, that number changed to about 63 pounds per person in 2001.

HFCS is a relatively unregulated source of fuel for the liver to convert to fat and cholesterol. Unlike glucose, which the body uses, large amounts of HFCS converts to fat more than any other sugar. It is also known to raise triglycerides significantly. Also, fructose does not stimulate insulin secretion or enhance leptin, a hormone thought to be involved in appetite regulation. Because insulin and leptin act as key signals in regulating how much food you eat and your body weight, this suggests that dietary fructose may contribute to increased food intake and weight gain.

A high blood level of triglycerides—the most common type of fat found in food—is a strong risk factor for heart attack among middle-aged and elderly men, independent of other factors such as total cholesterol levels. Researchers have concluded that blood triglyceride level is a stronger risk factor than total cholesterol and that such a test of blood triglyceride level taken after a patient had fasted should be included as a risk factor.

Something Old, Something New

Relatively few pharmaceutical newcomers greatly improve the health of patients over older drugs or advance the march of medicine. Last year, the FDA classified about three-quarters of newly approved drugs as similar to existing ones in chemical makeup or therapeutic value. Sadly, drug makers introduce what former *New England Journal of Medicine* Editor-in-Chief Marcia Angell, M.D., calls "me-too" drugs with similar ingredients, but taken in a different way or for a different disease—depending on what they ran their clinical trials for. Then they are advertised as vast improvements. This is how arthritis sufferers plunk down their money for pricey painkillers that unnecessarily expose them to higher heart risks, without relieving pain any better than older, cheaper brands. Let's face it, our society has been conditioned that newer is better, whether it's toothpaste, paper towels, or drugs.

On top of that, side effects often look like symptoms of diseases that doctors can't tell the difference between. This is why researchers agonized for months over how many heart attacks to blame on certain painkillers and how many on heart disease.

The attitude at the FDA can best be summarized by a statement by an FDA deputy commissioner, Dr. Janet Woodcock. She says allowing similar drugs for the same condition presents more options—and "choice is important."

While choice is important for toiletry items, not so with drugs, especially when their differences are negligible and their prices always seem to fall in line—coincidentally on the high side.

No End in Sight

The pharmaceutical companies are licking their collective chops over the future. When the Medicare drug benefit kicks in in 2006, it will stoke drug use and profits even more. Clever lads and lassies those drug companies. They sure knew that pitting two lobbyists for every member of Congress, and other parts of our government, and lavishing them with campaign cash and gifts would pay off. While we can get a quantity discount when we buy the aforementioned toothpaste and paper towels, not so with Medicare drugs. We the taxpayers will pay top dollar.

The drug industry has always worked hard to fan sales; the Medicare drug benefit is just their latest windfall. Their tried-and-true formula of dispatching sales representatives to medical offices, underwriting continuing education for doctors, and sponsoring drug research to help win government approval has paid dividends time and time again.

Greater use of medicines is a forgone conclusion in twenty-first-century America. The population is growing and living longer, and is contracting ailments of aging like cancer, heart attacks, stroke, and Alzheimer's disease. Then there are the other conditions that have proliferated, including asthma, diabetes, and obesity.

The FDA generally demands only that new drugs work—not that they work better than existing ones. As I've said, in recent years the FDA has accelerated standard drug-approval times while cutting back on safety inspectors and other support personal.

Despite what you've been told, safety problems aren't the domain of vitamins, minerals, and herbs such as ephedra, St. John's wort, kava, and others. It is now well documented that prescription drugs kill one hundred thousand or more persons in America even when they are correctly used. The danger of their interaction with other prescription drugs is also fairly well known, and the results of such interactions can be fatal.

Ironically, what has received little publicity or research is how prescription drugs disturb the body's ability to absorb nutrients, while reputable dietary supplements fortify our bodies' needs. So, when you use prescription drugs, not only are you increasing the load of possibly toxic chemicals in your body from which these drugs are made, you might be starving it of essential nutrients, thereby exacerbating the problem. This lengthens the period of recovery. Unfortunately, the FDA does not require any testing of drugs for nutrient depletion.

A good example of this is the depletion of coenzyme Q10 caused by most cholesterol-lowering drugs, particularly statins and beta-blockers used for lowering blood pressure. These drugs, as well as a number of others, including antidepressants, interfere with the body's synthesis of coQ10, a coenzyme essential for the heart's health. Older persons in good health have difficulty in synthesizing coQ10, so there is a real danger that the cholesterol-lowering drugs, while perhaps reducing the bad cholesterol count, could be damaging the heart's ability to function effectively because of a deficit of coQ10.

A 1995 study by Anatol Kontush of the University of Hamburg in Germany found that coQ10 "represents the first line of defense against oxidative modification in human LDL." He found the antioxidant protection of coQ10 was even stronger than that afforded by the well-known antioxidant vitamin E. And a combination of coQ10 and vitamin E enhanced the antioxidant effect of vitamin E alone. Kontush hypothesizes that coQ10 recycles vitamin E, prolonging its ability to fight free radicals. Kontush concludes that coenzyme Q10 plays a protective role in the very early stages of heart disease.

As more people take these drugs for longer periods of time, we may start to see increases in long-term adverse effects—some of which are already known and some not yet known. CoQ10 is also an essential element of the respiratory chain in our mitochondria, producing the necessary energy to power our cells. These include heart, brain, nerve, and muscle cells, to name just a few. There is scientific evidence to support the belief that dysfunction and death of mitochondria can lead to heart failure, Parkinson's, Alzheimer's, and many other chronic diseases of aging.

In the June 2004 edition of the journal *Archives of Neurology*, a study appeared regarding the use of Lipitor and its effect on coQ10. Conducted by the Department of Neurology at Columbia University, thirty-four individuals over the age of forty-five with elevated LDL cholesterol were studied. Serum coQ10 levels were drawn at baseline. Next, all thirty-four individuals were treated with Lipitor 80 milligrams daily. Fourteen days after starting treatment, thirty-two of the subjects had a decrease in their plasma coQ10 levels by 49 percent. By thirty days, the coQ10 levels had dropped even further.

In this very short study, the patients generally did not report any severe adverse effects, although one subject experienced weakness and tingling in the legs, which disappeared two days after the dose of Lipitor was cut in half. It's important to note that for that individual, their coQ10 level had dropped approximately 60 percent below the baseline level. This study was conducted at one of the most prestigious neurological institutions in the world.

The authors concluded that even brief exposure to Lipitor causes a marked decrease in blood coQ10 concentration. The authors further indicate that widespread inhibition of coQ10 synthesis could explain the most commonly reported adverse effects of statins, especially exercise intolerance, muscle pain, and muscle protein in the urine. It should be noted that another drug called Baycol was so effective at inhibiting coQ10 synthesis that it was actually removed from the market because of its many adverse effects, including numerous deaths.

Here's another important nutrient depleted by drugs: magnesium deficiency can result when using oral contraceptives, Premarin, Estratab, and corticosteroids. Magnesium deficiency is common, and can exacerbate osteoporosis, cognitive problems, and blood sugar regulation. Lack of magnesium can also trigger heart attacks, hypertension, and strokes.

Another very important mineral depleted by prescription drugs is zinc, which can be depleted by corticosteroids, oral contraceptives, oral estrogens, ACE inhibitors, diuretics, and many others. Zinc deficiency affects the activity of almost all enzymes in the body, as well as the synthesis of various hormones and insulin receptors. Typical symptoms of zinc deficiency include a weak immune system, poor skin, hair, and nails, anemia, and even joint pain.

Folic acid is another essential nutrient weakened by some prescription and over-the-counter drugs. Here aspirin, ibuprofen, certain antibiotics, and birth control pills, Celebrex, and methotrexate are some of the many drugs that reduce the potency of folic acid. Folic acid is already the most deficient vitamin in the average American, and the use of these drugs reduces it even more. A lack of folic acid is the cause of many serious birth defects, as well the build-up of unhealthy homocysteine levels in the blood.

Folic Acid and Heart Disease

Since I've been talking about possible causes of heart disease, you should be aware of another factor. A deficiency of folate, vitamin B12, or vitamin B6 may increase your level of homocysteine, an amino acid normally found in your blood. There is evidence that an elevated homocysteine level is a potential risk factor for heart disease and stroke, and high levels of homocysteine may damage coronary arteries or make it easier for blood clotting cells called platelets to clump together and form a clot

One out of every ten cases of coronary artery disease, which is the leading cause of heart attack, can be blamed on homocysteine. The good news is that the B vitamin folic acid is an easy and effective way to lower homocysteine levels and the risk of heart disease.

In a study appearing in the October 4, 1995 issue of the *Journal of the American Medical Association,* researcher Carol J. Boushey, Ph.D., examined data from thirty-eight earlier studies relating to homocysteine, folic acid, and heart disease. She found a strong, clear link between elevated homocysteine levels and the risk of heart attacks, strokes, and peripheral artery disease. She found a clear inverse relationship between folic acid and homocysteine in the blood, meaning that as levels of folic acid in the blood rose, levels of homocysteine dropped. Some of the studies administered high doses of folic acid, however, even small doses showed a remarkable ability to lower abnormal homocysteine levels.

For example, supplementing with 650 micrograms daily cut homocysteine concentrations by an average of 42 percent. A daily supplement of 400 micrograms of folic acid would reduce the risk of heart disease by the same amount as someone lowering their cholesterol levels by 20 milligrams/deciliter.

Folic acid supplements have a huge potential to benefit Americans, and nutritional surveys demonstrate that inadequate folic acid intake is all too common, while Dr. Boushey suggests that as many as 56,000 heart disease deaths each year could be prevented by simply boosting folic acid intake.

There is also some evidence linking low blood levels of folate with a greater risk of cancer. Several studies have associated diets low in folate with increased risk of breast, pancreatic, and colon cancer.

Fish Oil Can Combat Heart Disease

A study appearing in the *Journal of the American Medical Association* in November 1995 compared the incidence of cardiac arrest in men and women who consumed no fish oils to those consuming at least 5.5 grams of fish weekly. A 50 percent reduction in the risk of cardiac arrest was seen in the fish-eating group, while high levels of omega-3 fatty acids may also reduce the risk of heart diseases by preventing blood clots, lowering blood pressure, and reducing cholesterol levels.

Dietary intake of fish and red blood cell levels of DHA and EPA, the two key fatty acids in fish, were measured in 334 patients dying from cardiac arrest and 493 healthy controls. After controlling for factors that could affect heart disease risk, such as family history, tobacco use, hypertension, diabetes, weight, and exercise, researchers determined that omega-3 fatty acids guard against cardiac arrest. "When compared with no seafood intake, dietary intake of modest amounts of omega-3 fatty acids from seafood may . . . reduce the risk of coronary heart disease mortality," writes researcher David S. Siscovick, M.D., M.Ph., from the University of Washington.

New Tricks, Old Sleeves

But these simple-to-follow solutions to heart disease are drowned out by commercials for statin drugs that seem to run constantly. And now, we have lowered cholesterol standards that will ensure pharmaceutical cash registers will jingle even more. In 2001, the federal government published new rigorous cholesterol standards that, if followed, could have doctors writing prescriptions that would nearly triple—to 36 million people—the number of Americans on cholesterol-lowering drugs. The recommendations would put nearly 20 percent of American adults on statin drugs—some predict 50 percent or more.

Some heavyweight organizations are involved in setting and endorsing these new standards for statins and cholesterol. Officially, they come from the National Cholesterol Education Program's expert committee on cholesterol, and they are published in the *Journal of the American Medical Association.* The quasigovernmental group was appointed by the National Heart, Lung and Blood Institute, which is part of the National Institutes of Health. As you'll see in a later chapter stamps of approval from some of these organizations have lost some of their luster because of their growing dependency on corporate sponsors.

Under the guidelines, anyone who already has coronary artery disease and whose LDL, or "bad," cholesterol is above 130 generally should be on drug therapy. "We used to say to try lowering it with diet first, but now we say that if your LDL is above 130 and you have coronary disease, you should be on drug therapy," says the committee's chairman, Scott M. Grundy, director of the Center for Human Nutrition of the University of Texas Southwestern Medical Center at Dallas.

The new standard is similar for anyone with symptomatic peripheral or carotid artery disease, or with diabetes: Anyone with those conditions, and with LDL cholesterol above 130, should get drug therapy, the guidelines say. And even if the LDL cholesterol of these people is between 100 and 130, says Dr. Grundy, "We think the evidence justifies the majority of these people going on drugs." Also, people with multiple risk factors like smoking and high blood pressure should try dietary changes but then be on statin drugs if their LDL cholesterol remains above 130, the panel says.

The new standards don't change the overall guidelines for total cholesterol: Above 240 is still considered high, 200 to 239 borderline high, and below 200 desirable. But the latest guidelines focus more on components of cholesterol, and on groups of people with certain health risks.

For instance, HDL, or "good," cholesterol below 35 was previously considered too low. Now, below 40 is considered too low. Previously, people with coronary disease, symptomatic peripheral or carotid artery disease, or diabetes were considered in good shape if their LDL cholesterol was below 130. Now that target is below 100.

For people who are otherwise healthy, the recommendations are complex. But the panel says that anyone with LDL cholesterol over 190 should generally be on drug therapy regardless. No mention of exercise, lifestyle, or dietary changes.

Not surprisingly, the FDA, our watchdog, sits idly by. Coupled with the cover-ups and problems with the arthritis medicines and antidepressants, once again I have to ask: Is the FDA still part of the Public Health Service or is it a drug-sales-promoting adjunct to the pharmaceutical industry?

So What *Is* the Solution?

Modern medicine provides prescription and other pharmaceutical drugs—with the blessing of the FDA—that suppress the symptoms of the disease but do not cure it. While such treatment may be necessary in the case of life-threatening events most of what we take doesn't fall into that category.

Good nutrition, combined with a healthy lifestyle, is the basic necessity for lasting good health. Even in this modern contaminated world, good nutrition is attainable, but requires a serious personal commitment. Only then can our bodies build up a powerful immune system that is able to counter almost all attacks made on it by external influences.

In September, Lester Crawford, who had been acting FDA commissioner for three years, abruptly resigned as FDA chief only two months after being officially confirmed. His tenure was rocky at best. Besides the Vioxx controversy, the FDA was embarrassed when the U.K. had to shut down a supplier of tainted U.S. flu vaccine, the recall of malfunctioning heart devices grew, and his delay in approving nonprescription sales of emergency contraception. Rumor has it that despite all that, he was forced out because of his wife's vast pharmaceutical stock portfolio.

In a joint letter to the Senate Committee on Health, Education, Labor and Pension, three consumer groups criticized the nomination. They contended that the FDA's "high-profile missteps and failure to take timely action" in protecting the public against unsafe prescription drugs raise questions about Crawford's "leadership, his ability to manage interagency conflicts and willingness to act in the best interest of consumers."

The groups, Consumers Union, Consumer Federation of America, and the U.S. Public Interest Research Group, focused on the FDA's response to concerns raised about Vioxx, a painkiller that drug manufacturer Merck pulled from the market last year.

A day after he was nominated, Crawford announced his support for an independent board to oversee drug safety issues at the FDA. The board would consist of FDA employees and medical experts from other government agencies who would be appointed by Crawford. He also promised more openness in the agency's communications with the public.

Jeannine Kenney, senior policy analyst at Consumers Union, said the FDA already has an array of advisory boards. What it needs to do is to give an already existing office more authority and more resources to track and regulate drugs once they've been approved for the market, she said. Is it any wonder why U.S. Senator Judd Gregg from New Hampshire recently described the FDA as an "agency in crisis?"

Another Black Eye

It only gets worse. In June 2005, U.S. Representative Edward J. Markey released a staff report, *Conspiracy of Silence: How the FDA Allows Drug Companies to Abuse the Accelerated Approval Process.* The report reveals that the majority of pharmaceutical companies benefiting from the FDA's accelerated approval process haven't conducted the post-marketing studies that are required by law on a timely basis. Accelerated approval, which I discussed earlier in this chapter, is a mechanism—often abused—designed to expedite drugs for patients with life-threatening illnesses. Markey also took a swipe at the FDA since they're supposed to be the watchdog of the drug industry yet they haven't required companies to adhere to FDA policies on post-marketing testing.

In 1992, the Food and Drug Administration established a process that amounted to a tradeoff between its mission to ensure the effectiveness of the treatment and the need to speed promising new drugs to market to increase treatment options for life-threatening illnesses. This accelerated approval process allows the FDA to approve a drug on an expedited basis using promising but limited information about its safety and effectiveness, but only on the condition that the company agrees to conduct further studies to confirm the safety and effectiveness of the product. Under the law, drug companies are required to do additional studies to confirm that a drug is safe, effective, and works for its approved indication.

Markey found that of the ninety-one postmarketing studies required by the FDA, forty-two studies have not been completed and half of the unfinished studies have not even been started. "It is outrageous that drug companies and the FDA have been dragging their feet when it comes to conducting required postmarketing studies. Pharmaceutical products approved under the accelerated approval process are designed to treat patients with life threatening illnesses, so ensuring the effectiveness of these drugs is a life or death matter for many patients," said Representative Markey.

These treatments are expedited to the market on the premise that pharmaceutical companies must complete postmarketing studies—not raced through the process so that pharmaceutical companies might someday investigate the effectiveness of these drugs. It is outrageous that drug companies and the FDA have been dragging their feet when it comes to conducting required postmarketing studies. I will be proposing legislative solutions to address the failures of the drug companies and the FDA to keep their promises in order to protect patients and doctors across the country.

The importance of post-marketing studies is highlighted by the recent case of the drug Iressa, which was approved by the FDA in 2003 under the accelerated approval process for treatment of non-small-cell lung cancer. In early studies, Iressa caused significant shrinkage in tumors in about 10 percent of patients and was expedited to market. AstraZeneca, the company producing Iressa, complied with the FDA and conducted a follow-up study of approximately 1,700 patients. The study revealed that the cancer therapy showed no survival benefit in comparison to a placebo. The FDA shared the outcome of the study with the public and suggested alternative treatments.

The FDA's announcement of AstraZeneca's important trial prevented patients from spending $1,800 a month for a drug that is ineffective when there are alternative treatments available. The Markey report raises concerns that other companies that have failed to carry out similar commitments could have similar problems.

"It is very important that those drugs that hold the promise of helping to save lives and reduce pain and illness get to patients quickly. But this expedited approval process is done under the condition that a full review of their safety and effectiveness will be a priority for the drug company and the FDA," said Markey. "After all, a drug tested on a few thousand people for a few months cannot be assumed to be safe for millions of people to use over the years to come."

"The data in Markey's report is further evidence of the need for this Congress to make major reforms in the FDA's post market approval safety system," said Senior Policy Analyst Bill Vaughan of Consumers Union.

Clinical trials, and the lack thereof, are one of the raps against dietary supplements. Yet, the way the system is set up with the FDA and the drug industry there is little accountability, results are altered, exaggerated, or withheld, giving patients a false sense of security and safety. So much for the risk-versus-benefit equation. Maybe it ought to be changed to corporate accountability versus consumers' right to know.

Exhibit 4-A
Statin Studies

(*Source:* Compiled from Dr. Joseph Mercola, ["The Dangers of Statin Drugs: What You Haven't Been Told About Cholesterol-Lowering Medication"] and actual studies.)

Honolulu Heart Program (2001): This report, part of an ongoing study, looked at cholesterol lowering in the elderly. Researchers compared changes in cholesterol concentrations over twenty years with all-cause mortality. To quote:

> Our data accords with previous findings of increased mortality in elderly people with low serum cholesterol, and show that long-term persistence of low cholesterol concentration actually increases risk of death. Thus, the earlier that patients start to have lower cholesterol concentrations, the greater the risk of death. . . . The most striking findings were related to changes in cholesterol between examination three (1971–74) and examination four (1991–93).
>
> There are few studies that have cholesterol concentrations from the same patients at both middle age and old age. Although our results lend support to previous findings that low serum cholesterol imparts a poor outlook when compared with higher concentrations of cholesterol in elderly people, our data also suggest that those individuals with a low serum cholesterol maintained over a 20-year period will have the worst outlook for all-cause mortality.

MIRACL (2001): This study looked at the effects of a high dose of Lipitor on 3,086 patients in the hospital after angina or nonfatal myocardial infarction and followed them for sixteen weeks. According to the abstract: "For patients with acute coronary syndrome, lipid-lowering therapy with atorvastatin, 80 milligrams/day, reduced recurrent ischemic events in the first sixteen weeks, mostly recurrent symptomatic ischemia requiring rehospitalization." What the abstract did not mention was that there was no change in death rate compared to controls and no significant change in re-infarction rate or need for resuscitation from cardiac arrest. The only change was a significant drop in chest pain requiring rehospitalization.

Journal of the American Medical Association (December 2002): This study looked at the effect of statin drugs versus usual care (improving diet, exercise, etc.). While the statin group did lower their bad cholesterol levels significantly more than the usual care group, both groups had the same rates of death and heart disease.

But as Dr. Ravnskov has pointed out in his book *The Cholesterol Myths,* the results of the major studies up to the year 2000—the 4S, WOSCOPS, CARE, AFCAPS, and LIPID studies—generally showed only small differences and these differences were often statistically insignificant and independent of the amount of cholesterol lowering achieved.

In two studies, EXCEL, and FACAPT/TexCAPS, more deaths occurred in the treatment group compared to controls. Dr. Ravnskov's 1992 meta-analysis of twenty-six controlled cholesterol-lowering trials found an equal number of cardiovascular deaths in the treatment and control groups and a greater number of total deaths in the treatment groups. An analysis of all the big controlled trials reported before 2000 found that long-term use of statins for primary prevention of heart disease produced a 1 percent greater risk of death over ten years compared to a placebo.

ALLHAT (Antihypertensive and Lipid-Lowering Treatment to Prevent Heart Attack Trial) (2002): This was the largest North American cholesterol-lowering trial ever and the largest trial in the world using Lipitor. The study showed mortality of the treatment group and controls after three or six years was identical.

Researchers used data from more than ten thousand participants and followed them over a period of four years, comparing the use of a statin drug to "usual care," namely maintaining proper body weight, no smoking, regular exercise, etc., in treating subjects with moderately high levels of LDL cholesterol. Of the 5,170 subjects in the group that received statin drugs, 28 percent lowered their LDL cholesterol significantly. And of the 5,185 usual-care subjects, about 11 percent had a similar drop in LDL. But both groups showed the same rates of death, heart attack, and heart disease.

Heart Protection Study (2002): Carried out at Oxford University, this study received widespread press coverage; researchers claimed "massive benefits" from lowered cholesterol, leading one commentator to predict that statin drugs were "the new aspirin." But as Dr. Ravnskov points out, the benefits were far from massive. Those who took simvastatin had an 87.1 percent survival rate after five years compared to an 85.4 percent survival rate for the controls and these results were independent of the amount of cholesterol lowering. The authors of the Heart Protection Study never published cumulative mortality data, even though they received many requests to do so and even though they received funding and carried out a study to look at cumulative data. According to the authors, providing year-by-year mortality data would be an "inappropriate" way of publishing their study results.

PROSPER (Prospective Study of Pravastatin in the Elderly at Risk) (2002): Studied the effect of pravastatin compared to placebo in two older populations of patients of which 56 percent were primary prevention cases (no past or symptomatic cardiovascular disease) and 44 percent were secondary prevention cases (past or symptomatic cardiovascular disease).

Pravastatin did not reduce total myocardial infarction or total stroke in the primary prevention population but did so in the secondary. However, measures of overall health impact in the combined populations, total mortality, and total serious adverse events were unchanged by pravastatin as compared to the placebo and those in the treatment group had increased cancer. In other words: not one life saved.

J-LIT (Japanese Lipid Intervention Trial) (2002): This was a six-year study of 47,294 patients treated with the same dose of simvastatin. Patients were grouped by the amount of cholesterol lowering.

Some patient had no reduction in LDL levels, some had a moderate fall in LDL and some had very large LDL reductions. The results: no correlation between the amount of LDL lowering and death rate at five years. Those with LDL cholesterol lower than 80 had a death rate of just over 3.5 at five years; those whose LDL was over 200 had a death rate of just over 3.5 at five years.

American Journal of Cardiology (August 2003): This study found that lowering bad cholesterol with statin drugs may not reduce the rate at which plaque builds up in the arteries surrounding the heart. This finding contradicts the widespread belief that lowering LDL cholesterol levels is the best way to reduce arterial plaque. In the study, participants taking varying doses of a statin did generally lower their cholesterol. However, all the groups had an average increase in arterial plaque of 9.2 percent.

Meta-Analysis (2003): In a study of forty-four trials involving almost ten thousand patients, the death rate was identical at 1 percent of patients in each of the three groups—those taking atorvastatin (Lipitor), those taking other statins and those taking nothing. Furthermore, 65 percent of those on treatment versus 45 percent of the controls experienced an adverse event. Researchers claimed that the incidence of adverse effects was the same in all three groups, but 3 percent of the atorvastatin-treated patients and 4 percent of those receiving other statins withdrew due to treatment-associated adverse events, compared with 1 percent of patients on the placebo.

Statins and Plaque (2003): A study published in the *American Journal of Cardiology* casts serious doubts on the commonly held belief that lowering your LDL cholesterol, the "bad" cholesterol, is the most effective way to reduced arterial plaque. Researchers at Beth Israel Medical Center in New York City examined the coronary plaque buildup in 182 subjects who took statin drugs to lower cholesterol levels. One group of subjects used the drug aggressively (more than 80 milligrams per day) while the balance of the subjects took less than 80 milligrams per day.

Using electron beam tomography, the researchers measured plaque in all of the subjects before and after a study period of more than one year. The subjects were generally successful in lowering their cholesterol, but in the end there was no statistical difference in the two groups in the progression of arterial calcified plaque. On average, subjects in both groups showed a 9.2 percent increase in plaque buildup.

Statins and Women (2003): No study has shown a significant reduction in mortality in women treated with statins. The University of British Columbia Therapeutics Initiative came to the same conclusion, with the finding that statins offer no benefit to women for prevention of heart disease. Yet in February 2004, *Circulation* published an article in which more than twenty organizations endorsed cardiovascular disease prevention guidelines for women with several mentions of "preferably a statin."

ASCOT-LLA (Anglo-Scandinavian Cardiac Outcomes Trial— Lipid Lowering Arm) (2003): This study was designed to assess the benefits of atorvastatin (Lipitor) versus a placebo in patients who had high blood pressure with average or lower-than-average cholesterol concentrations and at least three other cardiovascular risk factors. The trial was originally planned for five years but was stopped after a median follow-up of 3.3 years because of a significant reduction in cardiac events. Lipitor did reduce total myocardial infarction and total stroke, however, total mortality was not significantly reduced. In fact, women were worse off with treatment. The trial report stated that total serious adverse events "did not differ between patients assigned atorvastatin or placebo," but did not supply the actual numbers of serious events.

Cholesterol Levels in Dialysis Patients (2004): Researchers found those with higher cholesterol levels had lower mortality than those with low cholesterol. Yet the authors claimed that the "inverse association of total cholesterol level with mortality in dialysis patients is likely due to the cholesterol-lowering effect of systemic inflammation and malnutrition, not to a protective effect of high cholesterol concentrations."

PROVE-IT (PRavastatin Or AtorVastatin Evaluation and Infection Study): This study compared two statin drugs, Lipitor and Pravachol. Although Bristol Myers-Squibb (BMS), makers of Pravachol, sponsored the study, Lipitor (made by Pfizer) outperformed its rival Pravachol in lowering LDL. The "striking benefit" was a 22 percent rate of death or further adverse coronary events in the Lipitor patients compared to 26 percent in the Pravachol patients.

PROVE-IT investigators took 4,162 patients who had been in the hospital following a myocardial infarction or unstable angina. Half got Pravachol and half got Lipitor. Those taking Lipitor had the greatest reduction of LDL cholesterol—LDL in the Pravachol group was 95, in the Lipitor group it was 62—a 32 percent greater reduction in LDL levels and a 16 percent reduction in all-cause mortality. But that 16 percent was a reduction in relative risk.

Red Flags Daily columnist Dr. Malcolm Kendrick said the absolute reduction in the death rate of those taking Lipitor rather than Pravachol was 1 percent, a decrease from 3.2 percent to 2.2 percent over two years. Or, to put it another way, a 0.5 percent absolute risk reduction per year—these were the figures that launched the massive campaign for lowered cholesterol in people with no risk factors for heart disease, not even high cholesterol. However, Kendrick said the study was seriously flawed because of "the two-variables conundrum." As this study presently stands, because they used different drugs, Kendrick said anyone can make the case that the benefits seen in the patients on atorvastatin (Lipitor) had nothing to do with greater LDL lowering, they were purely due to the direct drug effects of atorvastatin.

REVERSAL (2004): In a study similar to the one directly above, conducted at the Cleveland Clinic, patients were given either Lipitor or Pravachol. Those receiving Lipitor achieved much lower LDL cholesterol levels and a reversal in "the progression of coronary plaque aggregation." Those who took Lipitor had plaque reduced by 0.4 percent over eighteen months, based on intravascular ultrasound (not the more accurate tool of electron beam tomography). Dr. Eric Topol of the Cleveland Clinic claimed these decidedly unspectacular results:

> Herald a shake-up in the field of cardiovascular prevention. . . . the implications of this turning point—that is, of the new era of intensive statin therapy—are profound. Even today, only a fraction of the patients who should be treated with a statin are actually receiving such therapy. . . . More than 200 million people worldwide meet the criteria for treatment, but fewer than 25 million take statins.

But as outside investigators pointed out, the researchers looked at change in atheroma volume, not the change in lumen area, which is a more important parameter because it determines the amount of blood that can be delivered to the myocardium. Change of atheroma volume cannot be translated to clinical events because adaptive mechanisms try to maintain a normal lumen area during early atherogenesis.

5

So You Want to Be a Human Guinea Pig

"All NIH employees have a responsibility to assist in efforts to combat fraud, waste, and abuse in all NIH programs and have the responsibility to report such matters to the appropriate official."
—National Institutes of Health Policy Manual, Section 1754

Exhibit 1: Earlier this year, Eric T. Poehlman, a former researcher at the University of Vermont, pleaded guilty to submitting fabricated data to the National Institutes of Health in an application for a $542,000 research grant. Poehlman's plea ends a four-year investigation in research misconduct that started in 2000 when a researcher questioned data that Poehlman was encouraging the researcher to use as the basis of a paper.

Exhibit 2: Last year, the pharmaceutical giants Merck and Pfizer came under heavy criticism for endangering the lives of millions of people by failing to disclose the cardiovascular risks associated with two prescription painkillers, Vioxx and Bextra. Months later, the two companies are still hiding the risks of the drugs they market from the public by refusing to consistently publish the results of clinical trials.

The issues that first jumped out at me when I read these two stories were the dishonesty and how public safety was threatened as a result. We're told something is safe because it's been "clinically tested." Both these news items should raise some eyebrows on that score.

Then two other factors struck me. Once again, our government "watchdog" agencies dropped the ball, at least initially. Second, there were people who volunteered for these studies. They probably were paid and possibly paid handsomely. But since the data—which tests the efficacy of experimental drugs on human subjects and is a compilation of individuals' reactions and side effects—had been tampered with, they wasted their time, possibly risked their health, and were party to nefarious acts without their knowing it.

But there's an additional element drawing these two stories together. I suspect you'll probably catch it as you read along.

Our Sorry State of Affairs

You may wonder how the NIH and FDA can allow this sort of behavior. Even though the NIH—with a 2004 annual budget of $28 billion divided among twenty-seven institutes and centers—spends about as much money on research as does the pharmaceutical industry, it concentrates on basic research while sponsoring only about 10 percent of clinical trials. That seems backwards and shortsighted to me.

How many clinical trials are there? Actual numbers don't exist because not all trials are registered with the FDA and NIH. That's right—no one knows. CenterWatch, a Boston-based unit of the Thomson Corp., estimates that worldwide about eighty thousand clinical trials were underway in 2003. Presently they estimate there are 41,000 trials going on right now in the United States. They also estimate that up to 3.5 million people are currently enrolled in U.S. trials.

That figure is expected to grow briskly in the next few years, as drug companies propose scores of new medicines for the marketplace. Some experts favor tighter enforcement of existing rules and greater resources for the understaffed, overworked review boards that too often let shoddy research proceed. Others think patients need to be told more clearly and forcefully what the dangers and limitations of clinical trials really are. Still others are convinced that financial conflicts of interest—drug companies sponsoring trials and paying doctors—are the root of all evil. What's clear to nearly everyone, though, is that without uniform, federally mandated regulations, the situation will only get worse.

Prior to 1974, individual scientists and their financial backers could decide for themselves what constituted ethical research. Most of the time their judgment was sound, but there were plenty of appalling exceptions. In the 1950s, U.S. Army doctors gave LSD to soldiers without telling them what it was. In 1963, researchers injected prisoners and terminally ill patients with live cancer cells to test their immune responses; they were told only that it was a "skin test." In the 1950s, mentally retarded children at Willowbrook, a state institution in New York, were deliberately infected with hepatitis so scientists could work on an experimental vaccine. In perhaps the most infamous case on record, doctors at Georgia's Tuskegee Institute, starting in the 1930s, deliberately withheld treatment from syphilis-infected African-American men for forty years to monitor the course of the disease.

The revelation of these and other scandals led to the National Research Act of 1974, which required institutional review boards to approve and monitor all federally funded research. The Department of Health and Human Services followed up by creating what is now called the Office for Human Research Protection (OHRP), whose job was supposed to be to oversee Institutional Review Boards, or IRBs, which are a group of scientists, doctors, clergy, and consumers at each health-care facility that participates in a clinical trial to ensure that such trials meet federal standards for experimental design—including the obligation to inform participants of any safety issues. But the nature of medical research has changed dramatically in the past few decades. Back then, research tended to be a single investigator working at an academic institution conducting a small-scale clinical trial. As the medicine changed, however, the review system did not.

Until 2001, when the agency's budget tripled, the OHRP had just two full-time investigators to monitor more than four thousand federally funded research institutions. Since 1980, the agency has audited, on average, just four sites a year. The FDA does a bit better, making site visits to about two hundred of the approximately 1,900 IRBs that oversee research on FDA-regulated products.

Meanwhile, IRBs, which are supposed to be the first line of defense against unethical or badly designed studies, are often overwhelmed by the job. At some large research universities, a single IRB must supervise more than a thousand clinical trials at once. Indeed, a 1996 report by the General Accounting Office found that some IRBs spend only one to two minutes of review per study. Board members can't possibly be experts in every field; most are in-house researchers whose own studies are likely to come up for review some day. Says George Annas, a critic of clinical studies: "Researchers tend to approve research; they know this is how the institution makes its money. They rarely deny anything."

Unfortunately morally reprehensible studies like those at Willowbrook and the Tuskegee Institute still take place. Earlier this year, it was revealed that government-funded researchers tested AIDS drugs on hundreds of foster children over the past two decades, often without providing them a basic protection afforded in federal law and required by some states. According to an Associated Press review, the research funded by the NIH spanned the country. It was most widespread in the 1990s as foster care agencies sought treatments for their HIV-infected children that weren't yet available in the marketplace. While proponents argued the practice ensured that foster children—mostly poor or minority—received care from world-class researchers at government expense that slowed their rate of death and extended their lives, it also exposed a vulnerable population to the risks of medical research and drugs that were known to have serious side effects in adults and for which the safety for children was unknown.

The research was conducted in at least seven states—Illinois, Louisiana, Maryland, New York, North Carolina, Colorado, and Texas—and involved more than four dozen different studies. The foster children ranged in age from infants to late teens, according to interviews and government records.

Taking Care of Business

Let's face it: clinical trials have become big business and can lead to conflicts of interest. Researchers and universities hope for scientific breakthroughs bringing fame and fortune, and medical centers compete for trials to be at the forefront of cutting-edge medicine and the money that comes with it. But the cost of initiating trials can be prohibitive, so drug company sponsors pay institutions that serve as hosts for trials. The temptation to skew results to please your benefactor—especially if it's expected—can be daunting. Plus, drug companies are looking elsewhere, adding a level of competition for research dollars.

In 1991, universities, medical centers, and teaching hospitals carried out 80 percent of the clinical research underwritten by the drug companies, but by 2000 that figure had fallen to 34 percent. Even though clinical research is still largely funded by drug companies they don't conduct the clinical studies, which you may think is probably a good thing. With so many more trials being conducted today, and in their haste to get drugs to market, two-thirds of industry-funded clinical research is now performed by for-profit companies known as contract research organizations (CROs) that the drug companies hire to do their research.

In 2001 there were about a thousand CROs throughout the world. Eight to ten of them—the largest firms—capture about 35 percent of the business. CROs establish networks of doctors who are paid to administer the study drugs and collect information on their effects.

"For profit?" you might say. "Great, I'm all for wringing out the out-of-control costs from lazy spendthrift bureaucrats and getting someone in there who knows what they're doing. If they can make a buck, they deserve to."

If only that were true. Most clinical research is first and foremost commercial activity, says Robert Abramson, M.D., author of *Overdosed America*, camouflaged to look like public service, but really designed to maximize corporate profits. Abramson charges that commercialization as well as omissions and obfuscations and questionable comparisons of the drug under study have produced a world in which, "Doctors have to base their clinical decisions on scientific evidence, but the fundamental nature of that scientific evidence has become more like infomercials than objective science." Dr. Abramson spent two years as a Robert Wood Johnson Fellow learning to analyze and criticize research articles. He's also worked for more than twenty years as a family doctor.

Only Time Can Tell

One of the criticisms about dietary supplements is that they don't have to undergo the rigorous clinical trial regimen that pharmaceutical drugs and medical devices do. That's more baloney than I could ever slice through. The real clinical trial takes place after the drug or device is on the market.

Dr. Michael Traub, N.D., past president of the American Association of Naturopathic Physicians (AANP), chair of the AANP's Scientific Affairs Committee as well as director of the Lokahi Health Center of Integrated Care, says dangerous side effects don't necessarily show up in clinical trials even though testing involves large numbers of people. He says potentially dangerous side effects will not surface until many more people—even millions—are taking the drug in question.

The same holds true for medical devices. Here's an example. A couple of years ago, I wrote a feature article for *Focus on Healthy Aging* about the first FDA-approved drug-coated stent (the Cypher stent), a new technology for treating coronary artery disease. After balloon angioplasty is performed to clear an artery narrowed by fatty plaque deposits, the stent acts as a scaffold to keep the vessel from snapping closed. Medication then seeps out of the stent to prevent scarring that can close off the artery again, often leading to coronary bypass surgery or repeat angioplasties. One aspect I investigated had to do with the potential of restenosis, a re-narrowing or blockage of an artery at the same site where treatment such as an angioplasty had taken place.

I discovered a trial of the stent, known as SIRIUS, involved 1,058 people who were at high risk for restenosis due to the length of the blockage or the fact that they had diabetes. As reported in the October 2, 2003, issue of the *New England Journal of Medicine,* the researchers found the Cypher stent reduced restenosis among these patients from 35.4 percent (bare stent) to 3.2 percent (drug-coated stent). I thought that was impressive. Then I discovered that in July 2003, Johnson & Johnson sent a "Dear Colleague" letter to doctors across the United States warning of reports of blood clots (thrombosis)—and some actual deaths—after people received the Cypher stent. However, it was not clear that the stents were the cause of the clotting, which occurred in about one out of every thousand implantations of any kind of stent. As of November 21, 2003 the FDA had reports of seventy-five additional (more than 360 total) cases of thrombosis, including ten additional deaths (more than seventy total).

Still, the FDA concluded that blood clots appeared to be no more common in the drug-coated stents than in bare-metal stents and seemed satisfied that the stents were safe. In a letter, the agency emphasized that it considered the Cypher drug-eluting stent "a safe and effective product when used according to the labeling, particularly the sections of the labeling that deal with the selection of patients and the appropriate use of medication in patients receiving the Cypher stent."

Still, I checked with a couple of surgeons who had worked with the stents and they also gave them a thumbs-up. I reported it that way, trusting that our readers, now armed with information on the risks, would proceed with due caution.

Then two things happened. In July 2004, Boston Scientific Corporation, the second manufacturer of drug-coated stents, announced it was recalling approximately two hundred units of its stents since it found some of the delivery catheters were interfering with balloon deflation during a coronary angioplasty procedure. Impeded balloon deflation can result in significant patient distress, including emergency coronary artery bypass graft surgery and death. The FDA has received reports of one death and sixteen serious injuries associated with balloon deflation.

Then in the fall, a study published in *The Lancet* detailed four cases where patients experienced a heart attack from thrombosis of a drug-eluting stent about a year after implantation, and shortly after stopping antiplatelet therapy.

So, you never really know how safe devices or drugs will be until they've been on the market for a while. As in this case, problems never anticipated can arise.

This is not to use a deflection strategy. You know how that goes: "If you think supplements are bad, wait till you hear this." Rather it's necessary to show the weakness in many clinical trials and to dispel a false belief. Dr. Traub says that when people assume there isn't much scientific evidence backing many dietary supplements they're wrong. The problem is that most doctors—and people in the media who report on medical studies—generally read the high-profile medical journals, such as the *New England Journal of Medicine* (*NEJM*) and the *Journal of the American Medical Association* (*JAMA*). Doctors often also read one or two journals in their own specialty. However, most studies of natural medications do not appear in these publications. Rather, they appear in lesser-known specialty medical journals targeted to the naturopathic specialists, rendering the studies virtually unknown to the general public and mainstream doctors. This holds true even though they are peer reviewed in the same way as the more visible studies and are backed by many well-designed and well-conducted research studies. Plus, companies manufacturing dietary supplements don't receive the favorable publicity since they don't have the news-churning PR machines and lobby groups fanning out to twist arms and spread the word.

Although most studies on supplements do not have the huge sample size paid for by the pharmaceutical companies, many are indeed similar in size to a lot of mainstream studies. Remember, too, that these studies are in addition to the large quantity of anecdotal and observed evidence of natural medications that has accumulated over many, many years of product use. Still, it's odd that when a study reflects poorly on an herb or other supplement, *those* are the ones the mainstream media does report.

But Dr. Traub does not mean to imply that we should gobble anything at will. He believes no medication is harmless—even over-the-counter products of all types can have serious side effects when used improperly.

Things Have Radically Changed

I don't want to give you the wrong impression. Clinical trials are usually pretty safe, and most subjects complete the trials without incident. But serious problems have surfaced in recent years that many doctors and hospital administrators are starting to wonder whether there is something dangerously wrong with the clinical-trial system.

Nobody is suggesting that it be shut down completely. Clinical trials are a necessity. They are the primary way for testing potential drugs and separating the ones that work from the ones that are useless or harmful before they're sprung on the public.

Of course the first step is to wring out corruption. But even then, human testing involves risk; nobody can tell in advance whether a new medicine is dangerous. For each clinical trial, researchers must weigh and balance ethical and scientific considerations. If they make the rules protecting patients too lax, subjects may suffer and possibly die. Make them too strict, and lifesaving medications won't make it out of the lab and help the people who need them most.

Beyond outright corruption, where the balance lies is a matter of serious debate. At one extreme are those who believe that most trials are tainted because they play on the fears of desperately ill patients, involve some sort of subtle coercion like money or free medicine or fail to warn patients of the very real dangers they face. Some critics argue as well that there are simply too many trials, as pharmaceutical companies looking for a share of the blockbuster drug market pump out copycat medicines that no one really needs.

On the other side are clinicians who feel they are already burdened with too much regulatory paperwork. Tighter rules will just take time and energy away from what they should be doing—developing and testing desperately needed medications. A few mishaps today, they say, may be the price we pay to save thousands of lives tomorrow.

Still, something is clearly wrong with the system as it now operates. Over the past few years, more than sixty institutions, including several of the world's most prestigious research centers, have been criticized by the U.S. government for failing to protect human subjects adequately. Federal records show that since 1999 at least five people who entered clinical trials in reasonably good health wound up dead—including two infamous cases, at Johns Hopkins Medical Center and the University of Pennsylvania. (I'll cover another case in the next chapter.)

The actual number of such deaths is probably much higher, but nobody really knows. The monitoring of clinical research in the United States is so piecemeal, and the reporting of problems so haphazard, that it's almost impossible to find out what is really happening. Thanks to a patchwork regulatory system, perhaps a quarter of all clinical research has no federal oversight whatsoever. And even where oversight is mandated, it's often applied loosely, if at all.

Since they pay the freight, the pharmaceutical houses exert great influence over research at CROs. They design and carry out the studies, frequently withholding complete data even from the researchers responsible for analyzing and reporting the results. Studies with negative findings are far more likely to be delayed in publication, or not published at all. Making matters worse, the *New York Times* reports that large advertising agencies are buying up CROs. "The function of this research is to sell product—and who knows better how to do that than ad agencies?" says Dr. Abramson. "They'll do it soup-to-nuts: design the research and sell the drugs."

Unfortunately, conflicts of interest like this have become widespread throughout clinical research. Here's another disturbing fact: Studies published in major British and American medical journals show that corporate-sponsored research is 3.6 to 4 times more likely to be favorable about the product than non-sponsored research. "We're getting a distortion of our medical knowledge," says Abramson. "We look for new knowledge only in areas that offer the greatest potential return on corporate investment, while other knowledge is strongly suppressed."

Who's Watching "Our" Store?

It should come as no surprise that clinical trials are overseen by a fragmented and understaffed federal oversight system. The thirty-eight-person Office of Human Research Protection has jurisdiction over trials conducted or funded by the Health and Human Services Department. The FDA—with 276 U.S. clinical investigators in 2002, the most recent figure available—has oversight of any trial that spawns data submitted to put a drug or device on the market.

As I mentioned before, in practice, trials are largely overseen by local ethics panels called institutional review boards. The panels, which can be associated with an institution or be independent, are charged with ensuring that human subjects are protected and that the risks of an experiment are appropriate and in balance with the potential benefits for society as a whole.

But with federal oversight stretched thin, their performance isn't regularly reviewed by any outside authority. That became clear after the deaths of research volunteers Jesse Gelsinger at the University of Pennsylvania in 1999 and Ellen Roche at Johns Hopkins in 2001.

Gelsinger died in an experiment at Penn's gene therapy institute, whose director co-founded a company that hoped to market the discoveries. Roche, a Johns Hopkins lab technician, died after inhaling a chemical in a study of healthy lung function. Previous studies had shown that the chemical could cause fatal reactions.

An increasing number of academic medical centers and private clinical trials oversight boards are seeking accreditation. They hope that will increase both their efficiency and the public's trust—helping them attract more trials and patients. The two organizations that offer such accreditation—the Partnership for Human Research

Protection and the Association for the Accreditation of Human Research Protection Programs—require efforts to educate those who might enroll.

Alan C. Milstein, a Philadelphia-area attorney who represents clients harmed in research experiments, said accreditation will do little to improve safety, no matter how many questions the subjects learn to ask. "There's so much research going on, the money is so big, that I don't believe this is a measure that solves the problems that exist," Milstein said in a June 9, 2005 article appearing in the *Baltimore Sun*.

But let's be realistic. Even rigorous testing of the most promising drugs can't and won't provide absolute safety over the long term. And what gets reported to the public is not necessarily the entire truth, which is why the FDA is now revising regulations on full disclosure of research results.

The financial conflicts of interest can extend not only to the institutions but also to the researchers themselves. One of the reasons Jesse Gelsinger's death in the University of Pennsylvania's gene-therapy trial in 1999 seemed especially scandalous was that James Wilson, the principal investigator in the study, held a 30 percent equity stake in Genovo, which owned the rights to license the drug Wilson was studying; the university owned 3.2 percent of the company. When Targeted Genetics Corporation acquired Genovo, Wilson reportedly earned $13.5 million and Penn $1.4 million.

This doesn't mean that scientists are pushing bad drugs just to make money. Their interest is in research, and they often need the financial backing of corporate patrons just to get started. After Wilson's financial interests in the Gelsinger case came to light, he insisted that they played no role whatsoever in his decisions, that research was his driving motivation. Yet Marcia Angell, former editor of the *New England Journal of Medicine*, argues that such a link tends to bias the investigator, even if the bias is unconscious. A recent study by the University of Toronto analyzed 70 studies of a controversial heart drug. The results were telling: 96 percent of the researchers who were supportive of the drug had ties to companies that manufactured it, and only 37 percent of those critical of the drug had such ties. As more and more scientists either own stock in or get funding from for-profit companies, the ones who have no industry connections are increasingly rare.

Many critics also point to the consent forms people sign when they join a clinical trial. Even when the risks are clearly spelled out—and they frequently aren't—patients tend to misunderstand what's actually going on. The truth is that less than 5 percent of subjects in Phase I trials, which measure the toxicity of a new drug, will receive any health benefit whatsoever. Yet when a 1995 University of Chicago study quizzed patients about why they enrolled in their Phase I cancer trials, fully 85 percent answered, "Possible therapeutic benefit."

In another study of cancer patients, at Harvard Medical School, nearly 75 percent of the subjects did not understand that the trial was investigating a treatment that was not standard. Two-thirds said they did not know they might face additional pain or discomfort. Says Annas: "These trials involve a great deal of mutual self-deception. Patients really want to believe in the treatment, and doctors really want to believe they are curing somebody."

Insisting that patients be given the unvarnished truth about clinical trials might scare many away. But that doesn't bother Alan Milstein, an attorney who has represented Jesse Gelsinger's family, as well as many of the participants in McGee's study. "The biggest myth out there," Milstein says, "is that every one of these studies is essential to the advancement of medicine. That's just nonsense. Most have to do with the advancement of the researcher himself." If it were just a lawyer talking, that sentiment might be easy to dismiss. As Dr. Angell often points out, we have too many me-too drugs. "So much research is trivial duplication."

The Price of Honesty

It's not just an American problem, since the pharmaceutical companies' tentacles reach all over the world, as does their influence. (This also applies to dietary supplements, as you'll see later in the chapter on Codex.)

How a Drug Is Approved

Drug companies study thousands of compounds before settling on the very few that might eventually prove to have therapeutic value. During the six to seven years of preclinical testing (including animal testing), of five thousand compounds tested, approximately five will show enough promise for a company to file an Investigational New Drug Application (IND). If the IND is approved by the FDA and by an Institutional Review Board, the manufacturer can begin the first phase of development.

The IND stage consists of three phases:

Phase I: Clinical trials using healthy individuals are conducted to determine the drug's basic properties and safety profile in humans. Typically the drug remains in this stage for one to two years.

Phase II: Efficacy trials begin as the drug is administered to volunteers of the target population. At the end of phase II, the manufacturer meets with FDA officials to discuss the development process, continued human testing, any questions the FDA has, and the protocols for phase III.

Phase III: This is usually the most extensive and most expensive part of drug development, including additional human clinical trials.

(Note: During the phases of the IND, the manufacturer can obtain accelerated development/review of the drug.)

Once phase III is complete, the manufacturer files a New Drug Application (NDA). Review of the NDA typically lasts one to two years, bringing total drug development and approval (that is, the IND and NDA stages) to approximately nine years. During the NDA stage, the FDA consults advisory committees made of experts to obtain a broader range of advice on drug safety, effectiveness, and labeling. Once approved, the drug may be marketed with FDA-regulated labeling.

The FDA also gathers safety information as the drug is used and adverse events are reported, and will occasionally request changes in labeling or will submit press releases as new contraindications arise. If adverse events appear to be systematic and serious, the FDA may withdraw a product from the market.

Phase IV: Post-marketing Studies: The accelerated approval process allows the FDA to approve a drug on an expedited basis using promising but limited information about its safety and effectiveness, but only on the condition that the company agrees to conduct further studies to confirm the safety and effectiveness of the product. Under the law, drug companies are required to do additional studies to confirm that the drug is safe, effective and works for its approved indication.

Phase IV studies are also used to find new uses for older drugs and expand their markets. They're also used to generate publicity for the drugs.

Here's a story from our neighbor to the north.

Between 1996 and 2002, Dr. Nancy Olivieri lost her job four times, was sued for $10 million, and her scientific reputation was dragged through the mud. Why? All because she told the truth. Olivieri is a professor of medicine at the University of Toronto and a physician at the Hospital for Sick Children, where she is an award-winning specialist in the treatment of hereditary blood disorders, particularly a hemoglobin disorder known as thalassemia.

Patients who receive treatment for thalassemia must endure regular blood transfusions and run the risk of chronic toxicity from too much iron in the blood, called "iron loading." This can affect major organs such as the heart and liver. In the early 1990s, Olivieri wanted to continue studying a promising drug called deferiphone, which appeared to reduce iron loading in transfusion-dependent patients. To fund the research, Olivieri and her coworkers received sponsorship from Apotex, Canada's largest privately owned pharmaceutical company and matching funds from the Canadian Medical Research Council. At the time, Apotex also happened to be in the middle of complex negotiations with Dr. Olivieri's university about a $30 million financial donation, the largest in the university's history.

Olivieri signed two contracts continuing an already existing trial and starting a completely new one. However, Apotex had the right to withdraw funding at any time, and the contract for continuation of the existing trial also gave Apotex the right to control communication of the drug trial data for a year after the trial finished.

By 1995, Olivieri and her co-collaborator, Dr. Gideon Koren had identified an unexpected risk: in six of twenty-one patients studied, tissue iron burdens were higher than expected, meaning the drug lost effectiveness over time. By early 1996, the number of patients with high iron burdens had doubled to twelve.

This was not the outcome Olivieri expected, and her long-time hope that the drug would work seemed dashed. Nevertheless, she felt an obligation to inform patients in the clinical trials that there was a problem. In accordance with the hospital's ethics board, she told Apotex of this decision. Apotex disagreed. The company did "agree that some patients [were] responding inadequately," but stated that the trials should continue and wanted "no further action."

When Olivieri went ahead and informed her patients in May 1996, the company pounced. An investigation by the Canadian Association of University Teachers (CAUT) found that in response, Apotex showed "disregard for the interests and concerns of patients when without notice, it terminated both trials and stopped supplying the drug." Apotex also warned that it would "vigorously pursue all legal remedies," if Olivieri spoke to her patients or published anything.

According to CAUT, "Apotex acted against the public interest in issuing legal warnings to Dr. Olivieri to deter her from communicating about risks" of the drug trials. The company would subsequently deny ever having written any threat.

Showing just how intertwined corporate and public research had become, the person who terminated the trials was Apotex Vice President Dr. Michael Spino, who had been a full-time member of the University of Toronto Faculty of Pharmacy from 1975–1992, at which time he left to join Apotex. However, Spino still held a "status" professorship at the university.

By February 1997, Olivieri was worried that she had discovered an additional unexpected, but potentially far more serious, problem with the drug. She became concerned that it might cause liver fibrosis, findings that were backed up by other scientists working in England. Working with colleagues, she drafted a report for regulators warning of this "severe adverse reaction."

Meanwhile, the drug company began efforts to convince the regulatory authorities, patients, the hospital, and the wider scientific community that the drug was safe, while privately proposing to change the testing procedure to remove vital tests. They wrote to Olivieri warning that her results were "not scientifically valid" and threatened their business interests.

Throughout this three-year ordeal, Olivieri received no support from the Hospital for Sick Children or the University of Toronto. At the beginning of 1999, she was dismissed from her post as director of its hemoglobinopathy program. She and some of her close colleagues were later gagged by the Hospital for Sick Children. After mediation, she was reinstated and allowed to continue research in late January 1999. The hospital also belatedly promised to support her financially if Apotex sued her.

By 2000, the increasingly bitter feud had reached the courts. Olivieri sued Apotex for libel after the company accused her of making "false" statements. Apotex filed a counterclaim against Olivieri, asking for $10 million damages.

In January 2002, the CAUT published a supplement to its investigation, concluding that Dr. Olivieri had been exonerated by their inquiry and three others, including an inquiry conducted by the dean of the Faculty of Medicine of the University of Toronto. "Unless the lessons are learned," wrote the CAUT, "everyone will lose. It is important to recognize that the circumstances that gave rise to this case are not isolated—they illustrate a system-wide problem."

In November 2002, a settlement was reached that "resolved all outstanding litigation and arbitrations pending between all the parties." But Olivieri's case may only be the tip of the iceberg.

The *British Medical Journal* (*BMJ*) has warned about the "proliferation of stories of companies suppressing publication." A month before the Olivieri settlement, a paper in the *New England Journal of Medicine* concluded that universities "routinely" engage in lucrative industry-sponsored research that restricts academic freedom.

Dr. Kevin Schulman, of Duke University Medical Center, found that "academic institutions rarely ensure that their investigators have full participation in design of trials, unimpeded access to trail data, and the right to publish their findings." Schulman's team surveyed more than one hundred medical centers in the United States and found that only 1 percent involved in multi-center studies had independent access to all trial data.

In March 2001, the *BMJ* revelations that Wyeth Pharmaceuticals had "shelved" a study of its contraceptive pills that indicated "clear increases in the risk of developing deep venous thrombosis." Although Wyeth provided the data to regulatory authorities, it did not submit it for publication as "the study did not offer any new scientific information."

Six months later, the *BMJ* editorialized about problems that have arisen due to the "entanglement" of academia with industry, noting that "control lies in the commercial rather than in the academic or public sector." Methods used by industry included designing "studies likely to favor their products" and analyzing data "providing the spin—that favors them." This entanglement worries Olivieri deeply. "Commercialization of university research," she says, "benefits companies at the expense of the public good."

Blowing Whistles

Back to the Poehlman case that opened this chapter. The University of Vermont opened an investigation into the case in 2000 after a research assistant filed a formal complaint. Over the course of its investigation, which concluded in 2002, the university reviewed the data, which were contained in a series of spreadsheets, and concluded that they had been falsified, that they had been used as the basis for published articles and presentations, and that they had been used in support of grant applications.

In interviews with the University of Vermont panel investigating the misconduct, Poehlman provided a series of explanations for the misleading data. He claimed computer crashes, data input error both by himself and his assistant, and malicious tampering with the data designed to undermine him were to blame for inconsistencies. He reported that in some cases he had altered data in spreadsheets to create models to better understand the range of possible effects that various findings might produce. He may have substituted this simulated data for actual data and accidentally included it in some of his work.

Ultimately, the reviewers rejected his defenses and concluded that Poehlman had fabricated research data. While the review was taking place, Poehlman countered with a lawsuit against the university and then resigned, taking a position in Montreal.

After reaching its conclusions, the University of Vermont referred the case to the Office of Research Integrity and the Department of Justice, which conducted their own investigation, finding that Poehlman falsified data in several other studies and grant applications.

Then, Poehlman's research assistant who discovered the fabrications filed a whistle-blower suit, alleging violation of the False Claims Act because of Poehlman's inclusion of fabricated data on research grant applications. In addition to legal fees, the whistle-blower will receive $20,000 of the settlement.

Not every whistle-blowing case goes this smoothly. A whistle-blower at the Pennsylvania Office of the Inspector General (OIG) was escorted out of his workplace on April 28, 2005, and told "not to appear on OIG property ever again" after OIG officials accused him of talking to the press. The investigator, Allen Jones, who uncovered evidence that major drug companies sought to influence government officials, has been removed from his job and placed on administrative leave. The evidence Mr. Jones uncovered was widely reported in the *New York Times,* the *British Medical Journal,* and in other media outlets and showed that the pharmaceutical company Janssen had paid honorariums to key state officials who held influence over the drugs prescribed in state-run prisons and mental hospitals.

Mr. Jones filed a suit on May 7 against his supervisors charging that the OIG's policy of barring employees from talking to the media was "unconstitutional." Mr. Jones claimed, in the complaint filed in the Middle District Court of Pennsylvania, that he is being harassed by his superiors and Pennsylvania governmental institutions in order to "cover-up, discourage, and limit any investigations or oversight into the corrupt practices of large drug companies and corrupt public officials who have acted with them."

Three years earlier, Mr. Jones was appointed lead investigator when he uncovered evidence of payments into an off-the-books account. The account, earmarked for "educational grants" was funded in large part by Pfizer and Janssen Pharmaceuticals. Payments were made from the account to state employees who developed formulary guidelines recommending expensive new drugs over older, cheaper drugs with proven track records.

One of the recommended drugs was Janssen's antipsychotic medicine risperidone—a drug that has recently been found to have potentially lethal side effects. The Food and Drug Administration issued a warning letter to Janssen on April 27 saying that Janssen's "Dear Healthcare Professional" letter about risperidone was "false or misleading" because it failed to disclose or minimized risks of the drug relating to "serious adverse events including ketoacidosis, hyperosmolar coma, and death."

Don Bailey, Mr. Jones's attorney, said the case is a critical test of the right to a free press. "If they shut the employee up and they have all the documents locked up in a drawer there is no free press," he said.

Maybe We Need More Whistle-blowers

In May 2005, a survey of more than a hundred medical schools found that they vary widely in their standards for testing new medicines for drug companies, with some saying they would accept far more control from the companies than others would. In the survey, reported in the *New England Journal of Medicine*, almost none of the medical schools said they would allow private sponsors to quash publication of research findings. But they differed greatly on other standards, like whether researchers should be allowed to discuss trials publicly while they are underway or share raw research data with other scientists, and whether drug companies sponsoring the tests should be allowed to insert their own analyses into research reports, suggest revisions before they are published, or even draft reports in the first place.

The researchers, from the Harvard School of Public Health and the University of Massachusetts, Boston, said the variation in these standards might lead drug companies to channel their research money "to relatively permissive institutions." And they reported that 69 percent of the administrators surveyed said competition for research money "created pressure on administrators to compromise" with drug companies seeking to finance trials.

The researchers said 82 percent of the institutions surveyed reported they had experienced at least one dispute with an industry sponsor after a trial agreement had been signed. Usually the disputes involved money, the researchers wrote, but sometimes they exhibited "embedded ethical issues." One respondent told of commercial sponsors who refused to make the last payment for a drug trial "apparently because they did not like the results of the study."

Unfortunately, some researchers choose to go along. In the June 9, 2005 issue of the journal *Nature*, one-third of scientists surveyed said that within the previous three years, they had engaged in at least one practice that would probably get them into trouble, the report said. Examples included circumventing minor aspects of rules for doing research on people and overlooking a colleague's use of flawed data or questionable interpretation of data.

The survey, conducted by Brian C. Martinson of the Health-Partners Research Foundation in Minneapolis, included results from 3,247 scientists, roughly 40 percent of those who were sent the questionnaire in 2002. All respondents were researchers based in the United States who had received funding from the National Institutes of Health. Most were studying biology, medicine, or the social sciences, along with others in chemistry and a smaller group in math, physics, or engineering.

More than 5 percent of scientists answering the confidential questionnaire admitted to having tossed out data because the information contradicted their previous research or said they had circumvented some human research protections. And more than 15 percent admitted they had changed a study's design or results to satisfy a sponsor, or ignored observations because they had a "gut feeling" they were inaccurate.

Of the ten practices that Martinson's study described as the most serious, less than 2 percent of respondents admitted to falsifying data, plagiarism, or ignoring major aspects of rules for conducting studies with human subjects. But nearly 8 percent said they had circumvented what they judged to be minor aspects of such requirements. Also, nearly 13 percent of those who responded said they had overlooked "others' use of flawed data or questionable interpretation of data."

The new survey also hints that much scientific misconduct is the result of frustrations and injustices built into the modern system of scientific rewards. The findings could have profound implications for efforts to reduce misconduct—demanding more focus on fixing systemic problems and less on identifying and weeding out individual "bad apple" scientists.

"Science has changed a lot in terms of its competitiveness, the level of funding and the commercial pressures on scientists," Martinson said. "We've turned science into a big business but failed to note that some of the rules of science don't fit well with that model."

Just Say "No" to the Drug Safety Board

Many believe the new FDA Drug Safety Oversight Board (DSB), which was established to instill confidence in the nation's drug supply, will actually set back efforts to improve the safety of medications Americans take and will not make it any easier to take dangerous drugs off the market. In an article appearing in the *Washington Post* in June 2005, FDA safety officer David Graham criticized the Drug Safety Oversight Board for being "severely biased in favor of industry. Ironically, drug safety in the U.S. is worse off today than it was in November."

The FDA announced the fifteen-member board last fall in part to identify and review emerging drug safety issues that Graham and others said were not being treated seriously enough; it was formally established this spring. It consists largely of FDA managers, with some input from officials of the NIH and of the Department of Veteran Affairs.

The attacks on the panel come as a steady flow of bad news about safety problems with popular drugs has given rise to competing initiatives designed to reassure the public. The congressionally chartered Institute of Medicine has held public meetings to begin an FDA-requested study of its safety procedures, and Congress is considering bills that would more aggressively address drug safety.

Senator Chuck Grassley from Iowa sent a letter to the FDA critical of the agency's decision that the DSB will have private deliberations, requesting improved transparency and accountability and for the FDA to "explain in detail how it will ensure that the DSB is truly independent and objective."

The pharmaceutical companies are not amused. One answer they have is to move testing overseas, they say, in an effort to get drugs to market faster, at lower costs while testing drugs where they're likely to be sold. According to PhARMA, the industry spent more than $39 billion on research and development last year, with human drug testing accounting for the biggest cost. More than 21 percent of that was spent outside the U.S., versus 18 percent in 2000.

The Spin Zone

Post-market studies are designed to accomplish a couple of things. They can clear up some issues, and also generate publicity for the drug. They can also be slanted in such a way, so as to minimize a concern about the efficacy or safety of a drug. Some would call it "spin."

Here's an example with the number-three-selling drug in the U.S., Prevacid, and number seven, Nexium, and an over-the-counter version of Prilosec being sold to relieve heartburn/GERD. They all work by inhibiting the acid-producing proton pumps in our stomachs. The idea is by reducing the action of the pumps, there is less heartburn-causing acid, and acid backing up into the esophagus.

As I mentioned in chapter 2, the lining of our stomachs contains millions of these special cells or pumps. The acid they produce helps digest food and helps process it for the absorption of nutrients in the small intestine. The acid produced also kills infectious bacteria. In light of all this, do we *really* want to "turn off the pumps?" When there are lower levels of stomach acid, foods sit in the stomach much longer than normal. This extra "waiting time" means that the stomach acids that are present have a longer time to back up into the esophagus, causing heartburn. Eating slower, eating less and eating while under less stress can often eliminate many heartburn or GERD attacks.

So let's look at four recent studies:

1. When it comes to gastric cancer, too little stomach acid can be just as dangerous as too much, according to scientists at the University of Michigan Medical School. Both extremes create inflammatory changes in the stomach lining and a condition called chronic atrophic gastritis, which over time often leads to cancer. Their research appeared in the March 31, 2005 issue of the medical journal *Oncogene*.

2. A short course of proton pump inhibitor (PPI) therapy may result in a significant reduction in gallbladder motility and new-onset biliary symptoms, according to the results of a preliminary prospective study presented at the 2005 annual meeting of the Society of American Gastrointestinal and Endoscopic Surgeons in Fort Lauderdale, Florida. In other words, PPI drugs may reduce gall-bladder function.

3. Heartburn drugs increase the risk of pneumonia, probably because they reduce germ-killing stomach acid, reported researchers in a recent issue of the *Journal of the American Medical Association.* In a study of more than three hundred thousand patients, users of such drugs as Prilosec and Nexium faced almost double the risk of pneumonia compared with former users. And those taking another class of acid-fighting drugs, including Tagamet and Pepcid, were also at elevated risk.

4. Philip O. Katz, M.D., in a study reported in *Medscape Gastroenterology* in 2005 notes, "PPIs inhibit only active proton pumps. Because not all pumps are active at any given time, a single dose of a PPI does not inhibit all pumps and does not result in profound inhibition of acid secretion. Acid secretion by these proton pumps will therefore be inhibited with subsequent PPI doses, taking five to seven days to achieve a steady state with a PPI.

In other words, inhibiting the action of proton pumps is no big deal. We have plenty, so relax and supersize those fries.

OK, in light of what you just read, which study do you think received pharmaceutical cash? Take a wild guess.

Here's the score sheet:

1A. Research was funded by the National Institute for Diabetes and Digestive and Kidney Diseases (NIDDK) and the Michigan Gastrointestinal Peptide Research Center.

2A. The investigators report no pertinent financial conflicts of interest.

3A. The authors of the study, which took place in the Netherlands, report no pertinent financial conflicts of interest.

4A. Philip O. Katz, M.D., has disclosed that he has received grants for educational activities and research from AstraZeneca. Dr. Katz has also disclosed that he serves as an advisor for Ucyclyd Pharma and TAP and serves on the speaker's bureau of AstraZeneca, Janssen, and TAP.

Did you guess right?

According to the May 16, 2005 issue of *USA Today*:

• GlaxoSmithKline says 29 percent of its drug trials last year were outside the U.S. and Western Europe. In two years, that will hit 50 percent.

• Last year, 50 percent of trials for Wyeth Pharmaceuticals were outside the U.S. That'll be 70 percent in 2006.

• Merck's non-U.S. trials are at 50 percent, up from 45 percent five years ago, it says.

Drug manufacturers say cost is one factor. Trials in Eastern Europe, Asia, and Central and South America might cost 10 percent to 50 percent less than trials in the United States and Western Europe, says Ronald Krall, GlaxoSmithKline's head of development. Researcher and clinic/hospital costs are lower and patient recruitment is faster, which also lowers costs. Plus, bigger populations more in need of medical treatment make faster recruitment possible. The companies attempt to sell their drugs where tested, they say, and U.S. trials aren't declining as much as foreign ones are increasing.

Also driving the trend: some nations, such as Japan, want drugs tested in their populations before approving them to be sold, says Fred Fiedorek, vice president of clinical research for Bristol-Myers Squibb. Also, international standards for running clinical trials— including rules regarding consent—have been more widely adopted. The FDA expects companies to meet them, no matter where trials were done, to win approval to sell new drugs in the U.S.

The trend worries consumer groups. With more foreign trials, "They're further away from whatever scrutiny we have here," says Vera Hassner Sharav of the Alliance for Human Research Protection.

It's strange—when people try to import lower-priced (and perfectly safe) drugs from overseas, the pharmaceutical companies, with the blessing of the FDA, slap them down. Yet, when the pharmaceutical companies want to circumvent our rules for drug testing, they expect cooperation and understanding.

I guess they believe they're entitled to have it both ways.

A Little Transparency Could Go a Long Way

Scientists say drug companies have not kept their pledge to provide more information about their research on new medicines. Calls for more disclosure from medical journal editors and academic scientists in the last year have urged the industry to disclose more data after several drug companies failed to publish studies that showed their antidepressant medications were as effective as placebos.

In September 2004, the members of the International Committee of Medical Journal Editors announced that they will cease publishing studies that are not registered in an NIH database—ClinicalTrials.gov—at the time of their launches. Late in May, Jeffrey Drazen, editor in chief of the *New England Journal of Medicine*, said that GlaxoSmithKline, Merck, and Pfizer are not providing useful data on clinical trials they register on the government's Web site.

Within the drug industry, companies are sharply divided about how much information to reveal, both about new studies and completed studies for drugs already being sold. The industry lobby group PhARMA and three other major pharmaceutical associations earlier this year recommended to their members that they submit clinical trial information to the public registry beginning in July. I'm unimpressed. PhARMA makes a lot of requests but they're merely PR moves rather than a true effort to have their members—who pay for PhARMA's existence—to change their behavior.

Some have responded, at least in part. Eli Lilly and some other companies have posted hundreds of trial results on the Web and pledged to disclose all results for all drugs they sell, while Merck and Pfizer, among others, have released less information and are reluctant to add more, citing competitive pressures.

Academic researchers say that the result is that doctors' and patients' lack of critical information about important drugs has grown stronger since reports last year that several companies showing their antidepressants worked no better than placebos.

Merck and Pfizer have been particular targets for criticism for failing to disclose until this year's clinical trial results indicating that COX-2 painkillers like Vioxx might be dangerous.

Before we pat Eli Lilly too hard on the back for cooperating and posting trials, maybe we should take a look at one of their trial subjects, an attractive and bright nineteen-year-old college student—the late Traci Johnson.

So what's the other element I hinted at in the beginning of the chapter drawing the first two items together? Once again, we forget that it is *our* government, and we're supposed to be in control. Guess what? We're not.

6

So Sad

The campus at Indiana Bible College surrounds a former hospital. With only 260 students, the campus, located on the outskirts of Indianapolis, is a tight-knit community of pentecostals where TV is banned and girls are required to wear long skirts. It's not unusual to see students form a circle to pray for a sick aunt.

Near the campus sits one of Eli Lilly's human test clinics with students from the college often enlisting as subjects for clinical trials. Located at the University of Indiana Medical Center, it resembles a pleasant respite from the drab campus with a library, rooftop sundeck, and a panoramic view of downtown. The clinic itself sort of blends dorm living and medical quarantine, with subjects sharing meals and TV time.

The Eli Lilly Web site touts the drug trials as a great way for schools, churches, and community organizations to raise money. There are hundreds of similar test centers around the country, many of them near college campuses because of the ready supply of students looking for part-time work.

Lilly likes them because they make perfect subjects for studies requiring healthy people. The students sign up because it enables them to make hundreds, even thousands, of dollars for a few weeks' work.

Traci Johnson grew up in blue-collar Bensalem, Pennsylvania, but the center of her childhood was a pentecostal church in a dilapidated Philadelphia neighborhood some 15 miles away. Her pastor, Joel Barnaby, said that every Wednesday morning she would walk with him past bars and discount stores underneath the rambling elevated trains. As part of their mission, they huddled with prostitutes and drug addicts. He said Traci would pray so hard tears often rolled down her cheeks. On some evenings, Traci and other young people would gather neighborhood children for meals and entertainment. Barnaby said Traci planned to devote her life's work to inner-city missions.

In the summer of 2003, Traci announced that God told her to attend Indiana Bible College over six hundred miles from her home in Pennsylvania. Kathy DePalma, who ran the Christian day-care center where Johnson had worked, told the *Los Angeles Times,* "Traci went wherever the Lord was leading her."

When friends from Pennsylvania visited the nineteen-year-old freshman on campus, Traci beamed as she talked about the college, her new church, and the young men she found attractive. Traci's friends said she believed it was God's plan for her to leave her home in Bensalem to attend the college. They said she prayed every day for the Lord to show her how to get the $3,500 she needed for tuition, since her father had been laid off from his job as a machinist and she had little money. She told them she had faith that God would find a way. "It was in his hands," she also wrote in her diary.

Soon after, she told her friends back home that a clinical study Eli Lilly was recruiting for was her best hope to stay in school. Just before the semester began, a Lilly representative called. She was accepted into the trial for Lilly's new antidepressant, Cymbalta (duloxetine). She thought her prayers were answered. A month later, she was dead.

According to press accounts, this is how Traci became involved with the drug trial. After passing a physical and psychological screen, Traci was accepted as one of about twenty-five "healthy volunteers." There were seventy-five subjects at other sites taking part in the Cymbalta trials.

Johnson seemed like a good candidate for the study trial. At 5'4" tall, and weighing 130 pounds, she was physically fit and, by all accounts, reliable and upbeat. But during her interview, she told screeners that when she was fifteen, she had landed in the emergency room after overdosing on Tylenol pills. She said she had to have her stomach cleared, according to a psychiatrist studying duloxetine and who had read a report on Johnson's case. (The doctor spoke to the *Indianapolis Star* on condition of anonymity since the information was considered confidential.)

Johnson told the screeners she was not suicidal then or depressed now, the psychiatrist said. Later, a family acquaintance said the overdose occurred after Johnson's first boyfriend broke up with her, and involved a cholesterol-lowering medication used by her father, not the pain reliever. According to Lilly spokesperson Rob Smith, Traci was not considered depressed.

Before every trial, a Lilly official explained the risks and asked participants to sign a consent form, a legal document that protects both the subject and the company. It entitles participants to medical care for health problems arising from the trial, allows them to leave the study at any time, and warns of the danger of withholding information from researchers.

In Traci's case, they presented her with a consent form that listed side effects common in previous duloxetine trials, including insomnia, nervousness, and anxiety. It also noted rarer effects, such as fainting and an occasional feeling of indifference. Traci signed. Traci believed faith would protect her—faith that God had led her down a path to $7,000, that other people at the bible college wouldn't participate in an unsafe study, and that a company as huge as Eli Lilly would not let anything bad happen to her.

Drug History

Duloxetine, known best by its commercial name Cymbalta, is a selective serotonin reuptake inhibitor (SSRI). The theory is that by increasing the available amount of the neurotransmitter to the brain, SSRIs can help people suffering from depression. However, the full mechanisms of the medication's action are not entirely understood.

In 1972, a Lilly biochemist discovered that a patented chemical, fluoxetine, enhanced the action of the brain chemical serotonin, which affects mood. More testing showed the chemical could dissolve feelings of despair and sadness.

The FDA approved the drug, Prozac, in 1987 and since then, sales have totaled more than $21 billion. But by the late 1990s, the patent on Prozac was about to expire, and the company needed a sequel. Lilly began looking at duloxetine, a patented agent that not only affects serotonin, like Prozac, but also norepinephrine, another brain chemical.

Duloxetine had been shelved in the early 1990s, in part because low doses had no effect on depression. But higher doses, Lilly scientists discovered, relieved depression at least as well as Prozac. Subsequent testing proved the drug also curbed stress-related urinary incontinence. By 2003 Lilly had a trade name, Cymbalta, and industry analysts were projecting sales of $2.5 billion a year within five years for depression alone, approaching the success of Prozac.

The drug already had been tested in about nine thousand people, but the FDA wanted one last clinical trial to measure its effect on heart rhythm. Healthy subjects, free of the ailment for which the drug is designed, are typically used to measure a drug's side effects and health risks. By the time a drug has reached this stage, it has been extensively tested in animals, and the risk of death is considered minimal. To do this, the FDA approved duloxetine doses up to five times the recommended dosage for incontinence, and six times the dose for depression.

Lilly needed one hundred healthy females between eighteen and seventy-five (women are more prone to incontinence) for seven weeks. Traci Johnson was one of them.

At the time, a controversy was brewing over antidepressants that affect serotonin. Six months before the trial began, drug maker GlaxoSmithKline sent a letter to doctors in England warning that its drug Seroxat (known as Paxil in the U.S.) should not be prescribed to people under eighteen. It reported that in its own pediatric trial, subjects reported side effects including "crying, mood fluctuations, self-harm, suicidal thoughts and attempted suicide" when they stopped taking the drug. Two months later, drug maker Wyeth cautioned U.S. doctors that its drug Effexor—the FDA-approved antidepressant most similar to duloxetine—increased the risk in teenagers of "suicide-related adverse events such as suicidal thoughts and self-harm." Three months before Traci's death, British health officials effectively banned the use of most antidepressants in children and teens. Still, Lilly's chief medical officer, Dr. Alan Breier, said in an interview that the company was confident that duloxetine was safe. Previous trials did not reveal a statistically significant number of suicides, Breier said.

The trial's overseers agreed. Dr. Rafat Abonour, head of the University of Indiana board that approved the duloxetine protocol, said he did not recall that suicide was ever mentioned during the review process.

The truth was that five suicides had occurred among 4,124 depressed subjects in studies of the drug. One subject had taken only a placebo. In a more recent study of about a thousand depressed people taking duloxetine for up to a year, seven people attempted suicide and seven others reported that they'd thought seriously about it.

Breier said that was less than would be expected in a group of depressed patients. The annual suicide rate in the general population is about one in ten thousand. The risk in people diagnosed with depression can be ten to thirty times higher.

Lilly spokesman David Shaffer said that because data did not link duloxetine to suicide, a history of depression—even a past suicide attempt—would not necessarily disqualify somebody from the trial.

On January 10, 2003, Johnson, along with the bible college's secretary and another student, entered the Lilly lab, which occupies the fifth and sixth floors of an outpatient center on the campus of the Indiana University Medical School. Traci pocketed $150 a day plus meals during the seven-week trial.

In the study, subjects took duloxetine twice a day. At regular intervals, the medical staff took blood samples and checked heart rhythms. Each participant took the drug for twenty days: sixteen days working up to a dose of 400 milligrams of duloxetine, followed by a four-day weaning period in which the dosage dropped to zero. For the rest of the study, they were given a placebo.

Almost everyone had some odd reaction to the drug. Some couldn't sleep; others couldn't get out of bed. There was constant bickering. Several people in the trial had struggled with moodiness and despair.

One woman at the Glendale, California, site said she was stunned when she felt an overwhelming urge to run over her husband with the family car as he walked past.

After Traci took 240 milligrams, she began her withdrawal period, a time when brain chemicals can swing wildly. On February 3, Johnson took 120 milligrams of duloxetine before starting on the placebo.

People who saw her during that time said she seemed fine and even baby-sat three nights later, telling one mother she couldn't wait to get back to school. She talked with friends back home and was anxious to be there for the delivery of her sister's baby.

At three o'clock the next afternoon she spoke by phone with John Crompton, a church friend from Philadelphia, and told him she felt sick and needed to rest. Sometime in the next few hours on February 7, 2004, and without warning—or a note—the promising nineteen-year-old hung herself. According to the Indianapolis Police Department, Traci tied the multicolored scarf she often wore around her waist to a shower rod in a bathroom at Eli Lilly's Laboratory for Clinical Research and hung herself. A nurse found her body shortly after 8:30 p.m., her feet dangling close to the floor.

Todd Lappin, the Indianapolis police detective who investigated Johnson's death, told the *Indianapolis Star* that since she did not leave a note, her motive was undetermined. "I talked to her friends. They all said she was chipper," Lappin said.

Eli Lilly chose not to halt the clinical trial since the company didn't believe the drug put participants in danger. Incidents such as the suicide of a clinical trial participant often draw questions from the FDA and can delay the federal approval needed to bring a drug to market. Laura Bradbard, a spokeswoman for the federal Food and

Drug Administration, said at the time, "The agency is aware of this death and is concerned."

Lilly officials believed that their data ruled out a link between duloxetine and suicide, and that it wasn't necessary to tell subjects about the suicide controversy. At one of the other duloxetine trial sites in Glendale, California, clinic staffers tried to ease worries by telling subjects that Johnson had tried to commit suicide before, and that problems with money and other matters had pushed her over the brink, several subjects said. "The psychiatrist told me that she had a history of depression and that she had just broken up with her boyfriend," one study participant told the *Los Angeles Times*.

At another site in Evansville, Indiana, directors shut down the study, sending home all sixteen subjects, according to a Lilly spokesman. But enough people remained in the study to ensure the trial was still scientifically valid, the spokesman said.

While company officials declined to comment in detail on Johnson's death, they did say that they did not believe the duloxetine contributed to it—and that the reasons behind her suicide were a mystery.

Lilly asked test subjects to sign new consent forms and started daily psychological evaluations. It also doubled the weaning period from the drug to eight days. The new forms disclosed the suicide, saying that "at this point the sponsor believes that this event was not caused by duloxetine or the study."

It's All About Market Share, Baby

In August—six months after Traci's death—the FDA approved Cymbalta for treating major depressive disorder. Why the hurry? There were already more than twenty antidepressants on the market, with ten SSRI types alone. I doubt society was clamoring for another.

Plus, wasn't Eli Lilly supposed to be investigating "side effects?" Excuse me, but aren't attempted suicide *and* death considered side effects? The FDA responded by saying it may eventually approve a black-box warning about risks on the drugs' packaging. After dragging its feet and only after pressure from lawmakers did the FDA issue one to be placed on the packaging. The effects of black-box warnings are purely cosmetic. Few if any follow the warnings.

In February 2004, the *Philadelphia Inquirer* reported that David Shaffer, a Lilly spokesman, admitted that "over the years, there had been four other suicides in trials of duloxetine, but only among the more than 8,500 subjects who already had been diagnosed with depression." The next day, Shaffer said he had misspoken and that "more than 8,500" was the total number of trial subjects, both "depressed and not depressed." The *Indianapolis Star* then discovered that 4,142 patients were depressed. This raises further questions about who exactly were the four other subjects who committed suicide during duloxetine tests.

Shaffer claimed that he "was uncertain how many took part in each study and how long the studies had been under way." If the company is uncertain about such basic information about the trials and suicides, how reliable is Lilly's claim that "duloxetine was not associated with Johnson's death"?

Along with Traci Johnson's death, the previous suicides were never widely reported by the media. Even Traci's suicide was barely mentioned except in the Indianapolis and Philadelphia newspapers, along with the *Los Angeles Times*. No one seemed interested in investigating what with the Scott Peterson trial, Michael Jackson's ordeal, and the runaway bride garnering so many headlines, there simply wasn't any room about possible links between suicides and drugs prescribed for millions of people.

Could it be that media outlets were afraid of offending sponsors and running the risk that they might pull their ads? Nahh, everyone believes in freedom of the press, right? Right?

Of Course It's No One's Fault

Lilly spokesman Rob Smith said the toxicology tests "in all likelihood" won't definitively prove whether the impact of duloxetine or Johnson's withdrawal from it caused her to take her own life. "We have not seen any sign that the drug can be linked to any kind of suicidal behavior," he said. He said the company would "let facts guide us," but "it appears this is an isolated tragedy." He added, "As it relates specifically to duloxetine, we have not seen anything at all from the data that either being on the drug or being withdrawn would pose a suicide risk."

Traci Johnson's pastor and relatives, however, have hotly countered that contention. They noted Johnson's active participation in her church, the Greater Church of Philadelphia, where she led a Friday-night youth group and some singing during worship services. Her suicide, they said, was totally out of character. "Traci Johnson was one of the star young people of our youth group. Her death has taken the heart out of our church family," said Reverend Barnaby.

Barnaby told the *Philadelphia Inquirer*, "I am troubled to the core of my spirit that Eli Lilly has taken such a defensive posture and [has] been so quick to deny any responsibility" in Johnson's death, "throwing all the blame on this young lady. I am shocked that they have taken such a deliberate defense to distance themselves from any responsibility." Other people who knew Traci well could not accept the possibility that she freely chose suicide, since that would challenge the very foundations of her faith.

Their experience wasn't unique. There are numerous examples of families losing a loved one because of drug-induced hazardous effects encountering the exact same corporate stonewalling and buck-passing. Could it be because drug manufacturers are in a uniquely privileged position? It's as if their influence in government, medicine, and the health-care industry leaves them above reproach.

They say Lilly would have to conduct a thorough investigation of each suicide during the duloxetine trials to determine whether the drug was involved. Company officials, who knew few details about the previous suicides, said they now plan to study all six deaths. We're still waiting, as Cymbalta continues to be sold.

Reassuring Stockholders

After Traci's death, Eli Lilly assured stockholders that the suicide would not delay the drug's release later that year. The company also reported Johnson's earlier pill-swallowing episode to the FDA and the scientists who were studying duloxetine for Lilly.

Lilly has said it expected the FDA to approve duloxetine to treat both depression and incontinence in 2004. The Tuesday following Traci's death, shares of Lilly's stock hit a fifty-two-week high, rising $1.32 to close at $74.54.

The concerns over antidepressants were already serious enough that on March 22 of that year, the FDA warned that some patients could become suicidal upon first starting antidepressants or during withdrawal. The agency urged the makers of ten drugs currently on the market to include labels alerting doctors and consumers to danger signs such as anxiety, hostility, and agitation in patients of all ages.

Traci's suicide occurred one week after an FDA advisory committee had urged the FDA to issue warnings about prescribing antidepressant drugs for teens because of an increased risk in suicide.

Dr. Joseph Glenmullen, a Harvard University psychiatrist, author of *Prozac Backlash*, and an expert psychopharmacologist, told the *Indianapolis Star* that Traci Johnson's suicide, her lack of depression, her young age, and the time she had been off the drug suggests she was vulnerable to suicidal thoughts. "She's still a teenager. It does look that children or adolescents might be even more vulnerable to (suicidal thoughts while taking antidepressants)."

According to the *Journal of Clinical Psychiatry*, SSRI-type antidepressants boost serotonin activity in the brain, and have the potential to induce the very dangerous and potentially fatal hyperserotonergic state known as serotonin syndrome. This is a potentially lethal condition caused by excessive serotonergic activity and is diagnosed by the presence of at least three of ten symptoms: mental status changes (confusion, hypomania), agitation, myoclonus, hyperreflexia, diaphoresis, shivering, tremor, diarrhea, incoordination, and fever.

It should come as no surprise then, that, as reported in the *Wall Street Journal*, the *British Medical Journal*, and many other publications, a new FDA analysis of clinical trial data on antidepressants suggested a link between antidepressant use and suicidal tendencies in young people. To make matters worse, a Congressional investigation in September revealed that FDA officials forced a medical officer to delete material on the risks of antidepressants from records he was submitting to Congress—and then to conceal the deletions.

Cynics could say—and I count myself among them—that Eli Lilly put pressure on the FDA to approve the drug. Of course, there is no paper trail—there seldom is for an industry that advertises heavily, invests in political candidates, hires the most lobbyists, and has a cozy relationship with the FDA.

Avrum Geurin Weiss, Ph.D., a psychotherapist in Atlanta, says he's not surprised, adding that prescribing antidepressants is out of control. He says sometimes feeling sad or depressed is normal. "However", says Dr. Weiss, "the first thing doctors do is write a prescription rather than suggest professional counseling."

The FDA's policy on warning labels for antidepressants that are prescribed for children and adolescents is more than bizarre; it's downright dangerous. During congressional hearings in the fall of 2004, agency officials admitted they had urged drug makers on several occasions not to inform doctors or their patients that products such as Paxil and Zoloft, while helpful for adults, weren't proved to be any more effective than inert sugar pills in treating childhood depression. Even more startling is that they made those recommendations despite knowledge that some of the drugs increased "suicidal thoughts" in young people.

Even after studies of antidepressants involving thousands of people, the debate over their risk still rages. Most psychiatrists say antidepressants are more likely to prevent suicide than trigger it. But some researchers point out that suicide is inherently difficult to study. It occurs too rarely to provide reliable data, and too many factors, often deeply personal, can spark a plunge into depression.

In Case You're Wondering

You may be wondering why I spent so much time talking about the Traci Johnson story in a book entitled *Supplements Under Siege*. Allow me to explain. The FDA banned ephedra because it said it was too dangerous. This directly disputed what the RAND report, which the FDA trumpeted (at least up until its release, that is), discovered—that only a handful of deaths and other sentinel events occurred among millions of ephedra users and billions of consumed ephedra/ephedrine doses over more than a ten-year span. When the RAND report recommended clinical trials to test the safety of ephedra, the agency said it was too dangerous to even test. In comparison, with duloxetine we see the FDA push through a new antidepressant drug despite the cloud of controversy surrounding it, especially the risk of suicide by young people—a market that the drug companies are actively courting.

In light of what you just read in this chapter, do you see a pattern emerging?

Antidepressant drugs are a huge business already, with enormous potential for growth. They all see the youth market as an untapped gold mine. But besides that, drug manufacturers are always on the outlook for new markets, be it off-label for pain (as in the case of Milton Cole, which I described in chapter 2), or for incontinence, as in the case of Cymbalta. Want to quit smoking? Take Zyban. Suffer from "social anxiety disorder"? You have three choices: Paxil, Zoloft, or Effexor XR. Zoloft comes in at number eight on the list of most prescribed drugs, while Effexor comes in at number fourteen.

I'm sure there are people absolutely too terrified to venture out of their house and shun all social contact. These people not only have my sympathy but also my hope that they will seek professional help. But that's not what is driving the sales of antidepressants for social anxiety disorder or SAD (not to be confused with the other SAD, seasonal affective disorder, although that, too, is over-prescribed). Through their ads, drug companies are telling us we need a little pick-me-up when we're facing a new social situation. That's bunk.

If someone walks into a room full of strangers and is boisterous and way too effervescent, keep your eye on that person. He or she could be dangerous. It's normal to be shy and reserved when you first walk into a social setting. As the comedian Gallagher says (when he's not smashing watermelons), we're the ancestors of those who made it back to the cave, meaning we're naturally cautious.

But the drug companies want you to think being shy is a disease.

So You Think You're OK? Ha!

According to a study published in the June 2005 issue of *Archives of General Psychiatry,* about 46 percent of people surveyed said they had experienced a mental illness at some point in their lives, and about 26 percent said they had within the previous year. Many cases begin with mild, easy-to-dismiss symptoms such as low-level anxiousness or persistent shyness, but left untreated, they can quickly escalate into severe depression, disabling phobias, or clinical anxiety, said Ronald Kessler, a Harvard Medical School researcher involved in the study. Most mental illness hits early in life, with half of all cases starting by age fourteen, a survey of nearly ten thousand U.S. adults found.

Don't you believe it.

Also this year, the American Medical Association planned to take a stance against the FDA's decision to add stiff warnings about antidepressant use among teens and children at its conference in Chicago in June. Those behind the proposal say it is designed to combat a recent, rapid decline in prescriptions and ensure that children and adolescents are getting proper treatment for depression. But critics predict confusion will reign if the nation's largest doctors' group opposes the FDA and declares the agency has been too stern on antidepressants—especially during a time the agency is under criticism for lax oversight of drug safety.

Since the FDA began reviewing widely prescribed drugs such as Prozac, Zoloft, Paxil, and Celexa, antidepressant usage is down more than 10 percent among patients under age eighteen, according to a study by Medco Health Solutions, Inc. The pharmacy benefit company found usage down 16 percent for the same age group in the fourth quarter, "traditionally the time of the year when antidepressant use peaks," the study said.

How disingenuous. A black-box warning does not prevent doctors from prescribing a certain medication. It highlights risks and typically makes physicians think twice about using the product. Even though black-box warnings have little if any effect, the drug manufacturers don't want any deterrent, or questions raised in the minds of patients or parents, to pushing antidepressants.

This Is *Really* Depressing News

Unfortunately, many of us have been sold a bill of goods when it comes to mood-altering drugs. The truth is, drugs don't cure depression. They can temporarily mask the symptoms, of course, but they won't cure you or help you heal. On the contrary, their side effects can actually contribute to deteriorating health. A true cure must address the underlying cause of your symptoms.

An article published in the *Canadian Medical Association Journal* included negative data long withheld from public examination by the pharmaceutical industry, and claimed that four popular antidepressants being used to treat thousands of depressed American children are unsafe, ineffective, or both. Here's a direct quote: "An internal document advised staff at the international drug giant GlaxoSmithKline (GSK) to withhold clinical trial findings in 1998 that indicated the antidepressant paroxetine (Paxil in North America and Seroxat in the U.K.) had no beneficial effect in treating adolescents."

According to the comprehensive scientific review of all available studies, antidepressants proven ineffective or harmful include:

- Paxil
- Zoloft
- Effexor
- Celexa

Besides the *Canadian Medical Association Journal,* British medical journals are much more forthcoming than their American counterparts. For example, an editorial in Great Britain's *The Lancet* found:

• Research on SSRIs in children is marked by confusion, manipulation, and institutional failure.

• Despite these findings, the FDA continues to support these worthless antidepressants by claiming the failed trials don't necessarily mean the drugs are ineffective. Data has also confirmed that taking SSRIs wasn't any better for you than taking a placebo.

As a society, we *must* understand the implications. When drug companies find out that their drugs don't work, they still sell them to us and market them to children, despite the high risk of suicide. Unpublished studies of venlafaxine suggested the drug increased suicide-related events such as suicidal thoughts or attempts by fourteen times compared with placebo. When you get done rubbing your eyes in disbelief, try reading that sentence again. Then reread the AMA's stand on antidepressant warnings a few paragraphs above.

Two editorials in the *Canadian Medical Association Journal* bring up the following key points:

• The prescribing rate for antidepressants in young people has increased steadily in the past decade.

• Many studies show that antidepressants have little to no effectiveness compared to placebos.

• There is a large gap between the quality of evidence needed to get a drug to market and the actual treatment needs of patients.

• In addition to their weak or nonexistent evidence of efficacy, antidepressants may have serious side effects in children beyond suicidal behavior, including agitation and irritability.

• Patient reports of adverse drug reactions are commonly dismissed as anecdotal or unscientific.

• There has been no formal response to this crisis from leaders in child psychiatry, many of whom were investigators in both published and unpublished trials.

• All trial participants—and the broader public—should have access to the results of clinical trials.

• Study data must be subject to analysis by independent experts who are alert to conflicts of interest that may distort the interpretation of data.

• Guidelines for physicians need to be rewritten so they reflect the full body of evidence, both published and unpublished.

The use of antidepressants and other psychiatric medications among children has more than tripled in recent years and now approaches adult usage rates, according to a January 2003 study in the *Archives of Pediatric and Adolescent Medicine*, representing at least one American journal not afraid to speak out. Study author Julie Zito, an associate professor of pharmacy and medicine at the University of Maryland, estimates that more than one million American children used antidepressants in 2000.

Instead, we're more apt to get this blather. Last year a task force of the American College of Neuropsychopharmacology released its own preliminary review of published studies on antidepressants and suicide and stated it found no statistically significant increase in suicide attempts among children taking the drugs. "The most likely explanation for the episodes of attempted suicide while taking SSRIs is the underlying depression, not the SSRIs," said Graham Emslie, a child psychiatrist and researcher at the University of Texas Southwestern Medical Center in Dallas.

Now do you see why I spent so much time on the Traci Johnson suicide?

Unfortunately, the Beat Goes On

A few pages earlier I mentioned that during a Congressional investigation in September 2004, FDA officials forced a medical officer to delete material on the risks of antidepressants from records he was submitting to Congress—and then to conceal the deletions. Here's the rest of that story.

When FDA medical officer Andrew Mosholder was to present his report at an FDA advisory hearing it promised to be a contentious affair involving competing medical experts and parents whose children took their own lives while on the medications.

Prior to the hearings, Mosholder had been asked by the agency to perform a safety analysis of antidepressants after reports emerged in the summer of 2005 of high rates of suicidal behavior among children enrolled in clinical trials for Paxil, Effexor, and other antidepressants.

For his report, Dr. Mosholder, a child psychiatrist, reviewed data from twenty clinical trials involving more than 4,100 children and eight different antidepressants. His preliminary analysis, according to two FDA sources familiar with his report, concluded that there was an increased risk of suicidal behavior among children being treated for depression with Paxil and several other antidepressants.

The initial agenda for the hearing listed Mosholder and his findings, but his presentation was later removed. Mosholder was told that he could not present his findings at the hearing, an FDA official told the *San Francisco Chronicle*.

Seemingly, out of the blue, a senior FDA official said the study wouldn't be presented because it wasn't "finalized."

While Mosholder's safety analysis report may eventually be completed and made public, some FDA insiders fear that withholding it from the hearing indicates that the agency may be siding with the pharmaceutical industry in its long-running battle with critics of antidepressants. Industry critics, including consumer advocates and mental health professionals, argue that the drugs are often ineffective and dangerous and that the FDA has failed to fully investigate the risks to children. "The FDA is shielding the industry," said Vera Sharav, president of the Alliance for Human Research Protection, a consumer advocacy group.

Members of the Office of Drug Safety, who had prepared a thirty-seven-page safety report, were present at the hearing but also were not allowed to speak. It should come as no surprise, but a representative of the FDA division that originally approved the drug, along with the pharmaceutical company that makes Paxil, did most of the talking.

A documentary crew from the PBS series *Frontline* filmed the meeting and afterward, in the hallway, caught up with David Graham, M.D., a senior epidemiologist and associate director of the FDA's Office of Drug Safety. The producers had been denied previous requests to interview Graham, but the government scientist gave a brief interview without permission.

"We had a different perspective, and we really weren't given an opportunity to present our side of the story," Graham, on camera, told the producers. "And the people who did present, the reviewing division and the company, you know, they didn't see a problem. This was a very hostile process. And let's just leave it at that."

Painfully Unaware

Does Dr. Graham's name ring a bell, if you'll pardon the pun? His claim to fame—and rightly so—has to do with another recent drug scandal. In November 2004, in front of the Senate Finance Committee, Graham testified that the pain reliever Vioxx, used by many arthritis sufferers, was responsible for an estimated 38,000 excess heart attacks and sudden cardiac deaths. Graham also stated that this was a conservative estimate. He said that "a more realistic and likely range of estimates for the number of excess cases in the U.S." was between 88,000 and 139,000. "Of these," he added, "30–40 percent probably died."

Was this acceptable, as the drug manufacturers claim, by weighing risk versus benefit? That the deaths of some 55,000 people were worth it since these type of drugs eliminate the gastrointestinal problems from over-the-counter pain relievers? Sadly, that turned out not to be true.

The story gets worse. After being removed from the market, Vioxx was "reapproved" by an FDA panel. Their rationale was again risk versus benefit. But what ultimately came out was that ten of the thirty-two FDA drug advisers whose total votes favored the controversial painkillers Celebrex, Bextra, and Vioxx had financial ties to the industry. According to public records and disclosures in medical journals, the ten advisors had recently consulted with the drugs' makers.

While it's common practice for researchers who work with industry to serve on FDA advisory panels—the FDA says it balances expertise with potential conflicts of interest—the FDA often keeps such ties secret from the public, and experts say that studies have shown that money does influence scientific judgments. In this case the ten advisors had worked in some capacity for Merck, Vioxx's maker, Pfizer, which makes Celebrex and Bextra, or Novartis, which is applying to sell Prexige, a similar drug.

The FDA said that the committee members were "screened for conflicts of interest according to the same strict ethics guidelines FDA applies to all its advisory committees." No conflict of interest? You decide, since the FDA certainly didn't. Although eight of the ten members said their ties did not influence their votes, had they not voted, here's what the advisory committee results would have been:

- 14 to 8 to keep Vioxx off the market
- 12 to 8 to withdraw Bextra from the market

What about the advisors with company ties—what did their vote tally look like?

- 9 to 1 to bring Vioxx back to the market
- 9 to 1 to keep Bextra on the market

Their votes did not significantly influence the decision to keep Celebrex on the market.

The controversy and influence of the drug companies is not limited to our shores. In June 2005, the British newspaper *The Independent* reported that key data on prescription medicines found in millions of British homes has been suppressed by the FDA even though the information potentially threatened lives.

Their investigation shows that, under pressure from the pharmaceutical industry, the FDA routinely concealed information it considered commercially sensitive, leaving medical professionals in the dark and unable to evaluate the potential risks.

One team of investigators found that twenty-eight pages of data had been removed from the FDA files on one of a new family of painkillers because of confidentiality. One research study led by

Professor Julia Hippisley-Cox at Nottingham University, revealed that ibuprofen, the supposedly "safe" painkiller, increases the risk of heart attack by almost 25 percent. The finding was a shock to those who had switched from Vioxx, since it was shown that it, too, could increase the risk of heart attacks. Now researchers are questioning the reliability of the data about other drugs, including the full range of painkillers.

Dr. Peter Juni, one of the team of Swiss investigators who helped to expose the risk of the new-generation drugs, claims his efforts were obstructed by the FDA.

"As part of the Freedom of Information Act, the agency is required to make available its reports on all drugs that are approved. Unfortunately, these reports are not as useful as they could be," he and his team said in an editorial in the *British Medical Journal*. "For example, only 16 out of at least 27 trials of celecoxib that were performed up to 2002 in patients with musculoskeletal pain were included in the relevant reports. In the case of valdecoxib, we found that many pages and paragraphs had been deleted because they contained trade secret and/or confidential information that is not disclosable."

Dr. Juni, senior research fellow in clinical epidemiology at the University of Berne, is demanding that drug companies be legally required to make public any adverse effects as soon as they become available. Researchers also want more independent research, with financial firewalls between drug companies and doctors carrying out clinical trials.

In 2004, *The Lancet* published trial results showing that unacceptable heart risks linked to Vioxx were evident four years before it was finally withdrawn by its maker. *The Lancet*'s editor, Richard Horton, said, "Too often the FDA saw and continues to see the pharmaceutical industry as its customers, a vital source of funding for its activities, and not as a sector of society in need of strong regulation."

It was also revealed that FDA supervisors had again attempted to suppress a report by Dr. Graham showing that patients taking Vioxx suffered five times as many heart attacks as patients taking another pain reliever, naproxen. As with antidepressants, Dr. Graham's supervisors refused to allow him to present his conclusions at a meeting in France and later sought to interfere with the publication of his

For You Math Buffs Out There

Those of you who like to sit with a calculator at the ready may have noticed a mathematical discrepancy. If so, let me clear it up for you. In the last chapter, I mentioned that the government has admitted to "five" clinical trial deaths. Included in that tally, I suppose, since they don't give names, are Jesse Gelsinger at the University of Pennsylvania in 1999 and Ellen Roche at Johns Hopkins in 2001, whom I mentioned before. I added Traci Johnson to their total of four—the other two are unknown—making the number five. Now you just read of "four" or "five" deaths from an earlier trial of duloxetine. By adding those in, the total leapfrogs the official tally of five, even if two of those cover the "two unknowns" included in the official tally. If you picked up on this, kudos to you and shame, shame, shame on the government and the pharmaceutical companies for not being honest with us and for downplaying the relevancy. It also reemphasizes the secrecy surrounding deaths during clinical trials. Again, we don't know how many people die while taking part during such trials. The FDA does little to protect subjects, nor do they ensure that the risks are fully disclosed.

study results when they were scheduled to appear in *The Lancet*. Merck, the drug company behind Vioxx, subsequently acknowledged the risk of heart attacks, and the article was published.

What the FDA decides in cases like this filters all the way down to the front lines of health care, that is, to your doctor's office, and ultimately to you. The way the system is set up, they must rely on what the FDA and the drug companies—both directly and indirectly—tell them. You may be shocked by how much influence the drug companies have over the medical profession regarding their education. The drug companies have effectively drowned out competing, superior solutions for patients, as you'll see in the next chapter.

7

Take Two and Call Me in the Morning

No Free Lunch, an organization that encourages health-care providers to decline all industry largesse, requested a booth in the exhibit hall at this year's meeting of the American College of Physicians (ACP) in San Francisco. ACP, the nation's largest medical specialty society, denied the request. To combat the slight, University of California at San Francisco medical students wearing green "No Free Lunch" T-shirts wandered the exhibit hall handing out ACP's own guidelines on interactions with industry. The entire time, they were followed closely by San Francisco police officers.

No Free Lunch is a New York organization that encourages physicians to pledge to "accept no money, gifts, or hospitality from the pharmaceutical industry" and "seek unbiased sources of information" about which treatments are best for their patients—apart from drug company marketers. Likewise, the ACP's ethics manual strongly discourages doctors from accepting "gifts, hospitality, trips and subsidies of all types." But that didn't stop the ACP from financing its annual meeting—largely through the drug industry, including $60,000 worth of tote bags—after ACP promised them that the annual meeting would offer "an unparalleled opportunity to meet with physicians of power—prescribing power."

After a couple of days of pressure from corporate sponsors, the ACP distributed a memo reassuring exhibitors that the ACP had nothing to do with distributing the ethical guidelines. Huh? That's right, the ACP felt it necessary to reassure drug companies that the distribution of their own guidelines for declining gifts from drug companies was unacceptable and not their idea.

This type of conflict is all too common. I recently attended a press conference at a medical meeting in Orlando billed by the organizers— a well-known and respected medical association—as "An update on Irritable Bowel Syndrome (IBS) Treatments." It turned out to be five docs pushing a new drug. When pressed, all five grudgingly revealed their financial ties to the company producing the drug. When I asked, "You said this drug 'cures' IBS? Does that mean you found the mechanism that causes it?" One doctor tried to confound us with jargon until another doctor denied they ever said that. I looked at my notes, and read what they had said. They all looked at one another before one finally uttered, "Well, it's not really a cure but a new way to relieve the symptoms, which is a vast improvement."

Afterwards, as I glided down an escalator, there was a huge poster at the bottom stating, "We would like to thank 'XYZ Pharmaceuticals' for their generous contribution of 'X' million dollars for our capital fund."

Drug companies recognize that their top salesmen may very well be other doctors. As reported in the July 15, 2005 issue of the *Wall Street Journal,* hiring a doctor to speak about drug therapies to other doctors has proven to be a "highly effective" way for the pharmaceutical industry to market its drugs. "An internal study done by Merck & Co. several years ago calculated the 'return on investment' from doctor-led discussion groups was almost double the return on meetings led by the company's own sales force," the article states. "According to the document, doctors who attended a lecture by another doctor wrote an additional $623.55 worth of prescriptions for the painkiller Vioxx over a 12-month period compared with doctors who didn't attend. Doctors who participated in the more intimate discussions wrote an additional $717.53 worth of prescriptions for Vioxx, which Merck pulled from the market last year over concerns about cardiovascular side effects. That compared to an increase of only $165.87 in Vioxx prescriptions by doctors who attended a meeting with a salesperson."

Further, many doctors are routinely paid "consulting" fees to listen to the drug company talks at medical conferences typically held at deluxe resorts or at least in prime vacation spots. A typical medical conference features seminars, lectures, and required continuing medical education (CME) courses on the featured specialty or the diseases the organization focuses on, such as heart disease, gastrointestinal problems, cancer, and diabetes. Usually there are poster presentations ranging from a few dozen to hundreds, depending on the size of the conference.

Not so long ago, the posters focused more on independent research, often at the college level. Recently, I noticed more and more pharma studies featured and the college researchers nudged aside by marketing reps.

Needless to say, research on dietary supplements and other alternative treatments are rarely mentioned at these conferences. When an herb or vitamin is mentioned, it is usually to warn doctors that it should be avoided since they conflict with the drug under study. (Funny, it's never the other way around!)

Most conferences have strict policies against pharma reps entering the press rooms, yet many brazen reps set up shop not far from the entrances. Recently I saw one craft a makeshift desk out of one of those large round bussing trays perched on top of a folding stand. He latched onto every reporter on their way into the press room to make sure they had a copy of his company's latest brochure.

In addition, let's not forget the humongous corporate exhibit booths manned not only by sharply dressed drug reps, but also by (at the risk of sounding sexist, but there's no other way to describe them) "come-hither booth babes."

Dietary supplement associations also have conferences (including the ever-popular booth babes) but they're billed more as trade shows. There's a big difference.

Getting Educated

One of the most controversial issues with the pharmaceutical companies is their role in CMEs. Consider the following two choices faced by doctors specializing in diabetes management:

Course A is a five-day event sponsored by ABCPharma that includes golf and a series of lectures held at an upscale resort. Registration is only $125, and the airfare and hotel can be booked at a deep discount (sometimes it's free if you agree to speak).

Course B is sponsored by "XYZ University" in a college town in the Midwest. It costs $525 for three days, plus airfare and hotel accommodations at the Do-Drop Inn. The topic—managing diabetic patients with comorbidities—will be covered in multiple formats, including case-based workshops.

From a professional standpoint, Course B, given its more clearly defined objectives, should be the preferred course. But parasailing or blackjack tables can be a nice break from the day-to-day routine.

Obviously, the drug industry has its own interests, and there are lots of examples of so-called educational events whose real objective is to change prescribing behavior. On the other hand, a code of marketing practices does exist, and to be fair, many pharmaceutical companies are extra careful about distinguishing between CME and promotion. (Many of the big medical meetings have what are called "satellite" presentations geared toward particular drug brands.)

It actually gets *more* complicated. While drug company involvement in CME is obvious, medical school hosting is often a mixed bag of pharmaceutical and non-industry funding.

A recent survey of the Society for Academic Continuing Medical Education shows a growing trend among medical school providers of CME: over the period 1993–2001, while medical schools reported a modest 25 percent increase in the number of courses and a doubling of registration fees, they disclosed a quintupling of commercial support for CME. Does this automatically mean industry funding automatically leads to bias in medical school CMEs. Actually, yes. Research indicates that industry funding can skew CME content in various ways to match the goals of industry. This skewing may be felt in the subtle influence of industry on the selection of topics—maybe an emphasis on treatment over prevention.

"Free" online courses are not a solution to the problem. They're usually sponsored by pharmaceutical companies or device manufacturers.

Who's in Charge?

Conflicts of interest are increasingly common now that two-thirds of medical research at universities is funded by private industry. In his book *On the Take*, Jerome Kassirer, M.D., former editor in chief of the *New England Journal of Medicine* reports that the drug industry spent $2 billion in 2001 on events for doctors—double what it spent five years earlier.

In a 2002 review, the *Journal of the American Medical Association* found that 60 percent of doctors defending a drug's use had relationships with the drug's makers. Drug companies provide a significant portion of the budget for the FDA. One-third of the experts who recently recommended putting Vioxx and other arthritis medications recalled for increasing the risk of heart attack back on the market worked as consultants to makers of the drugs, according to the Center for Science in the Public Interest.

Consumers may not realize it, but this directly affects what our doctors prescribe for us. You don't have to have a doctorate in psychology to recognize that payments come with baggage—and expectations. Plus, the amount the pharma companies pour into direct-to-consumer advertising too often reduces us to lemmings asking for, or accepting whatever "sample" they push across their desk when something ails us. "The time has come to ask whether all of the money floating around medicine has created a pattern of corruption," writes Dr. Kassirer. "Clinical advice, like votes, should never be bought."

Sometimes this "partnership" gets much worse. In a practice known as "shadowing," drug company reps sit in on patients' visits with their doctors. Critics say the practice is an attempt to influence what medicines are prescribed. Drug companies say the practice is educational, but they sometimes pay hundreds of dollars a day to the doctors for these visiting rights. (The American Medical Association is trying to implement a rule to discourage the practice.)

Still, Big Pharma can usually count on its powerful friend, the AMA, which also campaigned to do away with ephedra. It's no secret many physicians feel threatened by dietary supplements. They see many of the claims as "hype" and worry about patients using unproven products in lieu of traditional medical treatments. From the outset, it was the clear intent of Congress in enacting DSHEA that consumers should be provided with products, information, and education that would help promote health and prevent disease. Yet, since Congress noted in its "findings" section of the act that "consumers should be empowered to make choices about preventive health-care programs based on data from scientific studies of health benefits related to particular dietary supplements," the AMA has balked. You may recall they also fought tooth-and-nail against acupuncture, until they could fight it no more.

Many doctors have little motivation—or time, for that matter—to investigate alternatives to prescription drugs. Reading scientific studies isn't in the standard course for doctors. While there are widely available sources of information on drugs not written by the drug companies, reading the literature dropped off by the drug reps, along with free sushi, is probably easier.

It's not much different from when Henry Ford said customers could have any color car they wanted as long as it was black. Today's slogan might as well be, "You can have any remedy you want as long as it's a prescription drug."

Get 'Em When They're Young

Did you ever wonder how our medical care became so wedded to pharmaceutical solutions? It starts early. Financially strapped and impressionable, medical students are easy marks for pharmaceutical companies. Unless their medical school or hospital has a strict policy against it, it's very easy to entice them with a free meal to hear a spiel about a company's drugs. Coupled with other goodies such as tote bags, and the resident or intern is an informed client when he's a full-fledged doctor.

The influx of drug reps into physicians' offices and hospitals has attracted the attention of both medical journals and the lay press. Newspapers including the *New York Times* and the *Wall Street Journal* have covered this issue. The *British Medical Journal* recently dedicated an entire issue to the topic, disclosing practices ranging from questionable gifts to near bribery. Much published research has also been conducted in this area, nearly all of it concluding that the interactions between drug reps and physicians are detrimental to doctors and their patients.

Simply, gifts, no matter how small, produce a sense of gratitude. This is why pharmaceutical companies provide pens, notepads, name badge holders, and the like. It's human nature for gift recipients to feel compelled to do something in return for the giver, even if it's something as simple as giving a patient a free drug sample. This creates a conflict of interest many doctors seldom consider: the desire to cure the patient versus the subconscious need to repay the drug company's generosity. It's quick and it's easy and seemingly doesn't cost the doctor or patient anything. Wrong! Because it's free doesn't make it the right solution, especially if the patient isn't cured or at best is wedded to a drug for the foreseeable future. Plus, someone is ultimately paying for those samples.

For too many doctors, providing free samples has become the path of least resistance and has changed the doctor's role. As Robert Scott Bell says, "The fact that they are good at chemically suppressing symptoms does not make them healers."

The pharmaceutical companies recognize their power and grease the skids before the patient even arrives, especially via direct-to-consumer ads. An increasingly common predicament for doctors is patients demanding a drug by brand name. Pharmaceutical companies exploit people's emotions in the ways they frame disease. Many anti-hypertensive drug ads carry emotional messages, such as one for Merck's Zocor that warns, "It's your future. Be there." If a doctor tries suggesting a different treatment, especially if it includes no drug at all, many patients feel shortchanged. They believe if it's on TV, it must be true, and feel slighted if they leave the doctor's office empty-handed.

The total marketing budget of U.S. pharmaceutical companies—everything from ads to sponsoring medical conferences to buying lunch for doctors—topped $22 billion in 2003, according to IMS Health, a company that tracks drug sales for its drug industry clients. The vast majority of that $22 billion went to directly influence doctors, primarily through $16 billion worth of free drug samples delivered to physicians' offices by drug reps bearing lunch. Fearful of losing market share, the industry has hired more drug representatives in order to contact more physicians. As a result, there are now ninety thousand pharmaceutical representatives in the United States. Numerous studies show this marketing affects physicians' prescription habits. Otherwise, why would they do it?

Dietary supplement companies don't have the budget, and probably the know-how to visit doctors to tout their products. And even if they did, they can't promote their products for curing diseases because they could technically be in violation of the law.

Doctors are less likely to see supplement success stories unless a patient explicitly says, "This supplement is really working for me!" Also, ads touting supplements for weight loss, muscle gain, hair regrowth, and breast enhancement—all of which sound too good to be true and all using products described as natural—bombard the public from radio stations and TV infomercials. Of course the FDA, FCC, and the FTC, which should be monitoring these ads and apprehending those who make bogus claims, seldom do. It's easier to claim you can't (which is not true) than to actually monitor the ads and product claims as they're supposed to for public safety.

Don't misunderstand me—there are plenty of valid studies supporting the use of a variety of nutritional supplements. But, most doctors don't have the time to read all the latest journals and can't possibly know unless someone tells them about it. Knowing this, drug reps bring studies touting their products to the busy doctors' offices. As sales people, drug reps are naturally biased. Among the studies conducted on a drug—it's not likely the drug rep will show every article, including the ones that prove it to be less effective than its competitor. The purpose of the drug rep is not to educate, but to sell.

The pharmaceutical companies defend their advertising as not only their right under "free speech" but also as a public service. Their ads, they believe, may alert patients of symptoms of serious diseases they might otherwise not recognize. Former *New England Journal of Medicine* editor in chief Marcia Angel disputes this. In her book *The Truth About the Drug Companies,* Dr. Angell says that drug company ads dupe many patients into believing they have "dubious or exaggerated ailments" such as "generalized anxiety disorder"—otherwise known as shyness, "premenstrual dysphoric disorder"—PMS—or "gastro-esophageal reflux disease"(GERD). As a result, thousands of Americans have prescriptions for Nexium—number four on the best selling list—or similar prescription drugs developed to treat stomach acid seeping back into the esophagus, which can become a precancerous condition.

Dr. Angell claims too many of the people clutching the prescriptions only have "normal" heartburn. She says that—as any responsible physician knows—for most people who have heartburn, the best way to treat it is probably to eat better, eat slower, lose weight, and exercise more. (But for some people, this "solution" is simply out of the question because it actually requires effort.)

On a flight from Atlanta to California, I read Dr. Angell's book. In it, she writes, and sources in great detail, how the pharmaceutical industry has become extremely wealthy—and thoroughly corrupt. She points out how they devote more money to marketing than research and development, despite claiming the opposite.

Dr. Angell, now a senior lecturer at Harvard Medical School, charges that while the top ten American drug companies in 2002 posted sales of $217 billion, only 14 percent ($30 billion) went to research and development, while they spent more than twice as much (approximately $67 billion) on marketing and "administration."

Dr. Angell also details how the drug companies are often in cahoots with members of the medical profession, showering them with gifts, trips, and free samples (to hook *you*), and how the FDA bends over backwards to accommodate the industry by approving new drugs on scant evidence. Naturally, I was pleased since her research echoed many of the same findings I reported in my own book, *Ephedra Fact & Fiction*.

Not surprisingly, after her book came out, Dr. Angell became a target. Imagine my dismay when I read a scathing book review attacking Dr. Angell appearing in the *Washington Times* and subsequently picked up by other media outlets. The reviewer, Elizabeth M. Whelan, is president of the American Council on Science and Health. She flat out misrepresents (OK, she lies) what Dr. Angell wrote.

For example, Whelan writes that Dr. Angell's arguments are "contradictory, inconsistent and often in error." She goes on and claims that Dr. Angell said "there are no truly innovative drugs out there." That's bunk, pure bunk.

On page 54, Dr. Angell writes that between 1998 and 2002, the industry introduced only twelve innovative drugs per year, or "14 percent of the total." Dr. Angell's point is that society is not served since the lion's share of new drugs are me-too drugs and simply duplicate what's already on the market.

Whelan also writes, "Dr. Angell recommends radical measures: in effect that the government takes over the industry and treat it as a public utility." Not quite. Rather, Dr. Angell argues that since the industry feeds so often at the government trough, "the pharmaceutical industry should be regarded much as a public utility."

For example, when the cancer drug Taxol was being developed the entire $183 million cost was borne by the taxpayer-funded National Institutes of Health. Then, in 1991 the NIH gave exclusive marketing rights to Bristol-Myers Squibb, netting them $1 to $2 billion per year. In effect, that means we paid twice.

I suspect Whelan wrote the review not to inform, but to keep people from reading the book. What most people don't know is the official-sounding American Council on Science and Health (for which Elizabeth Whelan works) receives financial support from drug and food companies, although they've refused to reveal their funding sources since the early 1990s.

It could be there's a more direct reason to keep us from reading the book. On page 214, Dr. Angell mentions a 2003 *New York Times* article based on confidential drug industry documents detailing the industries' plans to "buy influence" with government officials, economists, doctors, and others. Dr. Angell points out that "there would be $500,000 for placement of op-eds and articles by third parties." Apparently, Whelan and ACSH answered the call.

"According to Experts . . ."

We've all heard it before. A news anchor reports or a magazine writer states something to the effect of, "According to experts. . . ." And it's so common we don't even think about it. And we also assume that whoever this "expert" may be—a professor, doctor, or watchdog group spokesperson—must be on the level. But how do we really know? How often is it revealed who those experts are, where they get their funding, or with what organization(s) they're associated?

There are trade groups and lobbyists for every imaginable commodity. The beef, sugar, dairy—and yes, the dietary supplement—industries (including one for ephedra) all have organizations whose primary (or sole) function is to trumpet how wonderful their products are, as well as beat back and minimize any criticism.

Other organizations within the public relations industry also do a lot of product pushing for certain companies and industries, but you'd never know it from their names. The public relations industry has spent years and millions of dollars funding and creating industry front groups posing as dispensers of "sound" science. In reality, their "sound science" is simply product spin defined by the drug, tobacco, chemical, genetic engineering, petroleum, and other industries.

Here are examples of such "front" groups including the aforementioned ACSH:

• **American Council on Science and Health (ACSH)**: Receives financial support from about three hundred different sources, including foundations, trade associations, corporations and individuals.

- **Center for Consumer Freedom (CCF):** A front group for the tobacco, restaurant, and liquor industries that represents itself as an advocate for consumers' rights.
- **Consumer Alert (CA):** Funded by corporations, CA opposes flame-resistance standards for clothing fabrics issued by the Consumer Product Safety Commission, and defends products such as the diet drug dexfenfluramine (Redux), which was taken off the market because of its association with heart valve damage. In contrast with Consumers Union, which is funded primarily by member subscriptions, Consumer Alert is funded by the industries whose products it defends—companies like Pfizer Pharmaceuticals, Philip Morris, Eli Lilly, Monsanto, Upjohn, Chemical Manufacturers Association, Ciba-Geigy, the Beer Institute, Coors, and Chevron USA.
- **International Food Information Council Foundation (IFIC):** The IFIC—which receives its financial support from the food, beverage, and agricultural industries—says the mission of its foundation is to convey science-based information on food safety and nutrition to consumers, health professionals, educators, journalists, and government officials. While the IFIC says its goal is to bridge the information gap by collecting and disseminating scientific information, what the IFIC fails to reveal are the names of the companies that finance it. It's an impressive list and includes Coca-Cola, Pepsi, Hershey, M&M/Mars, and Procter & Gamble.

All these groups (and there are many, many others) support research and publish results favorable to their clients and those who finance their operations. What kind of findings do you think they would support? Those disparaging what they sell?

Quietly financed by the industries whose products they—ahem—evaluate, these "independent" research agencies churn out "scientific" studies and press materials announcing "breakthrough" research to every radio, television, and print media outlet in the country, endeavoring to create the image their underwriters want.

Many of these carefully scripted reports are molded in a news format and can be read like straight news. This saves journalists the trouble of researching the subjects on their own, especially on topics about which they know very little. Entire sections of the release can be used intact with no editing, given the byline of the reporter or newspaper or television station.

Does this really happen? According to research by the Center for Media and Democracy (CMD), a nonprofit public-interest organization that conducts investigative reports on the public relations industry, sometimes as many as half the stories appearing in an issue of the *Wall Street Journal* are based solely on such press releases. These types of stories are mixed right in with legitimately researched stories. Unless you have done the research yourself, it's nearly impossible to tell the difference.

Among the "ask your doctor" television ads running in recent months, one tells viewers that although they may think they have their cholesterol under control, they should think again since the definition of high cholesterol has been changed. As I've mentioned before, eight of nine experts who sat on the government National Cholesterol Education Program panel that recommended the new guidelines had financial ties to companies marketing cholesterol-lowering drugs. In a letter of complaint, the Center for Science in the Public Interest noted no studies had proven that increasing use of such drugs helped elderly men likely to take them, but the drugs were known to increase the risk of cancer.

Same goes for high blood pressure. The average person doesn't know that drug companies pay one-third of the budget of the American Society of Hypertension (ASH) and it wouldn't be far-fetched to think that might influence what doctors are told. At their last convention in San Francisco doctors were ushered into rooms full of drug company literature and salespeople. It was a great opportunity to "educate" doctors about the new "condition" known as "prehypertension."

For years, doctors considered 120/80 to be ideal and anything under 140 to be OK. But a change took place in May 2003, when American doctors got new advice from a government-sanctioned medical panel called the Joint National Committee on Prevention,

Detection, Evaluation, and Treatment of High Blood Pressure. Systolic pressure as low as 120 could be unsafe, the panel said. It also established a new condition, called "prehypertension," systolic pressure from 120 to 139, and said millions more people should take hypertension drugs to save their lives. As I already pointed out—but it's worth repeating—nine of the eleven authors of the guidelines on the NIH panel recommending broader use of hypertension drugs to lower blood pressure had ties to the drug companies. I can assure you that at the ASH meeting there wasn't a big push (or any push, for that matter) for supplements such as vitamin E or coenzyme Q10.

As the drug industry marketed them vigorously and compliant doctors followed the new guidelines and treated hypertension at lower readings, sales of the newer drugs increased. According to IMS Health, in 2004 patients and their insurance companies spent $16.3 billion for blood-pressure pills, up $3 billion from five years earlier.

Image Is Everything

Under pressure from doctors, the drug companies' lobbying association, the Pharmaceutical Research and Manufacturers of America came up with a new code of ethics in 2002 instructing member companies in the ways of influencing doctors. Under the rules, giving doctors cash for writing prescriptions is bad—not to mention illegal. Paying doctors a handsome "consulting" fee to come to a resort golf course for training as company "speakers," however, is just fine.

So, while pharmaceutical companies cannot bribe docs directly, they can form alliances with them in plenty of other ways, just as political lobbyists often form alliances with elected officials. One maker of a popular erectile-dysfunction drug paid doctors cash after they wrote prescriptions. Ostensibly the money was to compensate doctors for time spent enrolling the newly prescribed patients in a study.

The practice is perfectly acceptable under PhRMA's ethical guidelines and there is no formal regulation. The rules are purely voluntary. But the more drug companies advertise products, the worse the public's view of the industry, polls show. In fact, their image only got worse following last year's scandals of allegedly dangerous—but widely advertised—drugs being pulled off the market.

PhRMA now recognizes that the industry as a whole needs promotion. As the industry struggles with its public image, PhRMA is getting ready to counter with institutional ads to polish their image. In the new ads, PhRMA and its clients discuss the innovation of the industry and promote its efforts to get drugs into the hands of the one-fourth of Americans who don't have drug coverage. A new wave of drug industry commercials already has aired touting drug giveaway programs for the indigent, to whom PhRMA member companies provided about forty million free prescriptions during the past two years.

I've been kind of hard on the medical profession in this chapter and to some degree, I believe they've earned it. However, they do play a critical role in our health-care system. In fact, as you'll see in the next chapter I think they should have even more responsibility— despite what members of the U.S. Congress say.

8

Bad Reactions:
Who Are You Going to Call?

When I was twenty years old and home from college, I went to the family doctor for an allergy test. Dr. Goldstein's office in Merrick, Long Island, was on a pretty tree-lined street in an old colonial-style house, set back about fifty feet from the curb.

The test consisted of a grid of pin pricks on the arm. After about fifteen minutes, Dr. Goldstein checked the site for a reaction, such as redness, itching, or raised bumps signifying an allergy to something. After a half hour or so, I was free to go.

Rather then go home, which turned out to be a good thing, I headed in the opposite direction to a local music store about a mile from the doctor's office. The store was closed, which turned out to be the second good thing.

The route to my home took me past the doctor's office. About a half mile from there, my throat became itchy, my eyes began to water, and it became harder to breath. My heart also started to palpitate. After covering another quarter mile, breathing became even tougher, my heart beat even harder and faster, and I was virtually blinded by my tears. Suddenly, I had an overwhelming urge to scratch my entire body, to the point I had to choose to either scratch like mad or keep my hands on the steering wheel. By the time I rolled to a stop in front of the doctor's office I was a complete zombie.

I stumbled from the car, staggered to the front door, and hammered once before I collapsed in a heap. I vaguely remember two elderly women hooking me under their arms and dragging me over the threshold yelling for the doctor. Despite my condition I remember the shock on his face just before he scampered away and quickly returned with an injection, possibly epinephrine, a form of adrenaline. After about an hour, with my heart still beating stronger than normal, but otherwise much improved, I once again was released.

Apparently I had either an anaphylaxis attack, or an anaphylactoid reaction, which are serious and rapid allergic reactions usually involving more than one part of the body. If severe enough, it can kill.

I shudder when I think what would have happened if I had driven home—since my mother didn't drive—or if the music store was open. Since I felt like I was five minutes from literally jumping out of my skin—with my heart leading the way—I may have been dismissed as an overzealous Grateful Dead fan and left to freak out on my own. (The truth be told, I was after an album by The Association, the group that sang "Along Comes Mary," "Cherish," "Never my Love.")

I tell you this story because during my time of distress I had a choice to make. I could either go back to the doctor's office or find a phone to complain to the maker of the allergy test. Of course the second option seems silly, but that's what current legislation proposes to do, only not for drugs or medical devices but for dietary supplements.

Let's say this happened today, which is possible, since skin tests are still administered. But whether a skin test or a prescribed drug, after witnessing my reaction, Dr. Goldstein would be expected to notify the FDA. Same thing if my reaction happened at a hospital. If my reaction was milder, I might have contacted my local poison control center, which would then pass the information on to the FDA.

I had no intention to contact the manufacturer of the test and I certainly wouldn't expect Dr. Goldstein to pass the information to a pharmaceutical sales rep between bites of a complimentary pastrami on rye during lunch. What would the rep do? Make note of it on a cocktail napkin and call it in to his office later? What guarantee would there be that the information would ever reach the FDA?

The issue here is public safety and part of that is building an accurate database of possible adverse reactions, especially serious events (including death). This should be the case for food, drugs, and—yes—dietary supplements.

I bring this up because there are those who think one of the big problems with dietary supplements is the poor system for reporting adverse reactions. In April 2001, the Office of Inspector General, which is part of HHS, reported that, unlike new prescription and over-the-counter drugs, the FDA does not have the authority to require that supplements undergo pre-market approval for safety and efficacy. Instead, it relies mostly on its adverse event reporting system to identify safety problems. They said the system is flawed partially because reporting adverse events is entirely voluntary. The report admitted the FDA's adverse event reporting system detects only a small portion of the events that actually occur. It stated an earlier FDA-commissioned study that estimated the FDA received less than 1 percent of all adverse events associated with dietary supplements. They concluded that among the factors that may contribute to the under-reporting are that many consumers presume supplements to be safe, use these products without the supervision of a health-care professional, and may be unaware that the FDA regulates them. It never occurred to them—or at least they weren't willing to admit—that maybe they were safe and there wasn't a whole lot to report. Or, if there were problems, that having the manufacturers reporting—voluntary or not is a system not in the best interest of consumers.

One solution proposed by a prominent U.S. Senator—Dick Durbin and others—makes no sense. Specifically, Senator Durbin from Illinois proposes that manufacturers accumulate, tabulate, and report adverse reactions. One of the big complaints against ephedra was sloppy recordkeeping of adverse reactions by Metabolife, the biggest seller of ephedrine-containing products.

Senator Durbin has proposed a mandatory adverse event reporting system for some time now. The latest version of his proposal is called the "Dietary Supplement and Nonprescription Drug Consumer Protection Act." First introduced on the heels of the ephedra ban in 2003, the bill, known as S-722, has not died as some people say, but is still rattling around in the bowels of the Senate and could come up at any time. Even if it did die, or Senator Durbin withdrew it, I'd be willing to bet it would be replaced by a similar bill.

The bill, as written by Senator Durbin and co-sponsored by three other senators, requires anyone selling dietary supplements to report "serious" adverse events to the government within fifteen days. It also requires that they maintain records about these events for at least seven years. Similar bills have also been introduced in the U.S. House, including one identified as HR 3377.

Let's step back and look at Senator Durbin's bill for a minute. If you have an allergic reaction to food, maybe shellfish or peanuts, who's the first person you'd want to call? Charlie the Tuna? Mr. Peanut? I would guess your first thought would be to call a doctor, maybe 911, or a poison control center. Then, once you receive treatment, be it from a doctor or a hospital emergency room, you'd be right to expect them to notify the local health department and the FDA, not to add your name to a list (reports are supposed to be anonymous). It would also be reasonable to expect them not to ban the food or slap warning labels on every lobster or peanut, but to build a database of symptoms and treatments to warn and help future sufferers. The same is true for the drug surveillance system that is in place for prescription drugs.

Isn't that logical? Doesn't that make sense? It's supposed to be all about protecting the consumer. Expecting the manufacturer to be the main source for compiling and reporting adverse events is just not the best way to identify dangerous products. It does little to protect us.

No, since dietary supplements have an exemplary record for overall safety (there are a few exceptions, of course), there's something else at work here.

Dick Durbin's Blind Spot

Senator Durbin is very popular with most voters in Illinois. After being reelected to the U.S. House of Representatives continuously since 1983, he successfully ran for the U.S. Senate seat vacated by Paul Simon in 1996 and won reelection in 2002. He's smart and funny, and outside of the recent flap over statements he made about prisoner abuse, he seems to garner respect from his peers on both sides of the aisle. There's no doubt he cares about public safety. After meeting with the mother of a Chicago six-year-old who died after eating contaminated hamburger, Durbin led the effort to modernize the fragmented federal food safety system under a single food-safety agency. He also fought to implement new safety standards that protect patients from injuries related to reuse of medical devices that are intended to be used only once.

But then came ephedra and the death of a sixteen-year-old constituent, Sean Riggins from Lincoln, Illinois, in the fall of 2002. Young Mr. Riggins was a high school wrestler and football player. Coroner Charles Fricke from Logan County, Illinois, testified before the U.S. Senate Subcommittee on Oversight of Government Management that Riggins died from myocardial infarction, and had traces of ephedra in his urine. I'll cover young Mr. Riggins' death in greater detail later on, but suffice it to say that there were other circumstances that may or may not have contributed to his death. For example, it hasn't been widely reported that Mr. Riggins' doctor administered a prescription drug to him (Reglan) that same day. (I wonder if the death was added to that drug's adverse event database?)

After the death, Senator Durbin appeared with Riggins' parents and fought to have ephedra removed from the market. Obviously, he—along with others who fought tooth-and-nail (some behind the scenes) against ephedra—was successful.

But Senator Durbin hasn't stopped there. While he fights to treat nutritional supplements like drugs, he stops short when it comes to reporting adverse events. Further, he wants to shift the burden and cost of tracking safety from the FDA to the manufacturers. It makes no sense.

There are other provisions in the bills floating around that are also wrongheaded, all of which I'll cover later. For now, I'd like to focus on the aspect of adverse event reports. It might be helpful to provide some definitions.

What Is a Serious Adverse Event?

According to the FDA, an adverse event is, "Any undesirable experience associated with the use of a medical product in a patient." Basically, this could be a consumer complaint or negative experience. Something as simple as "it makes me cough" to "it killed my wife" would qualify. The FDA says a "serious" event should be reported when the patient outcome is:

Death
Report if the patient's death is suspected as being a direct outcome of the adverse event.

Life-Threatening
Report if the patient was at substantial risk of dying at the time of the adverse event or if it's suspected that the use or continued use of the product would result in the patient's death.

Hospitalization (initial or prolonged)
Report if admission to the hospital or prolongation of a hospital stay results because of the adverse event.

Disability
Report if the adverse event resulted in a significant, persistent, or permanent change, impairment, damage, or disruption in the patient's body function/structure, physical activities, or quality of life.

Congenital Anomaly
Report if there are suspicions that exposure to a medical product prior to conception or during pregnancy resulted in an adverse outcome in the child.

Requires Intervention to Prevent Permanent Impairment or Damage
Report if you suspect that the use of a medical product may result in a condition that required medical or surgical intervention to preclude permanent impairment or damage to a patient.

Unfortunately, Senator Durbin's bill doesn't spell out what a "serious" event is. Supplement retailers and manufacturers could be deluged with calls about things such as coughs, itchy throats, or other minor problems. These, which would represent the vast majority of complaints, real or imagined (we all know people who complain about everything) keep manufacturers occupied with the lesser issues rather than focusing on more serious problems. Also, how is a manufacturer supposed to filter out fraudulent reports? There are those who would love nothing better than to burden and defame the dietary supplement industry.

Also, what if one manufacturer decides a particular problem isn't serious enough to report while a competitor does. What if a manufacturer provides different details or delays reporting the events? The one that reports quickly and accurately could find itself at a competitive disadvantage, a deterrent to report in the first place.

Doesn't it make more sense for complaints to go to the FDA via the health services industry? Or course if someone does have a specific complaint with a manufacturer, he should by all means tell the manufacturer about it.

But it doesn't end with the manufacturers. Durbin's bill requires every party involved with dietary supplements—the manufacturer, packer, distributor, and retailer—to report each complaint of a serious adverse event to the FDA. Odd, but it exempts over-the-counter medicines and doesn't apply to foods at all. OTCs are exempt from reporting as long as they spell out potential problems on their labels. Why this distinction? It's obvious that dietary supplements are being singled out.

I guess some would argue that the dietary supplement industry has gotten away with "murder" already because of lax standards. Nonsense. As you'll see later, the FDA proved with ephedra that it has the power to remove any product it wants despite a lack of evidence.

Consumers have other protections. The Federal Trade Commission has the power to remove products guilty of false advertising. Also, Durbin's bill does nothing to improve the safety of products. The Food Drug and Cosmetic Act already prohibits product adulteration and misbranding and gives the FDA civil and criminal powers to punish those responsible for harm to the public.

And consider this: irresponsible companies that sell adulterated and misbranded products—the ones most responsible for potential harm to the public—are already risking civil and criminal liability for their wrongdoing. It is naïve to expect that they will report evidence of their shoddy business practice, in essence making the government's case against them even easier. In other words, the very reports that matter most—those revealing intentional harm to public health—are the least likely to be received by the government under this proposed bill.

Plus, there's plenty of evidence that foods cause far more adverse events than supplements, partly because the total quantity consumed is higher, but partly because many adverse events are simply allergic reactions to a particular food such as peanuts or shellfish. It's as if dietary supplements, which are derived from foods, are being singled out. If the real reason for a mandatory adverse event reporting system is to protect the public, doesn't it make sense that foods and drugs, whether prescription or OTC, be included? This is just creating a new bureaucracy and added confusion.

I do suggest you tape the above FDA list of adverse events near your phone, because if Senator Durbin's bill or one like it ever passes, you're going to need to call in the problem to the product's manufacturer.

But That's Only Part of It

Senator Durbin wants us to think the poor FDA has no control over dietary supplements. A press release his office issued states, "The burden is currently placed on the U.S. Food and Drug Administration to prove that they are unsafe before the agency can take any action against dangerous dietary supplements." And according to Senator Durbin, "this places an unreasonably high hurdle in the path of effective agency action." Senator Durbin should know that's not true. The FDA currently has the power to pull any product off the market that it deems to be unsafe.

Under his bill, the FDA will have the power to remove an entire class of supplements from the market if there is *even a single* serious adverse reaction complaint filed. This will be the case even if the complaint comes from someone who used the supplement contrary to the instructions and warnings of the manufacturer. Doesn't matter. The burden shifts to the manufacturer to demonstrate the safety of the supplement, placing a heavy financial burden on accused manufacturers—heavy enough to drive some out of business. For those supplements that do reach the evaluation stage, the FDA will set the standards for the evaluations and then determine if the standards are met while the accused manufacturers foot the bill.

I guess the most important question is, if implemented, will the bill save lives? Not likely. Besides the already inherent safety of dietary supplements, the regulations for prescription drug safety hasn't prevented the thousands of deaths that already occur every year. All it does is hinder the dietary supplement industry and guarantee greater power for regulators.

Let's Be Realistic

The FDA already complains that it lacks the resources to investigate every instance of alleged product adulteration and misbranding. The increased volume of adverse event reports flowing from the provisions of this act are unlikely to be met by an adequate army of federal agents to investigate all alleged incidents. Despite their verbosity about the importance of public safety, Congress isn't going to appropriate more money. Instead, as the industry saw with ephedra, the FDA will likely allow claims to accumulate over many years. When political pressure grows, they'll ban the class of ingredients that is the subject of adverse event reports, regardless of any proven risk.

Here's a solution. It's so simple, it's almost scary, which probably dooms it from serious consideration by the federal government.

Include on the label and packaging of all substances people consume—be it a drug, food, or dietary supplement—a toll-free number for adverse events reporting to the FDA. Combined with reports filed by the medical community and poison control centers, this will streamline the system, provide one method for all substances, and—bottom line—offer the best protection for the public.

Too simple, I know.

Where the Real Focus Should Be

Why don't Senator Durbin and other critics of dietary supplements—and proponents of public safety—focus on a more serious problem? In 1998, the *Journal of the American Medical Association* reported that between 60,000 and 106,000 deaths per year in the United States are caused by prescription drugs. For some strange reason, that doesn't seem to alarm too many people. It should.

I have a great place to start. By sheer coincidence, I'm sure, it's a prescription diet drug named Meridia, a former competitor of ephedra. I say former, since ephedra, which the RAND report could only link to a handful of serious adverse events, has been effectively banned at dose levels that aid weight loss.

When first introduced, Meridia got off to a rocky start. The most troubling side effects encountered included increases in blood pressure, heart rate, and abnormal heart rhythms (arrhythmias) in some participants during clinical trials.

In September 2003, the consumer watchdog group Public Citizen sent a letter to then–FDA Commissioner Mark McClellan, calling for the banning of Meridia (sibutramine), which was first made by Knoll Pharmaceuticals and is now made by Abbott Laboratories. They pointed out—with proof—a rising number of cardiovascular events associated with the drug. In his letter, Sidney Wolfe, director of Public Citizen's Health Research Group, cited nineteen deaths from cardiovascular disease that had been reported to the FDA from the time of sibutramine's launch in February 1998 through the end of September 2001. Dr. Wolfe pointed out that ten of the nineteen cardiac deaths struck people fifty or younger, including three women under the age of thirty. He also noted that he had not received a decision on a petition Public Citizen had sent to the FDA on March 19, 2002, nearly a full year earlier. "Since then," Wolfe continues, "from reviewing subsequent FDA adverse event data, we have become aware of an additional thirty cardiovascular deaths in people using Meridia, for a total of forty-nine cardiovascular deaths. Twenty-seven of the forty-nine (68 percent) were in people less than fifty years old."

Dr. Wolfe also mentioned that his organization found a total of 124 serious cardiovascular adverse events requiring hospitalization. "These 124 hospitalizations are in addition to the 49 cardiovascular adverse events that resulted in death."

Of course, if you measure risk versus benefit as the FDA likes to do, Meridia must be a very effective drug, right? According to the *Los Angeles Times*, no. The last two prescription diet drugs to reach the market, Meridia in 1997 and Xenical in 1999, were introduced with a lot of hype but have attracted only a modest following. In studies, Meridia, which works by creating a sensation of fullness and curbing hunger, has been linked to increases in blood pressure and heart rate, and—along with Xenical—produces only modest weight loss, an average of eleven pounds compared with a placebo and *only* when combined with dietary recommendations.

When he testified in front of the Senate in the fall of 2004 about the problems with Vioxx, FDA whistle-blower Dr. David Graham listed Meridia among five potentially dangerous drugs the FDA needed to evaluate. "There are at least five drugs on the market today that I think need to be looked at quite seriously to see if they belong there," said Graham, associate director for science in the FDA's Office of Drug Safety. Specifically, he singled out Abbott Laboratories, Inc.'s, weight-loss drug Meridia, AstraZeneca's cholesterol fighter Crestor, Pfizer Inc.'s arthritis treatment Bextra, Roche's acne drug Accutane, and GlaxoSmithKline's asthma drug Serevent. "Naturally, Abbott Labs disagreed," Tim Lindberg, a spokesman for the company said, "science continues to support the safe use of Meridia to treat obesity, the leading health epidemic in the U.S." His view is supported by the American Obesity Association, which, in a letter to the FDA on December 8, 2004, criticized Graham's testimony on minor points about side effects and how long people should take the drug. Their letter totally ignored the safety issue. Here's something you should know about the American Obesity Association: One of its many corporate sponsors is Abbott Laboratories.

As for the FDA, well, it stands by past statements that Meridia is safe and effective if used according to its label. If anything, they questioned Graham's conclusions and defended the FDA's actions on Meridia and the four other drugs he named.

In a November 19, 2004 article posted on the Health and Human Services (HHS) Web site attributed to *HealthDay Reporter*, author Amanda Gardner wrote, "The FDA's top officials on Friday defended the agency's drug-review process, saying they took all possible steps to ensure the public's safety. 'Dr. Graham's congressional testimony does not reflect the views of the agency.'"

Dr. Steven Galson, acting director of the FDA's Center for Drug Evaluation and Research, said:

> The five specific drugs that Dr. Graham identified in his oral testimony are currently approved as safe and effective for use in the United States. The FDA evaluates the safety and effectiveness of all drugs independently on a case-by-case basis before they are approved to enter the marketplace, and also evaluates reported adverse events with all drugs already on the market to assess whether unforeseen safety concerns need to be addressed.

A little defensive, wouldn't you say?

And so, two years after Dr. Wolfe's letter, the FDA is expected to issue an advisory that could result in a stiffer warning, restricted use, or something minor such as updated prescription guidelines for use of Meridia, with no ephedra-type ban.

Up to this point, I've tried to show you the erratic—some would say underhanded—behavior of the FDA along with its principal benefactor—the pharmaceutical industry. In the next part of the book, I will show you specific cases of how the FDA—along with other regulatory agencies and outside interest groups, coupled with a compliant media corps—is working to undermine the dietary supplement industry.

The best place to start is with ephedra, since many think it was a test case for the removal of other dietary supplements, which threaten the "sickness industry" and its supporters. But before I talk about ephedra, I'd like to leave you with a list, a compilation put together by Public Citizen of those harmed by Meridia. I hope you keep this list in mind as you read the remainder of the book and see if you agree that dietary supplements are under siege.

Meridia Adverse Events
(*Source:* PublicCitizen)

Table 1. Sibutramine-Associated Cardiac Deaths
(10/2001 through 3/2003)

Age/sex	Adverse Event
28/F	Cardiac arrest
30/F	Myocardial infarction
37/F	Cardiorespiratory arrest
37/F	Cardiorespiratory arrest
37/F	Cardiac arrest
39/F	Cardiac arrest; tachycardia
39/F	Cardiac arrest
40/F	Myocardial infarction
40/M	Myocardial infarction
42/F	Myocardial infarction
43/M	Myocardial infarction
43/M	Sudden death unexplained
45/M	Myocardial infarction
47/M	Chest pain
48/M	Cardiomyopathy
48/M	Myocardial infarction; palpitations
50/M	Myocardial infarction
50/F	Cardiomegaly
50/M	Myocardial infarction

51/M	Myocardial infarction
61/F	Cardio-respiratory arrest
65/M	Myocardial infarction
65/F	Ruptured cerebral aneurysm
66/F	Arrhythmia
67/F	Myocardial infarction
67/M	Myocardial infarction
U/F	Arrhythmia
U/F	Hypertension
U/M	Myocardial infarction
U/F	Cardio-respiratory arrest

Table 2. Sibutramine-associated Cardiac Adverse Events (all outcomes excluding death) (10/01 through 3/03: chronological order)

Age/Sex	Adverse Event	Outcome
31/M	Chest pain	Hospitalization
64/F	Myocarditis	Required intervention
42/M	Myocardial infarction	Required intervention
61/F	Arterial aneurysm	Hospitalization
54/F	Cerebral infarction	Hospitalization
U/F	Tachycardia; cardiac failure	Required intervention
55/M	Tachycardia; atrial fibrillation; cardiomyopathy	Life threatening
17/F	Intracranial pressure increased	Hospitalization
29/F	Hypertension	Hospitalization
69/F	Tachycardia; hypertension	Required intervention
48/F	Hypertension; tachycardia	Required intervention
40/F	Sinus tachycardia; pulmonary hypertension	Required intervention
62/F	Cardiac failure; pulmonary hypertension	Hospitalization

Age/Sex	Adverse Event	Outcome
62/F	Cardiac disorder; chest pain	Hospitalization
31/F	Blood pressure increased; chest pain; pulmonary hypertension	Hospitalization
41/F	Heart rate increased; blood pressure increased	Required intervention
U/F	Arrhythmia; syncope	Required intervention
62/M	Hypertension aggravated	Hospitalization
U/F	Cardiac disorder	Hospitalization
68/M	Transient ischemic attack	Required intervention
57/F	Cardiomegaly; chest pain; arrhythmia	Hospitalization
47/M	Hypertension	Disability
U/F	Pulmonary hypertension	Hospitalization
50/F	Cardiac failure congestive	Required intervention
42/M	Chest pain	Required intervention
70/F	Cerebrovascular accident	Hospitalization
44/F	Arrhythmia; tachycardia; atrial flutter	Required intervention
39/M	Atrioventricular block; atrial flutter; atrial fibrillation	Hospitalization
34/F	Cerebrovascular accident	Hospitalization
35M	Hypertension	Hospitalization
27/F	Chest pain	Unknown
U/F	Cerebrovascular accident	Other
31/F	Blood pressure increased	Hospitalization
56/F	Blood pressure increased; chest pain	Required intervention
31/F	Myocardial infarction	Hospitalization
47/F	Cardiac disorder; arrhythmia; blood pressure increased	Hospitalization

Age/Sex	Adverse Event	Outcome
49/F	Sinus arrhythmia; cardiomyopathy; ventricular tachycardia	Hospitalization
U/F	Arrhythmia; heart rate increased	Hospitalization
U/F	Heart rate increased; blood pressure fluctuation	Required intervention
68/M	Cerebrovascular accident	Life-Threatening
29/F	Chest tightness	Required intervention
50/F	Heart rate increased; Blood pressure increased	Hospitalization
U/F	Cerebrovascular accident	Other
42/M	Blood pressure increased	Other
50/F	Chest pain; blood pressure increased; palpitations	Hospitalization
52/F	Transient ischemic attack	Other
51/F	Tachycardia	Life-Threatening
13/M	QT prolonged	Other
32/F	Hypertension	Hospitalization
35/F	Pulmonary hypertension primary	Hospitalization
46/M	Blood pressure increased	Hospitalization
53/M	Ventricular extrasystoles	Other
U/F	Cardiac arrest	Required intervention
32/F	Cardiac murmur; palpitations	Other
U/U	Cardiac failure	Hospitalization
48/F	BP increased; tachycardia	
44/M	Chest pain; heart rate irregular	Required intervention
60/M	Cardiac arrest; acute myocardial infarction	Hospitalization
42/F	Chest discomfort; ECG PR shortened	Life threatening

Age/Sex	Adverse Event	Outcome
38/F	Cardiac failure; ventricular fibrillation	Hospitalization
47/M	Chest pain; vasovagal attack	Hospitalization
47/F	Hypertension; hemorrhagic stroke	Hospitalization
59/F	Cardiac failure	Required Intervention
47/F	Palpitations; collapse	Hospitalization
U/F	Diastolic dysfunction; hypertension; tachycardia	Required Intervention
44/F	Cerebrovascular accident; hypertension	Hospitalization
73/F	Vasovagal attack	Required Intervention
48/F	Cerebral infarction	Hospitalization
63/F	Pulmonary hypertension; aortic valve stenosis; cardiomegaly	Hospitalization
48/M	Chest pressure sensation; ventricular extrasystoles	Hospitalization
38/F	Cardiac arrest	Hospitalization
53/F	Acute myocardial infarction; cerebral infarction	Hospitalization
U/M	Cardiac failure congestive	Hospitalization
39/F	Accelerated idioventricular rhythm	Hospitalization
41/M	Chest pain; ST-T ECG change	Hospitalization
63/F	Left ventricular hypertrophy	Required Intervention
42/M	Hypertension	Life threatening
38/F	Cardiac failure	Hospitalization
U/M	Arrhythmia; ejection fraction decreased	Required Intervention
63/F	Pulmonary hypertension; cardiac disorder	Hospitalization

Age/Sex	Adverse Event	Outcome
29/U	Hypertension	Required Intervention
37/F	Blood pressure increased	Required Intervention
47/F	Blood pressure increased; Cerebral hemorrhage	Hospitalization
62/F	Cardiac failure; cardiomyopathy; tachycardia	Required Intervention
54/M	Syncope	Required Intervention
35/F	ECG: P wave abnormal; Palpitations	Required Intervention
51/F	Cardiac murmur; cardiomyopathy	Required Intervention
48/F	ECG abnormal; tachycardia	Required Intervention
U/M	Atrial tachycardia	Required Intervention
U/F	Atrial tachycardia	Required Intervention
41/F	Blood pressure fluctuation	Hospitalization
U/F	Arrhythmia	Life threatening
U/F	Cerebrovascular accident; stroke	Hospitalization
34/F	Blood pressure increased; palpitations	Hospitalization
48/F	Hypertension; tachycardia	Required Intervention
37/F	Hypertension	Life threatening
42/F	Chest pain; dizziness	Hospitalization
42/M	Hypertensive crisis	Required Intervention
53/U	Atrial fibrillation; palpitations	Hospitalization
41/M	Myocardial infarction	Hospitalization
49/M	Atrial fibrillation	Hospitalization
35/F	ECG: P wave abnormal; palpitations	Required Intervention
42/M	Hypertension	Required Intervention
22/F	Chest pain; dizziness	Hospitalization
42/M	Hypertension	Required Intervention

Age/Sex	Adverse Event	Outcome
61/F	Arrhythmia; chest pain	Hospitalization
U/F	Chest pain; cerebrovascular accident; tachycardia	Hospitalization
54/F	Cerebral infarction; tachycardia	Hospitalization
U/F	Heart rate increased	Required Intervention
54/F	Cerebral infarction; tachycardia	Hospitalization
22/F	Chest pain; dizziness	Hospitalization
40/F	Heart rate increased	Required Intervention
U/M	Tachycardia	Required Intervention
34/F	Blood pressure increased; palpitations	Hospitalization
U/F	Chest tightness; clamminess	Required Intervention
34/F	Transient ischemic attack	Hospitalization
40/F	ECG abnormal; chest pain; heart rate increased	Hospitalization
30/F	Ischemia	Required Intervention
U/F	Supraventricular tachycardia	Hospitalization
45/F	Hypertension	Required Intervention
55/M	Cardiovascular disorder	Required Intervention
40/F	Chest tightness	Hospitalization
60/F	Myocardial ischemia	Life threatening
58/M	Chest pain	Hospitalization
38/F	Chest pain; dyspnea	Required Intervention
66/F	Atrial fibrillation; right ventricular failure	Hospitalization

Table 3. Effects on fetus in patients using sibutramine (Meridia) February 1998 through March 2003 (chronological order)

Maternal Age/ Fetal or Infant Sex	Adverse Event	Outcome
43/F	Premature baby	Hospitalization
U/F	Abortion missed	Other
U/M	Aortic valve stenosis; disorder neonatal congenital anomaly	Hospitalization
31/F	Abortion spontaneous	Other
21/F	Stillbirth; omphalitis	Other
33/F	Intra-uterine death; abortion spontaneous	Other
30/F	Musculoskeletal disorder; abortion induced	Other
34/F	Abortion spontaneous	Other
U/M	Death neonatal; congenital heart disease	Death
U/M	Erb's palsy; shoulder dystocia; delayed delivery	Disability
U/M	Pre-auricular sinus congenital; C-section	Congenital anomaly
U/F	Ovarian disorder	Other
30/F	Abortion spontaneous	Other
32/F	Vaginal hemorrhage; abortion threatened	Other
30/F	Abortion spontaneous; cervical incompetence	Other
39/F	Abortion induced	Required Intervention
32/F	Ultrasound antenatal screen abnormal; aborted pregnancy	Required Intervention

Maternal Age/ Fetal or Infant Sex	Adverse Event	Outcome
30/F	Unwanted pregnancy; abortion induced	Required Intervention
U/M	Congenital foot malformation; eye deformity; intrauterine death; hydrocephalus	Death
29/F	Congenital hydrocephalus; abortion induced	Unknown
U/U	Down's syndrome; abortion induced	Death
37/F	Neonatal disorder; premature baby	Hospitalization
U/F	Pulmonary edema neonatal; sleep apnea syndrome	Hospitalization
U/F	Ventricular hypoplasia	Death
12/U	Fetal growth retardation; premature baby	Death
32/F	Premature baby; preeclampsia	Hospitalization
U/U	Premature baby	Death
38/F	Spontaneous abortion	Required Intervention
39/F	Spontaneous abortion	Other
29/F	Congenital hydrocephalus; chromosome abnormality	Required Intervention
U/M	Congenital foot malformation; hydrocephalus; syndactyly	Death
37/F	Fetal disorder; abortion induced	Required Intervention

Maternal Age/ Fetal or Infant Sex	Adverse Event	Outcome
37/F	Down's syndrome; abortion induced	Required Intervention
U/F	Chiari malformation; nervous system anomaly; spina bifida; abortion	Death
38/F	Abortion spontaneous	Required Intervention
U/U	Fetal growth retardation; hypertension	Death
39/F	Abortion spontaneous	Required Intervention
28/F	Abortion induced; congenital heart disease	Required Intervention
U/U	Cardiomegaly; congenital abnormality	Death
40/F	Abortion spontaneous	Required Intervention
38/F	Neonatal apneic attack; testicular disorder; premature baby	Hospitalization
39/F	Abortion induced	Required Intervention
25/F	Unknown	Required Intervention
31/F	Unintended pregnancy	Required Intervention
U/M	Cardiac murmur; hemoglobin decreased; premature baby	Hospitalization
U/M	Bicuspid aortic valve; cardiac murmur; premature baby	Hospitalization
21/F	Unintended pregnancy	Required Intervention
U/U	Congenital anomaly	Cerebellar tumor
U/F	Congenital abnormality; brain neoplasm; abortion induced	Required intervention

Maternal Age/ Fetal or Infant Sex	Adverse Event	Outcome
U/F	Pyelocaliectasis; C-section	Congenital anomaly
U/M	Renal agenesis	Required intervention
21/F	Chiari malformation; abortion induced	Unknown
U/U	Chiari malformation; abortion induced	Congenital anomaly

PART 2

". . . When First We Practice to Deceive."

—Sir Walter Scott, Marmion, Canto vi. Stanza 17

9

Ephedra Redux

On April 13, 2005, a federal judge in Utah struck down the FDA's ban on all sales of ephedra ruling that the FDA failed to provide proof that ephedra was unsafe in low doses. Soon after, companies started advertising 10 milligram pills of the herb. Nutraceutical Corporation, which filed the suit, was not among them. Their purpose when they filed the suit was not to sell ephedra, but to preserve the Dietary Supplement Health and Education Act (DSHEA). The fear was—and is—that if the FDA could ban a dietary supplement without proof, they'd be emboldened to do the same with any dietary supplement they targeted.

No proof you say? You may recall that the newspapers provided plenty of proof that ephedra was very dangerous. If you think that, you've been conned, just like the reporters who regurgitated what the FDA told them without performing any real digging on their own.

Let's back up. In February 2003, Baltimore Orioles pitcher Steve Bechler collapsed and died while at a spring training workout session. Soon enough, it became known that Bechler may have been using an ephedra-based supplement. Almost immediately, newspaper headlines across the country blared: "Ephedra Kills Baseball Player!" or similar incendiary words, and pundits, critics, and regulators worked themselves into a collective frenzy, many of them calling for tighter regulations and others for an outright ban of the controversial herb.

Prior to that, ephedra had been both widely hailed for its supposed benefits and roundly criticized for its alleged dangers. Depending on who you talk to, ephedra could be a fantastic weight-loss tool or an evil poison waiting to kill you, just like it did Steve Bechler.

The debate over the safety and efficacy of ephedra is a classic example of how misinformation portrayed in the media and from various special interest groups can cause a political and legal firestorm over a dietary supplement. Although a significant body of scientific evidence indicates that use of synthetic ephedrine or herbal ephedra can safely promote weight loss when used as directed in overweight but otherwise healthy individuals, there have been unprecedented efforts made to see that ephedra is banned for sale in the United States.

Those favoring a ban on ephedra pointed to adverse events voluntarily reported to several poison control centers and adverse event monitoring systems, suggesting that some people who took ephedra-containing supplements experienced mild to severe side effects. They also pointed to several recent deaths among high school, college, and professional athletes who were believed to have taken ephedra-containing supplements as evidence that ephedra is dangerous, even though:

• Ephedra has been used as an herbal supplement for thousands of years.

• An estimated twelve to seventeen million people consumed approximately three billion doses of ephedra-containing dietary supplements annually.

• Available clinical trials showed ephedrine or ephedra supplementation can be safely used to promote weight loss and/or improve performance in healthy populations.

• Definitive conclusions about the safety of ephedra cannot be made based on available adverse events reported because many are incomplete and reveal a number of additional contributing factors.

• Millions of people in the United States consume over-the-counter cold medications containing pseudoephedrine at equivalent or higher doses than found in dietary supplements.

• The safety profile of ephedra is much better than many over-the-counter and prescription medications.

Most everyone is aware that nothing sells newspapers or attracts TV viewers better than a good, old-fashioned health scare. When Steve Bechler died, many were quick to blame as the main culprit the ephedra-based fat-burning supplement he was taking. Since ephedra was already under fire, it was easy for irresponsible (or lazy, or naïve—take your pick) headline writers to push the ephedra connection, probably causing many people to rummage through their son's gym bag and their own medicine cabinet searching for the substance.

While there's reason to believe that the ephedra product Bechler was taking, Cytodyne's Xenadrine RFA-1, might have contributed to his death, there were certainly other contributing factors. Because he was some ten to fifteen pounds overweight, and due to pressure from the team to lose this weight and get in shape quickly, Bechler embarked on a low-calorie liquid diet. Reports indicate that he hadn't eaten any solid foods in two days. He also had a history of borderline high blood pressure and undiagnosed liver abnormalities, and he had experienced episodes of heatstroke earlier in his life. Bechler was also wearing multiple layers of clothing as part of his efforts to sweat off the extra pounds, despite it being quite hot and humid. And, needless to say, almost no one is questioning the guidelines of teams and organizations that oversee workout conditions and procedures. Neither is anyone asking if his existing liver condition or history of heatstroke had anything to do with his death.

It's obvious that these and other red flags never received the level of publicity the ephedra connection received—not by a long shot. So why has all the heat focused on the ephedra connection?

As you'll see, there's more going on here than just hand-wringing over a controversial herb. When you learn about ephedra and the uproar surrounding it, you stumble upon hypocrisy and inconsistency. After all, in a country focusing on the alleged dangers of ephedra, little is said about the painkiller acetaminophen, which has claimed many more lives, or aspartame, which comprises the majority of all the complaints directed to the FDA regarding AERs and side effects from drugs, supplements, and food additives (some reports put this number as high as 75 percent). Compare that to the deaths that some say were caused by ephedra (and which occurred over several years, for that matter), and you have to ask yourself why so much fuss is made about ephedra and not things like acetaminophen or Meridia as I mentioned in the last chapter.

We should realize that no matter what we take, whether it is an over-the-counter medication, a prescribed drug, or a dietary supplement, there will probably be risks. And yet, we hear the loudest condemnation of and demand for restrictions on a variety of herbs, while we seem to think it's just dandy there's only token regulation for tobacco and alcohol. (And then there's the issue of medicinal marijuana, which reportedly has never killed anyone.) Where is the consistency?

I believe Richard B. Kreider, Ph.D., professor and chair, Exercise and Sport Nutrition Laboratory at Baylor University, has it just about right: "Sometimes, we focus on obscure problems—particularly in the media—that in reality have little risk compared to many common activities. The pharmaceutical, alcohol, and tobacco industries have huge political lobbies. The pharmaceutical lobby also has an interest to see supplements that may work as well as some drugs be regulated."

Dr. Kreider points out that even though the RAND report—which I cover later in the book—pointed out there may have only been five "sentinel" cases of death related to ephedra use over an approximate ten-year period, many clamored for action to ban it yet ignore the risks of severe side effects and even death from much more common products. "It is my view that policy should be based on science not speculation. Unfortunately, in politics the latter often dictates action," says Dr. Kreider, who is also president of the American Society of Exercise Physiologists.

There's no question that at its peak, ephedra was very popular. Although there is no complete tally on how many people have used it, a study of fourteen companies manufacturing and marketing ephedra-containing supplements by the American Herbal Products Association (AHPA) between 1995 and 1999 shows that sales increased 700 percent during that five-year period. The reported 425 million servings sold in 1995 rose to three billion in 1999.

According to M. McGuffen of the Department of Health and Human Services at a hearing on the safety of ephedra products on August 8, 2000, there were a total of only sixty-six serious adverse events during that period reported by these same companies, or fewer than ten reports per billion servings sold.

As you'll see, the issues surrounding ephedra use are quite complex, and they certainly involve money, politics, and a lack of common sense. Part of the problem is that ephedra products made fantastic profits for manufacturers promising quick energy and slimmer torsos. These people will do whatever it takes to defend their markets—just as major pharmaceutical, cigarette, and alcohol companies do. In this case, several pharmaceutical companies may have lost millions of consumer dollars to the ephedra manufacturers. Add to that prescription-writing doctors, prescription-filling pharmacists, politicians (a few grandstanding, some dependent on political contributions from lobby groups opposing ephedra), overreacting consumer groups, the media—which vacillates between unquestioned stenography to sensationalism—and you have a chorus of condemnation drowning out reason.

Who suffers? You and I, of course, who depend on all these groups for honest and accurate information. There's no question outside help is needed. Ideally, this would be provided by the U.S. Food and Drug Administration; that is, if they're up to the task.

It should be obvious that it's very easy to manipulate numbers to get them to say what you want. Is this what's happened with ephedra? Did opponents place great weight on the numbers of adverse reactions, while the herb's defenders pooh-pooh them? Possibly.

And here's another point. Just as with anything we put in our bodies there are potential risks to using ephedra products, and self-prescribing is never a good idea. Each person's condition is unique and the guidance of an appropriately trained health practitioner should be sought. For example, ephedrine stimulates the central nervous system and increases heart rate. If you already have high blood pressure, ephedra could raise it even more.

As I alluded to earlier, it seems that the controversy surrounding ephedra isn't just about the herb. Could it be that ephedra is only the outer ring of this high-stakes archery match? Could it be that the real bull's-eye—the one politicians, special interests, and their allies in the media are aiming for—is DSHEA, the current legislation governing dietary supplements?

Ephedra Facts

Ephedra is an adrenaline-like stimulant that affects the heart, nasal passages, lungs, and nervous system. Ephedra has been used for medicinal purposes for over three thousand years, originating in Mongolia and the bordering regions of China.

There are several varieties of ephedra, with *Ephedra sinica* or *Ephedra sinensis* being the most commonly used in nutritional supplement products. In the United States, it's generally just called "ephedra" or by its Chinese name "ma huang" (which means "hemp yellow" because of its color).

The most common historical medicinal use of ephedra was to relieve symptoms of the common cold, asthma, and related conditions. In more recent times, synthetic versions of its active ingredients—namely ephedrine and pseudoephedrine—have found worldwide use as ingredients in over-the-counter cold and allergy medications. But it was from the more modern notion that ephedra helps promote weight loss and improvement in athletic performance that this big hubbub has developed. A number of popular weight-loss and energy products include either the whole herb, extracts of the herb, or pure concentrates of its alkaloids, ephedrine and pseudoephedrine. To varying degrees, these products can stimulate the nervous system and increase metabolism by stimulating the thyroid gland, all of which theoretically result in more burned fat.

In addition, the ephedra alkaloids also stimulate the heart, cause blood vessels to constrict, and dilate the airways. Manufacturers of diet and energy products claim when blended with "tonic" herbs that help to counteract its side effects, ephedra is safer to use than other popular stimulants such as coffee, kola nut, or guaraná, all of which contain caffeine.

While there is evidence ephedra-containing products can help people lose weight and provide energy, there are possible dangerous side effects. Some people using ephedra have reported the following:

- poor digestion
- increased blood pressure
- sleeping difficulties
- nervousness
- anxiety attacks
- general weakness and lethargy
- muscular tremors
- urinary retention (in men with prostate enlargement)

There are some other problems with ephedra supplements. First, as we just mentioned, some manufacturers add other "tonic" herbs to help counteract some of these negative reactions. We don't know how or if these herbs truly interact, and how they influence the effect of ephedra or its alkaloids. More importantly, many ephedra products also contain caffeine, itself a stimulant, which seems to amplify some of ephedra's effects. Funny thing is, Senator Durbin wants to regulate *all* stimulants—except caffeine, since many of the major food manufacturers sell products containing this stimulant.

Finally, as with any medication or supplement, everyone has a different tolerance to ephedra and its main constituents. It is difficult to predict how each individual will respond.

Not only should people with heart disease and hypertension avoid taking ephedrine-containing products, but those with diabetes or hyperthyroidism should use it cautiously as well. Ephedrine can also contract the uterus, meaning it should not be used during pregnancy. (By the way, there are no studies regarding adverse effects on a developing fetus.) And since it passes through the mother's milk to the infant, ephedra should not be taken when breast feeding. In addition, ephedra should not be taken with monoamine oxidase inhibitors (MAOIs), such as isocarboxazid, phenelzine, and tranylcypromine, which limited research shows may heighten the stimulating effects of ephedra.

Animal studies have not demonstrated carcinogenic or mutagenic potential for ephedrine. In addition, the alkaloid is rapidly eliminated from the human body. It has been shown that 88 percent of an oral dose is excreted in the urine within twenty-four hours; 97 percent after forty-eight hours.

Despite the number of side effects listed for purified ephedrine in therapeutic doses, studies show that the whole herb ephedra has a very low toxicity and potential for side effects, especially when used in recommended amounts.

While the FDA tried to ban ephedra for at least a decade, they received little traction because they were unable to make a case. Then in spring 2003, Major League baseball teams gathered in Arizona and Florida for spring training so players could get in shape and teams could pare their rosters for the upcoming season. For some it was a chance for established veteran players to become reacquainted with teammates, and for rookies to wow managers and make a positive impression. For some, though, it was possibly their last chance to make a team. It was their make-or-break time.

10

The FDA Gets Its Poster Boy

Steve Bechler had high hopes of making the Baltimore Orioles opening-day roster. Problem was, the twenty-three-year-old needed to shed between ten and fifteen pounds quickly to improve his chances of making the squad. Instead of making the team, he ended up in the morgue.

Toxicology reports released soon after he died showed that Cytodyne's diet supplement Xenadrine RFA-1, which contains ephedrine, was present in his system. While the official cause of his death was heatstroke, there is still considerable speculation about the role ephedra played in his death.

Here's why. Shortly after he performed the autopsy, Broward County, Florida, medical examiner Dr. Joshua Perper said in his official report that the toxicology analysis "revealed significant amounts of ephedrine" in Bechler's blood, along with smaller amounts of two other stimulants, pseudoephedrine and caffeine. The amount he found is consistent with taking three tablets of the weight-loss supplement Xenadrine.

However, the autopsy—and the investigation into his death—showed other very pertinent and revealing facts. First, Bechler had virtually no food or liquid in his gastrointestinal tract. He also wore extra layers of clothing to induce extra sweating, which in the Florida heat actually impedes sweat evaporation and reduces cooling. As a result, his self-imposed hypohydration (less than normal total body water) negatively affected his thermoregulatory responses, resulting in sweating, shivering, a rise in heart rate, an extremely high core temperature (reports say he collapsed with a core temperature reportedly of 106 degrees Fahrenheit before being removed from the field), and a decrease in overall performance. Plus, some teammates said he took much more of the Xenadrine product than is recommended—which also elevates heart rate—and probably degraded his condition.

A Puzzle Piece Ignored

When Bechler died, H. J. Roberts, M.D., called Dr. Perper and asked him how many diet drinks Bechler was in the habit of drinking. Dr. Perper didn't even know why he asked. Dr. Roberts is director of the Palm Beach Institute for Medical Research and an emeritus member of the medical staffs of the Good Samaritan Hospital and St. Mary's Hospital in West Palm Beach. He is a member of the American College of Physicians, the Endocrine Society, the American Academy of Neurology, and the American Federation for Clinical Research. He is also author of the book *Aspartame Disease: An Ignored Epidemic.*

In his book, Dr. Roberts points out that aspartame is a seizure-triggering drug, and four different types of seizures are listed on the FDA's report of ninety-two documented symptoms triggered by this artificial sweetener, including death. It triggers strokes, can damage the cardiac conduction system, and cause sudden death. It also triggers an irregular heart rhythm and interacts with all cardiac medication.

It's quite likely that people trying to lose weight would use drinks containing aspartame, which is estimated to be consumed by two-thirds of the population. Besides soft drinks, it also is an ingredient in natural and artificial flavors.

At the time, the *Idaho Observer* wrote a story, "Aspartame Poisoning Cover for Ephedra," which revealed Steve Bechler would go without eating for a couple of days and then drink diet pop with aspartame all day. Could it be because he had a family history of heart problems, and because aspartame destroys the heart, that Steve Bechler did not die because he was using ephedra, but possibly because of aspartame, or the combination of ephedra and the sweetener? Due to his lack of knowledge about aspartame and Bechler's habits, Dr. Perper could only conclude that ephedrine "probably contributed" since he was unaware that that Steve Bechler was using the sweetener.

During the investigation of his death, Bechler's teammates reported that he was listless during practice—typical telltale signs of dehydration and heat exhaustion. One report stated he was able to complete only 60 percent of the team workout two days before he died. To top it off, Bechler suffered from hypertension and liver problems, and had a prior history of heat illness episodes while in high school, all of which only increased the possibility for tragedy.

In response to the public uproar surrounding Bechler's death and the alleged link to ephedra, researchers from Baylor University, led by Richard B. Kreider, Ph.D., professor and chair, Exercise & Sport Nutrition Laboratory, released a statement that included their observations and interpretation of what happened to Mr. Bechler.

In addition to the points I've already raised, the Baylor researchers also said the media was guilty of over-sensationalizing the dangers of ephedra use:

"Unfortunately, these media reports may mislead some to conclude that simply prohibiting athletes from taking ephedra supplements will eliminate the risk of heat fatalities," wrote the Baylor University team. Instead, they say, those in charge should be stressing the importance of properly educating athletes, coaches, and athletic trainers about the risks of training in hot and humid environments when participants are poorly conditioned, have not acclimatized to the heat and humidity, have engaged in dehydration practices, and/or have questionable medical histories. The Baylor researchers continue:

It seems that Major League Baseball and others want to blame ephedra for the death of Mr. Bechler, rather than admit that they may have been negligent in screening, conditioning, and supervising their athletes. Closer examination of contributing factors related to Mr. Bechler's death reveals that even if Mr. Bechler did consume the supplement, it was probably the least of the contributing factors leading to his death—and it may not have been a factor at all.

Is Ephedra Safe?

Suppliers of ephedra products, most experts in alternative medicine and herbalism, and even some "conventional" health experts, believe that when used as directed, ephedra is safe. On the opposing side, the Food and Drug Administration says it has compiled a list of over eight hundred adverse events for ephedra, including heart attack, stroke, tremors, insomnia, and death. One report lists at least seventeen deaths due to supplements containing ephedra.

Here's a list of some of the statements made and actions taken by organizations and entities in response to the ephedra "scare":

• The American Heart Association says the supplement should be banned, saying it does more harm than good.

• In April 2003, the American Society of Health-System Pharmacists (ASHP) urged the FDA to ban the sale of dietary supplements containing ephedra because of significant risks to public health. ASHP warned the labeling changes proposed by the FDA will not protect the public from the dangers of these products.

• A study by the RAND Corporation reports two deaths, four heart attacks, and nine strokes among 16,000 adverse event reports.

• Other research, appearing in the journal *Annals of Internal Medicine* in 2003, shows ephedra is responsible for 64 percent of all adverse reactions reported to poison control centers from herb use, although it accounts for less than 1 percent of such supplements sold.

• In March 2003, Senator Jackie Speier introduced a law to ban diet supplements containing ephedra in California.

• In March 2003, the editors of the *Journal of the American Medical Association (JAMA)* called for more stringent regulations on dietary supplements, citing the potentially dangerous effects of ephedra.

• In early 2003, Napa County, California, prosecutors sued Cytodyne Technologies, Inc., the maker of Xenadrine RFA-1 (the Steve Bechler supplement of choice), alleging the company had failed to disclose the link between the stimulant and health hazards, including myocardial infarction, strokes, and death.

• Ephedra is prohibited by several professional and amateur sports-sanctioning bodies, including the NFL and the International Olympic Committee. After Steve Bechler's death, Major League Baseball banned the herb.

• On May 25, 2003, Illinois Governor Rod Blagojevich signed the nation's first statewide ban on ephedra, flanked by the parents of a sixteen-year-old football player who died of a heart attack after taking a product that contained ephedrine.

At first glance it's easy to believe ephedra is one troublesome herb and a public relations nightmare for the companies that sell it. That is, until you compare it to findings in various reports regarding over-the-counter and prescription drugs.

For instance, a study published in the *Journal of the American Medical Association* in 2000 showed that more than two million American hospital patients suffered a serious adverse drug reaction (ADR) within the twelve-month period of the study and, of these, over one hundred thousand died as a result. (Note: Sometimes ADR and AER are used interchangeably when referring to drugs.) The researchers found that over 75 percent of these ADRs were dose-dependent, which suggests they were due to the inherent toxicity of the drugs rather than to allergic reactions. It's also important to note that the data did not include fatal reactions caused by accidental overdoses or errors in administration of the drugs. If these had been included, it is estimated that another one hundred thousand deaths would be added to the yearly total. The researchers concluded that ADRs are now the fourth leading cause of death in the United States after heart disease, cancer, and stroke.

Pretty scary numbers, yet the report elicited nothing like the outrage swirling around ephedra. (In fact, I'd be willing to bet big bucks that you've never heard of this risk associated with prescription drugs.)

Ephedra and Weight Loss

So, what does all of this have to do with ephedra? Plenty, but before moving on, we need to look at the principal reason why ephedra products are used in this country. As I've mentioned, one of the main uses for ephedra today is to lose weight. And let's face it, if we look around (and perhaps into a mirror), many of us need to lose a few pounds. How bad is the problem?

According to the American Public Health Association (APHA), two-thirds of all American adults and nine million children between the ages of six and nineteen are overweight. Approximately three hundred thousand deaths in the U.S. each year are directly related to obesity. The condition is associated with an increased risk of heart disease—the leading cause of death in the U.S.—as well as the currently surging rates of diabetes, certain cancers, and other chronic ills.

Enter Ephedra

As a society, we have learned to crave quick results as much as we do excess calories. We want to lose weight with little or no discomfort, and many of us want chiseled muscles quickly without the pain. When we compete in sports, we want that extra edge pushing us to the victory stand, and we're willing to get there by just about any means necessary. Rather than doing a few more crunches or push-ups or walking an extra mile, we opt for a medicated edge. In short, we want results with the lowest possible sacrifice.

Two crosscurrents are at work here. Our own internal fortitude and natural abilities versus our willingness—or unwillingness to be precise—to change our behavior. It's no wonder that weight loss is a multibillion-dollar industry.

Because of the orchestrated media frenzy over the dangers of ephedra use, The market for the herb nosedived. Several major manufacturers discontinued their products, and numerous retailers pulled ephedra products from their shelves due to safety concerns.

But when ephedra weight-loss products were taken off the market people just sought other remedies, many with scant evidence of effectiveness or safety. Despite such risks, people are seeking a simple way to lose pounds fast, and will simply turn to other stimulants, says Katherine Beals, a nutrition professor at Ball State University. "Americans are looking for a quick fix," said Beals, a dedicated distance runner. "Rather than eating healthfully and exercising, which take time and effort, we would rather pop a pill to lose weight. A pill is thought to be infinitely easier and potentially quicker.

"Unfortunately, as we saw with fen-phen in the 1990s and now with ephedrine, it is also risky," she said. "Yet, a good many Americans are willing to take that risk and forsake their health in the name of looking good."

Fen-phen became a dieting craze in the 1990s after research found a positive slimming effect from combining two appetite suppressants, fenfluramine and phentermine. Beals added that even the fallout caused by several deaths linked to ephedra products has hardly put a dent in the nation's hunger for weight-loss pills.

There's no doubt many of us need an attitude adjustment. But beyond that, why the differing levels of concern regarding problems with prescription drugs—which you rarely hear about—and ephedra, which generated bold headlines? Is it simply a question of not wanting the risks of an "unnecessary" medication, even though the chances of these risks are very small? Is that why we look the other way when the AMA reports numerous deaths from the popular non-steroidal anti-inflammatory drug (NSAIDs) ibuprofen, five hundred annual aspirin deaths, or when the American Association of Poison Control Centers says more than one hundred people die from acetaminophen use? Is it because we believe all these medications are "safe" if taken as directed, and doctors and patients are completely aware of potential side effects?

If it's a question of safety versus benefit, why are we considering banning ephedra when we all know that tens of thousands of people die or are injured each year because of alcohol-related accidents, tens of thousands more suffer physical abuse at the hands of alcoholics, and cigarette smoking causes an average of 430,700 deaths a year? While both these substances have sale restrictions of sorts, you don't hear much noise about outright bans, do you? Could it be the way the "substances" are regulated and by whom?

Still, there were charges that the FDA dragged its feet in banning ephedra because of the influence of powerful lobby groups and the amount of money at stake. Compared to the ultra-powerful drug lobby PhARMA, that point is laughable.

Here's something you probably never heard when Steve Bechler died and the effort to ban ephedra hit full throttle:

"At the time Mr. Bechler collapsed from heat stroke, much of the ephedrine he had swallowed was still in his stomach and had not yet entered his bloodstream. [The unabsorbed ephedrine] could not have caused or contributed to Mr. Bechler's death." This came from a letter that forensic pathologist Dr. Michael Baden, former New York City chief medical examiner wrote to the Subcommittee on Oversight and Investigations Hearing on Issues Relating to Ephedra-Containing Dietary Supplements, July 23, 2003. It was never mentioned by the committee, and was buried along with other evidence in the bowels of the House of Representatives. But this wasn't the first time important evidence and testimony about ephedra was stifled.

In Defense of Ephedra

In August 2000, a group of scientists, government officials, industry experts, and interested parties gathered at the Office of Women's Health (OWH), a part of the Department of Health and Human Services (HHS). They were in Washington, D.C., for two days of hearings about the safety and risks of ephedrine alkaloids. The FDA and the Center for Food Safety and Applied Nutrition (CFSAN) sponsored the meeting.

The hearings were spurred by the FDA's recent change in its proposed policy announced in 1997, which would have drastically curtailed the use of ephedra. Specifically, the proposal called for limiting intake of ephedra to 8 milligrams of total ephedra alkaloids per dosage, and a total daily dosage of 24 milligrams for a duration of use not to exceed seven days. It also required an extensive warning label, banned any combinations with products containing caffeine or other stimulants, and prohibited any claims that would encourage use for more than seven days, including claims for weight loss or sports performance. The FDA claimed that its proposed rules were based in part on hundreds of adverse event reports associated with the use of ephedra—including alleged deaths—received by the agency.

After a flurry of complaints from Congress and the dietary supplement industry over the scientific accuracy of the safety data supporting the FDA's position of stricter controls, the FDA withdrew its proposal. The clincher was a report from the General Accounting Office (GAO) criticizing the manner in which the FDA's policy was developed, especially the adverse event reports allegedly associated with ephedra.

When the GAO report came out, members of Congress were appalled. "I am concerned about the apparent lack of scientific data behind the FDA's actions," said House Science Committee Chairman F. James Sensenbrenner, Jr. "For the FDA—one of the most important regulatory agencies in government—to use such poor science for a dietary supplement raises warning flags for the other products the agency regulates."

There were similar comments from the other side of the aisle. "According to the GAO report, FDA missed the mark in their proposed regulation," said Congressman Ralph Hall. "Documentation of FDA's work was inadequate, they failed to record key steps in their analysis, they neglected to review the AERs for reliability, they arbitrarily inflated the benefits of their regulation and all of this fed into their proposed rule." Hall added, "I would suggest that FDA withdraw the proposed rule, do their job right, and see whether we can't come up with a rule that everyone can support grounded in real science and reliable data."

The GAO found that the FDA's rule-making regarding ephedrine alkaloids relied almost exclusively on adverse event reports that were not reviewed for linkage to ephedra or for reliability by the FDA. For example, the FDA relied on just thirteen AERs as the "sole source of support for specific dosing levels," yet the GAO described those critical AERs as "poorly documented." Examining the thirteen AERs, the GAO noted that, among other problems, three AERs included reports where the physician explicitly noted that the cause of the event was not related to dietary supplements. The GAO added that the FDA, "did not perform a causal analysis to determine if, in fact, the thirteen AERs it used to set dosing levels were caused by supplements containing ephedrine alkaloids."

On February 25, 2000, the FDA associate commissioner for legislation, Melinda K. Plaisier, sent a letter to members of Congress concerned with drug and dietary supplement regulation announcing the agency planned another attempt to evaluate the "the potential health risks associated with those products." CFSAN's Joseph Levitt described the withdrawal as a "mid-course correction" and not a surrender or capitulation. Levitt noted that the agency had new information to review, that it would hold a public hearing, and "follow that data, wherever it leads us."

Then, on April 3, 2000, the FDA released a report entitled "Assessment of Public Health Risks Associated with the Use of Ephedrine Alkaloid-Containing Dietary Supplements." In the report, the FDA used four types of evidence to show that the unrestricted use of ephedrine constituted an ongoing public health menace:

• A summary of 140 adverse event reports submitted between June 1, 1997 and March 1, 1999, which purport to demonstrate medical complications caused by ephedrine.

• A systematic analysis of these adverse event reports.

• A literature review summarizing the existing peer-reviewed literature on ephedra toxicity.

• An analysis of the first three items provided by a panel of independent reviewers.

After reviewing the accumulated data, FDA analysts felt that there was a clear connection to ephedrine alkaloids in sixty of the cases, approximately one-third of which involved the cardiovascular system. The sixty cases were submitted to medical reviewers who analyzed them separately, and then jointly, before determining that a connection existed between the episode described and the use of ephedrine alkaloids.

What the FDA did not refer to was criticism leveled at it a year earlier during a hearing of the Committee on Government Reform. Congressman Dan Burton indicated his committee identified six problem areas in the FDA's adverse events monitoring systems, including "causality not established." Burton said, "Ironically, this is done for veterinary drugs. For instance, if a dog takes a medicine and a dog has a heart attack and dies, the FDA evaluates this report to see if the death was related to the drug or not. . . . With people and dietary supplement events, the FDA has not done this analysis."

Representative Burton brought up two specific cases regarding ephedra. He pointed out that one death attributed to ephedra was actually attributable to hypothermia. The other was the death of a woman who had been using an ephedra supplement and who died after driving her automobile the wrong way on a one-way street and striking a pole going ninety miles an hour. "Her blood alcohol limit was .212, more than twice the legally intoxicated limit in most states," said Burton. "Are these two cases really ephedra deaths?"

Now, back to the hearings at the Office of Women's Health. Some people suspected the FDA might have orchestrated the meetings to give it an excuse to remove ephedra from the market. Their fears lay specifically in the fact that under the Dietary Supplement Health and Education Act of 1994 (DSHEA), the FDA has the authority to pull an unsafe dietary supplement from the market if the Secretary of Health and Human Services—and not the FDA Commissioner (who reports to the Secretary of HHS)—deems it an "imminent hazard" to public health, as long as HHS can justify its actions in an administrative hearing. If the recommendations by OWH, based on testimony provided at the hearing, convinced the secretary that ephedra dietary supplements posed an imminent hazard, then at least some of the procedural requirements for removal might be met and therefore doom ephedra.

Whether that was a formal strategy or just paranoia, we'll never know. If it was a strategy, testimony presented at the hearing provided a more difficult challenge than the people involved had anticipated.

A panel at the meeting, comprised of a group of seven scientists hired by the Ephedra Education Council (EEC), reported its findings after performing a comprehensive review of all the studies to date, along with the AERs compiled by the FDA.

And what did the seven scientists report? They clearly stated that there was no supporting data proving a link between the use of dietary supplements containing ephedrine alkaloids and serious adverse events when used according to the recommendations made by the industry. These recommendations included:

• Serving limits of no more than 25 milligrams of total ephedrine alkaloids.

• Limits on daily consumption of not more than 100 milligrams of total ephedrine alkaloids.

• Appropriate warnings consistent with other available over-the-counter ephedrine alkaloid products.

Maybe you're thinking, "Ah-hah! What would you expect people hired by the ephedra lobby group to say?" However, it's important to point out a few things. First, they have been completely above board about their relationship—nothing, as far as I have been able to determine, has been hidden or subverted; no scientists have been pulled off the panel because they disagree with the industry (at least as far as I discovered); and they've laid out their credentials—and reputations—for all to see. The panel included the following experts:

• Stephen E. Kimmel, M.D. An expert in cardiovascular epidemiology from the University of Pennsylvania, Dr. Kimmel is a leading researcher in the effect of drugs on the heart.

• Stephen B. Karch, M.D. Dr. Karch is a cardiac pathologist and medical examiner from San Francisco with specific expertise in the cardiac toxicity of catecholamines, including ephedrine and ephedrine alkaloids derived from ephedra.

• Norbert P. Page, M.S., D.V.M. Dr. Page has thirty years experience in chemical and radiation toxicology, and was previously director of Scientific Affairs for Toxic Substances and Pesticides at the EPA and director of the NCI's Carcinogen Testing Program.

• Theodore Farber, Ph.D., D.A.B.T. Dr. Farber has over twenty years of experience as a toxicologist and pharmacologist with the federal government, including senior positions as director of the Division of Drug and Environmental Toxicology in the Center for Veterinary Medicine at FDA and the director of the Health Effects Division at EPA.

• John W. Olney, M.D. A leading researcher in the effects of food ingredients and other chemicals on the brain from Washington University Medical School in St. Louis.

• Grover M. Hutchins, M.D. A researcher and author in pathology and cardiac pathology from Johns Hopkins University.

• Edgar H. Adams, M.S., Sc.D. An expert in substance abuse, Dr. Adams worked for seventeen years at the National Institute on Drug Abuse (NIDA), during which time he supervised several data collection and analysis initiatives as the head of the Division of Epidemiology and Prevention Research, including the Drug Abuse Warning Network (DAWN) and the National Household Survey on Drug Abuse.

After studying the AERs, the FDA submitted in April, Dr. Karch noted that a detailed review of all four elements clearly showed the FDA had failed to make a case for the toxicity of ephedra-containing dietary supplements—though it has made a stronger case against over-the-counter drugs such as phenylpropanolamine (PPA) and pseudoephedrine (PE). PPA is an ingredient used in prescription and OTC nasal decongestant and appetite-control drug products. PE is a common decongestant in a variety of cold and cough products.

Along with Drs. Page and Farber, Dr. Karch prepared an analysis of the entire case series where he dealt only with FDA claims of cardiovascular toxicity.

Dr. Karch said that two general considerations about AERs were important enough to mention. The first is the AER system itself.

The detection of adverse drug reactions has traditionally been the role of the medical community and of peer-reviewed medical journals. He said from his experience, the medical community is usually more observant than any government agency, and very few case reports describing ephedrine-related toxicity have been published in the peer-reviewed medical literature.

Dr. Karch said one explanation for the disparity in the number of case reports published in peer-reviewed journals and the very large number of case reports received by the FDA is papers submitted to peer-reviewed medical journals are scrutinized far more critically than those submitted to the FDA.

Dr. Karch also said an equally plausible explanation is that significant numbers of ephedrine-related complications are simply not occurring, and therefore no one is writing papers about them. The likelihood of the alternate explanation is reinforced by the lack of evidence to be found in government surveys not commissioned by the FDA, particularly surveillance of drug abuse patterns and complications sponsored by the Substance Abuse and Mental Health Services Administration. "Neither the Medical Examiner nor the Emergency Room components of the Drug Abuse Warning Network, nor the National Household Drug Abuse Survey contain any data suggesting that ephedrine toxicity is nearly the problem which FDA perceives it to be," said Dr. Karch.

Dr. Karch noted that of the fourteen reported cases of cardiac arrest, the FDA panel placed only four in the "attributable" or "supporting" groups. In three of these four cases, other much more plausible explanations for the adverse event seemed the likely cause. In one case, that of a dieting and overweight woman who had been fasting, vital information (her electrolyte status) was never reported. Case by case, the panel showed how the FDA confusion, inaccuracy, and outright errors undermined the whole AER set. As for the literature cited, Dr. Karch said it, "consists of many references that are either irrelevant or inappropriate to an analysis of the safety of ephedra products."

One citation was not even a case report. Instead, it was a letter to the editor describing a case where an episode of angina was thought to have been the result of pseudoephedrine (PE) ingestion. Of the eight cases the FDA presented to prove that ephedrine caused angina and/or infarction, there was only one ephedrine case cited—that of a chronic ephedrine abuser.

Dr. Stephen E. Kimmel, the panel's chair, summarized his group's findings: "Conservative estimates suggest no greater risk for adverse events than the risk in the general population," he continued. "The number of reported adverse events are consistent with what would occur in the general population, even after accounting for possible under-reporting of events. Such findings represent the efforts of the panel to step back from the emotional impact that individual adverse reports can have and look objectively at the available scientific information."

Not Really What the FDA Wanted to Hear, Wouldn't You Say?

The EEC panel members weren't the only ones who found ephedra to be safe. George Bray, Boyd Professor of Medicine at Louisiana State University and executive director of the Pennington Biomedical Research Center, discussed the results of completed clinical trials that show that dietary supplements containing ephedrine alkaloids are effective and safe as weight-loss products. He reported that, in his view, ephedra products offered a safe, effective, and affordable option for losing weight. He concluded that, "the balance of the risk-benefit fulcrum is clearly on the side of benefit."

Dr. Arne Astrup of Copenhagen, Denmark, a well-respected researcher in the treatment of obesity, discussed data from his own research supporting the safety and efficacy of ephedrine/caffeine combinations in weight loss. More experts provided evidence in support of ephedra. Drs. Patricia A. Daly and Carol Boozer, who conducted two clinical trials of ephedra/caffeine combination products at hospitals associated with Harvard and Columbia Universities, presented data from an eight-week study showing that ephedra products could produce safe and significant weight loss. They also announced that a longer-term, more comprehensive follow-up study had been completed and was currently being prepared for publication. These researchers reported that there were no serious adverse events seen in their latest study.

There were also consumers and several treating physicians who testified as to their experience and success using ephedra products for weight loss. Dr. Gary Huber of the Texas Nutrition Institute reported in his own research data on ephedra used alone or in combination with caffeine that these products are safe and effective for weight loss. Dr. Huber was accompanied by three patients who recounted their personal experiences with the products and the physical and mental health benefits that resulted from their loss of weight.

Dose Dependent

Ephedra doses in the studies presented during the hearings varied between 8 and 25 milligrams total alkaloids per dose, ranging from 72 to 150 milligrams total per day, sometimes in combination with caffeine, sometimes not. There was a consensus that larger, randomized controlled clinical trials for weight loss, endurance, and body building were needed. They noted the few trials and studies reported at the meeting consisted primarily of small groups—fewer than 150 people, and of short durations of use—between six and eight weeks. They also noted that data on long-term weight loss and maintenance were scarce and might have as much to do with calorie-restricted diets as the ephedra products themselves.

A Call to Inaction

Based on the statement issued by Dr. Wanda Jones, deputy assistant secretary for women's health at the National Institute of Health, things didn't seem quite as dire as we hear today. "The available evidence for adverse effects, particularly from the adverse event reports submitted to FDA, is very circumstantial," said Dr. Jones. "While these reported adverse events give cause for concern, the AER data set is not robust."

Jones noted that experts at the meeting pointed out inherent weaknesses of a passive reporting system. Also, while some rare adverse events "plausibly and temporally" might be related to use of ephedrine alkaloids, she noted that opinion was divided on the value of the AER system in assessing the strength of the association. "Information presented at, and contained in the transcript of, this meeting indicates a need for enhanced AER capability, including engaging industry to improve the quality of the system."

In her concluding remarks, Dr. Jones added, "Given the current widespread use of EADS [ephedrine alkaloid dietary supplements], a consumer education campaign about these products is warranted. Good manufacturing standards are needed, reasonable dose and duration levels determined, and warnings and contraindications clearly indicated on labels." She added, "A research agenda should be established. Therefore, the research community should take the next logical step by conducting a systematic review of the world's literature on ephedra."

Jones recommended that after compiling the state of the science and identifying the limitations and gaps of the current research, an appropriate agenda could be established. "In this regard, the National Center for Complementary and Alternative Medicine of the National Institutes of Health already is requesting proposals to study herb-drug interactions," said Jones.

A few presenters suggested the results of newer studies to be published the following year might show EADS to be effective and safe—or not—for short-term weight loss, but there were no large-scale studies forthcoming.

Soon after the meeting, an industry coalition of four leading dietary supplement trade associations formally petitioned the FDA to adopt a national standard for the labeling of dietary supplements containing ephedra. The petition was filed on October 25, 2000 by the American Herbal Products Association (AHPA), Consumer Healthcare Products Association (CHPA), National Nutritional Foods Association (NNFA), and the Utah Natural Products Alliance (UNPA)—organizations whose members comprise many of the manufacturers and distributors of dietary supplements containing ephedra. The group also suggested that the current industry label warning on ephedra be adopted as the official national standard. The warning would state that the product not be used by anyone under the age of eighteen and would mention possible drug interactions and preexisting conditions.

Journal Entries

Seven months after the hearings at the Office of Women's Health, the Boozer-Daly clinical study appeared in the March 2001 issue of the peer-reviewed *International Journal of Obesity*. The study showed a commercial product, Metabolife 356, produced significant weight loss over an eight-week period. The study, conducted by researchers from St. Luke's-Roosevelt Hospital Center and the Department of Medicine at the Columbia School of Medicine, included sixty-seven subjects with thirty-two taking a placebo and the rest taking 73 milligrams a day of ephedrine alkaloids and 240 milligrams per day of caffeine from guaraná.

The researchers concluded that the ephedrine-caffeine combination did, indeed, promote short-term weight loss—an average of 4 kilograms for the treatment group—but recommended further studies be conducted to determine if there would be sustained weight loss over a longer term.

During the study, none of the placebo group withdrew, while eight of the treatment group did. The most common reasons for withdrawal were dry mouth, headache, and insomnia. Funding was provided by Science Toxicology and Technology Consulting, Metabolife, and a National Institutes of Health grant.

This is probably a good place to discuss AERs a little more. Shortly after the Boozer-Daly study came out, the FDA released a statement on the AER issue regarding ephedra. The seven-member panel agreed with their findings: in essence, that there was no proven association between ephedra consumption and serious adverse events.

Basically, they said AERs cannot be viewed as scientific "data," and it is not possible to use AERs to establish whether an event is attributable to ephedra, or whether ephedra increases the risk of adverse events. They also said the industry would be willing to review all new AERs that the FDA receives for ephedra products to help monitor whether the current national standard for these products is working, which they hoped would promote a more cooperative approach with the FDA concerning the regulation of the supplements.

Added Dr. Kimmel, one of the "EEC 7": "These conclusions are also consistent with a quantitative risk study submitted to the FDA in December 2000 by Cantox Health Sciences International, and with data from clinical studies on ephedrine and ephedra products, including the recently published abstract of the Harvard and Columbia study."

Oh, Canada!

The "Cantox Report," was the first formal risk assessment on dietary supplements containing ephedra and ephedra alkaloids. Who is Cantox? Canadian-based Cantox Health Sciences International provides scientific consulting services, specializing in safety and regulatory issues related to products and processes affecting human health and the environment. For more than twenty years, Cantox has worked with clients and projects in over one hundred countries. Cantox's president, Ian Munro, Ph.D., is a regulatory toxicologist and Chairman of the UL Subcommittee, Food and Nutrition Board (FNB), U.S. National Academies. Cantox's principal investigator on the ephedra risk assessment project was Earle Nestmann, Ph.D., a recognized authority in toxicology with extensive experience in regulatory issues and risk assessment. The ephedra risk assessment was contracted and funded by the Council for Responsible Nutrition (CRN), which in turn is funded by a broad spectrum of companies, not only firms selling ephedra products.

The objective of the Cantox Report was to determine the risk of ephedra taken as a dietary supplement, by reviewing and interpreting existing data and determining a safe Upper Limit (UL) for the herb. They did this by using using the Tolerable Upper Intake Level (also called Upper Limit, or UL) method developed by the Food and

Nutrition Board, Institute of Medicine, National Academies. They did not attempt to perform a risk-benefit analysis.

Based on the evidence, particularly the results of nineteen clinical trials, including the preliminary results of the Boozer study scheduled to appear in the *International Journal of Obesity,* the Cantox study pegged the "No Observed Adverse Effect Level" (NOAEL) for ephedra at 90 milligrams per day taken in three equal doses of 30 milligrams. And the "Lowest Observed Adverse Effect Level" (LOAEL) was set at 150 milligrams per day. At these levels, they found the adverse effects were of "moderate intensity and are not life-threatening or debilitating."

They also said AERs were not conclusive, they were not useful in identifying limits because they did not prove blame, and therefore were not an adequate basis for identifying appropriate limits. They found the overall rate of adverse effects was low, considering the amount of ephedra sold and consumed.

The Cantox Report determined there were other factors in the AERs that made them less reliable:

• Most of the reports focused on the product identity and characterization of the adverse event.
• Many contained little information of reliable quality.
• Others lacked critical information needed for any possible assignment of cause.
• Most reports lacked reliable dosage information.
• Some are confounded by preexisting conditions and others by concomitant intakes of other substances that may have caused or contributed to the adverse effect.

Based on the scientific evidence, Cantox also made recommendations for the safe use of ephedra supplements, including limiting daily dosages to 90 milligrams per day, with no more than 30 milligrams per dose, and an age limit or eighteen years or older.

Numbers Don't Lie—Unless You Want Them To

After the FDA and Cantox reports came out, the seven-member EEC panel pointed out why, as with past reports, this batch of AERs shows why frequent media reporting of the raw number of AERs is meaningless and only confuses consumers. (Just think of the headlines after baseball player Steve Bechler died.)

The researchers found the AERs included had no relationship to ephedra use. Included were reports on products that did not contain ephedra, reports where no adverse event was even listed, and cases where the event occurred well prior to any ephedra consumption. Also included were cases medically unrelated to ephedra, such as gallstones, small bowel obstruction, and fat feet, as well as absurd reports including one where a married woman had an affair with a student, and blamed ephedra for her behavior. (She eventually faced criminal prosecution.)

The only experts who had reviewed the entire FDA collection of AERs have consistently found that the AERs, when considered in the context of scientific data from clinical studies, do not represent a public health concern when dosages of ephedra products did not exceed 90–100 milligrams per day.

The EEC panel went even further. They claimed that not only did independent researchers and leading academic experts consulting with industry prove the AER database was not useful from a scientific standpoint, but also that the FDA had seriously mischaracterized the published literature. They also claimed that the FDA and its consultants had ignored data regarding the benefits of these products.

Return to the Lab

A year later, some of the same researchers involved in the March 2001 clinical study reported above published new findings after a six-month trial of ephedra use. Appearing in the April 2002 issue of the *International Journal of Obesity*, the researchers described it as "the first reported long-term, clinical trial of a herbal preparation containing ephedrine alkaloids and caffeine in combination." The researchers involved including Dr. Carol Boozer, the director of the New York Obesity Research Center at St. Luke's-Roosevelt Hospital and Columbia University, and Dr. Patricia Daly, formerly a professor at Beth Israel Medical Center at Harvard Medical School.

The study followed thorough protocols: it was a prospective, two-arm, six-month, randomized, double-blind, placebo-controlled, clinical safety and efficacy trial conducted at two sites.

Recruited for the study were 167 overweight subjects, with eighty-four assigned to the placebo group and the remaining eighty-three assigned to the ephedra/caffeine alkaloid group. For six months, the subjects were given daily either a placebo or 90 milligrams of ephedrine alkaloids (from herbal ephedra) and 192 milligrams of caffeine alkaloids (from kola nut) in three divided doses, along with diet and exercise counseling. All the subjects were instructed to eat normally—but to limit intake of dietary fat to 30 percent of calories—and to exercise thirty minutes per day, three times a week.

After the study was completed, the researchers found that compared with placebo, the tested product produced no adverse events and minimal side effects consistent with the known action mechanisms of ephedrine and caffeine. They also noted there were "no significant differences between treatment groups in self-reported chest pain, palpitations, blurred vision, headache, nausea or irritability at any point."

None of the subjects suffered from a serious adverse event, and the side effects in both groups were transient and mild.

The researchers also concluded that "herbal ephedra/caffeine herbal supplements, when used as directed by healthy overweight men and women in combination with healthy diet and exercise habits, may be beneficial for weight reduction without significantly increased risk of adverse events."

I thought a note on Dr. Boozer's background might be helpful, since she will be mentioned again in the next chapter. Dr. Boozer is a nutrition scientist with primary research interests in the area of energy metabolism. She received her doctorate from Harvard's School of Public Health. In 1994, she joined the New York Obesity

Research Center with an appointment as assistant professor of nutrition at the Institute of Human Nutrition, Columbia University. Her research is supported primarily by grants from the National Institutes of Health, with some secondary funding from industry. She is active in several professional organizations and is currently the membership chair of the North American Association for the Study of Obesity.

Exercise in Futility

On February 28, 2003, the Department of Health and Human Services (HHS) issued a press release titled "HHS Acts to Reduce Safety Concerns Associated with Dietary Supplements Containing Ephedra." In the statement, the HHS said, based on new evidence, including a study by the RAND Corporation, that dietary supplements containing ephedra "may present significant or unreasonable risks as currently marketed," and announced a series of actions designed to protect Americans from these risks."

Huh? I have read the RAND report and that's not what it says. Perhaps a little background would be helpful.

The RAND report, commissioned by the National Institutes of Health, reviewed recent evidence on the risks and benefits of ephedra and ephedrine. After searching published reports, journal articles, conference presentations, and various sources of unpublished studies, they identified fifty-two controlled clinical trials of ephedrine or herbal ephedra for weight loss or athletic performance in humans. The FDA provided them with copies of over one thousand adverse event reports related to herbal ephedra and 125 AERs related to ephedrine. These reports often included interviews with patients and/or family members, extensive medical records, and copies of product labels. They also identified sixty-five case reports in the literature and received a disk of 15,951 reports containing 18,502 cases from Metabolife, a prominent manufacturer of ephedra products.

The study reviewed over sixteen thousand adverse events reported after ephedra use and found about twenty sentinel events, including two deaths, four heart attacks, nine strokes, one seizure, and five psychiatric cases involving ephedra that occurred in the absence of other contributing factors. Now here's an important distinction in the RAND report—it called such cases sentinel events, because they may indicate a safety problem but do not prove that ephedra caused the adverse event.

The HHS statement said the study "also found limited evidence of an effect of ephedra on short-term weight loss, and minimal evidence of an effect on performance enhancement in certain physical activities."

So there is no misunderstanding, I'm going to quote pertinent passages of the RAND study. Here is what it says:

Efficacy for Weight Loss
We identified 44 controlled trials that assessed use of ephedra or ephedrine used for weight loss. Of these, 18 were excluded from pooled analysis because they had a treatment duration of less than 8 weeks. Six additional trials were excluded for a variety of other reasons. Of the remaining 20 trials included in the meta-analysis, only five tested herbal ephedra-containing products.

Together, these 20 trials assessed 678 persons who consumed either ephedra or ephedrine. The majority of studies of both ephedra and ephedrine are plagued by methodological problems (particularly high attrition rates) that might contribute to bias. These methodological limitations must be considered when interpreting any conclusions regarding the efficacy of these products.

Nevertheless, the evidence we identified and assessed supports an association between short-term use of ephedrine, ephedrine plus caffeine, or dietary supplements that contain ephedra with or without herbs containing caffeine and a statistically significant increase in short-term weight loss (compared to placebo).

Adding caffeine to ephedrine modestly increases the amount of weight loss. There is no evidence that the effect of ephedra-containing dietary supplements with herbs containing caffeine differs from that of ephedrine plus caffeine: Both result in weight loss that is approximately 2 pounds per month greater than that with placebo, for up to 4 to 6 months. No studies have assessed the long-term effects of ephedra-containing dietary supplements or ephedrine on weight loss; the longest duration of treatment in a published study was 6 months.

Can you see the difference? As I've stated, HHS said the study "also found limited evidence of an effect of ephedra on short-term weight loss." But the actual report said, "Nevertheless, the evidence we identified and assessed *supports an association between short-term use of ephedrine, ephedrine plus caffeine, or dietary supplements. . . .* Both result in weight loss that is approximately 2 pounds per month greater than that with placebo, for up to 4 to 6 months" [emphasis added].

When HHS states that there is "limited evidence" of the herb's effectiveness for short-term weight loss and performance, do they mean more studies are needed or that the studies conducted so far haven't proved its effectiveness? After all, it doesn't say "showed limited or no effectiveness."

This is when I began to become suspicious.

Let's go to the next point, "Efficacy for Physical Performance Enhancement." The RAND researchers stated:

The effect of ephedrine on athletic performance was assessed in seven studies. No studies have assessed the effect of herbal ephedra-containing dietary supplements on athletic performance. The few studies that assessed the effect of ephedrine on athletic performance have, in general, included only small samples of fit individuals (young male military recruits) and have assessed the effects only on very short-term immediate performance. Thus, these studies did not assess ephedrine as it is used in the general population. The data support a modest effect of ephedrine plus caffeine on very short-term athletic performance. No studies have assessed the sustained use of ephedrine on performance over time. The only study that assessed the additive effects of these agents reported that ephedrine must be supplemented with caffeine to affect athletic performance.

. Again, HHS said, ". . . and minimal evidence of an effect on performance enhancement in certain physical activities."

This made me perk up even more. While technically true, what the RAND researchers reported was that it was difficult to evaluate because of a lack of data, not a lack of evidence supporting the contention that ephedra improved physical performance. A subtle difference in the use of words, but that subtle difference has enormous impact in what the words convey.

And it gets worse.

HHS also said the report concluded that "ephedra is associated with higher risks of mild to moderate side effects such as heart palpitations, psychiatric and upper gastrointestinal effects, and symptoms of autonomic hyperactivity such as tremor and insomnia, especially when it is taken with other stimulants."

HHS further states, "In conjunction with other recent studies of serious adverse events involving persons taking ephedra, the RAND study adds significantly to the evidence suggesting that ephedra as currently marketed may be associated with unreasonable safety risks."

Here's what RAND *really* stated:

> The data on adverse events were drawn from clinical trials and case reports published in the literature, submitted to the FDA, and reported to Metabolife, a manufacturer of ephedra-containing supplement products. The strongest evidence for causality should come from clinical trials, however, in most circumstances, such trials do not enroll sufficient numbers of patients to adequately assess the possibility of rare outcomes. Such was the case with our review of ephedrine and ephedra-containing dietary supplements. Even in aggregate, the clinical trials enrolled only enough patients to detect a serious adverse event rate of at least 1.0 per 1,000.
>
> For rare outcomes, we reviewed case reports, but a causal

relationship between ephedra or ephedrine use and these events cannot be assumed or proven. Evidence from controlled trials was sufficient to conclude that the use of ephedrine and/or the use of ephedra-containing dietary supplements or ephedrine plus caffeine is associated with two to three times the risk of nausea, vomiting, psychiatric symptoms such as anxiety and change in mood, autonomic hyperactivity, and palpitations.

The majority of case reports are insufficiently documented to make an informed judgment about a relationship between the use of ephedrine or ephedra-containing dietary supplements and the adverse event in question.

For prior consumption of ephedra-containing products, we identified two deaths, three myocardial infarctions, nine cerebrovascular accidents, three seizures, and five psychiatric cases as sentinel events; for prior consumption of ephedrine, we identified three deaths, two myocardial infarctions, two cerebrovascular accidents, one seizure, and three psychiatric cases as sentinel events. We identified forty-three additional cases as possible sentinel events with prior ephedra consumption and seven additional cases as possible sentinel events for prior ephedrine consumption. About half the sentinel events occurred in persons aged thirty years or younger. Classification as a sentinel event does not imply a proven cause and effect relationship.

Did you notice of the sixteen thousand adverse events reported, only twenty instances caused alarm? Besides not flat-out blaming ephedra directly, the sentence by HHS that, "ephedra as currently marketed may be associated with unreasonable safety risks," is also wide open to interpretation. It's not saying ephedra is dangerous, but rather that it could be a danger "as currently marketed." Can you see the distinction?

As for the future, here's what the RAND report recommended under "Future Research":

Our analysis of the evidence reveals numerous gaps in the literature regarding the efficacy and safety of ephedra-containing dietary supplements.

Evidence regarding the effect of herbal ephedra or ephedrine on physical performance that reflects its use in the general population (repeated or long-term use by a representative sample) is (also) needed. In order to assess a causal relationship between ephedra or ephedrine consumption and serious adverse events, a hypothesis-testing study is needed.

Continued analysis of case reports cannot substitute for a properly designed study to assess causality. A case-control study would probably be the study design of choice.

Spinning the Un-Spinnable

So, has the RAND report spurred the FDA to evaluate fairly whether ephedra is safe or effective?

To the contrary—it has had the opposite effect.

Did HHS take the RAND report and say "we need to find out if ephedra provides long-term benefits by approving a large-scale study?"

No.

Did HHS take the RAND report and say "we need better studies?"

No.

Did HHS take the RAND report and say "we need to find out if the sentinel events imply a proven cause-and-effect relationship?"

Again, no.

Instead, HHS has stated that dietary supplements containing ephedra, "may present significant or unreasonable risks as currently marketed," and announced a series of actions designed to protect Americans from these risks.

Besides the publication of the RAND study, what happened to implement the recommendations from the Office of Women's Health, the Cantox Report, and other studies in the last three years?

Virtually nothing. Nada. Zilch.

What the heck is going on here? In reality, a lot. As FDA Commissioner Mark B. McClellan, M.D., Ph.D., stated in the HHS press release, "The standard for regulating the safety of dietary supplements is largely untested, but we are committed to finding the right public health solution."

As you'll see in the next chapter, the FDA's interpretation of and response to the RAND report points to bigger issues than just the safety of ephedra. With the help of dramatic newspaper headlines after a couple of tragic incidents—dutifully reported by a compliant press—the next big meeting in July 2003 wasn't to gather information. It was more like a witch hunt.

11

Pushing for a Ban

It was a heartbreaking scene reported by television stations and newspapers across the country. On May 25, 2003, inside DePaul University's Athletic Center, Illinois Governor Rod Blagojevich signed into law a statewide ban on ephedra. "The FDA, I hope, will take notice of the fact that we, through the legislature and the governor signing a bill, have done what the FDA should have done a long time ago," said Governor Blagojevich. "And, hopefully, now they'll see a trend coming and they'll act to either regulate or, more importantly, ban the sale of ephedra."

Nearby were Debbie and Kevin Riggins, who had lost their son Sean, age sixteen, to a heart attack. They attribute his death to Yellow Jackets, an ephedra and caffeine product sold by New Jersey-based NVE Pharmaceuticals that Sean allegedly bought repeatedly. Yellow Jackets were displayed near the cash register at a local convenience store, undoubtedly near the chewing tobacco and steps away from the beer cooler. He and other athletes at his school were suspected of taking the product for some time. While tobacco, alcohol, and ephedra products all have warning labels, only the beer and tobacco are backed up by state law. Reports say store clerks seldom—if ever—checked the ages of the Yellow Jacket buyers.

The bill that Governor Blagojevich signed made it a misdemeanor to sell ephedra, punishable by up to a year in jail and a $5,000 fine. The measure passed both Houses unanimously, and the Illinois Retail Merchants Association has warned members to stop selling ephedra.

Mr. Riggins, who along with his wife pushed for the ban, also spoke. "I do have one message for the industry, and that is that ephedra's time is over. It is at an end," said Riggins, who has lobbied for the ban since his son died the previous fall, a day after playing middle linebacker for his Lincoln High School sophomore football team. For the Riggins family, the death toll from ephedra was 100 percent.

Piling On

Consumer watchdog groups also joined the fray. On October 8, 2002, while giving testimony before the Senate Governmental Affairs Committee Hearing on Dangers of Ephedra, the director of the Public Citizen Health Research Group, Sidney M. Wolfe, M.D., said the ephedra issue is not and has never been simply a question of scientific or medical evidence. Instead, he said, "It is a question of politics and the extraordinarily dangerous political cowardice of the FDA and HHS Secretary Thompson in the face of massive lobbying by ephedra-makers in Washington. Is the FDA still part of the Public Health Service or is it a drug-sales-promoting adjunct to the pharmaceutical and dietary supplements industries? De facto drug pushers include those who refuse to use their legal authority to remove a well-documented hazard to the public health from the market."

The following February, Bruce Silverglade, director of legal affairs for the Center for Science in the Public Interest (CSPI), said, "Ephedra has probably caused far more deaths and serious adverse reactions than any other dietary supplement on the market. If the FDA cannot restrict the sale of ephedra, there is little hope that it could protect consumers against other dietary supplements that pose substantial health risks." Silverglade said it was up to Congress to enact legislation, "making it easier for the FDA to restrict the sales of ephedra and other herbal medicines that should not be used without a doctor's prescription."

League Limits

The United States Army, Marines, and Air Force, Canada, the National Football League, Major League Soccer, Minor League Baseball, the National Collegiate Athletic Association (NCAA), and the International Olympic Committee had already outlawed the use of ephedra-based products followed by Major League Baseball.

The NFL banned ephedra after the death of Minnesota Vikings offensive tackle Korey Stringer during training camp in 2001. A bottle of Ripped Fuel, which contains ephedra (and guaraná, a source of caffeine), was found in Stringer's locker after he died, although Stringer's remains weren't tested for the substance—nor were any traces found inadvertently—during investigations of his death.

Fearful of legal repercussions, the NFL consulted with several experts and held a series of discussions and seminars about ephedra before training camp opened in 2002. The league banned all products containing ephedra and began random testing for it.

Not all football players are happy about the ephedra punishments. Shortly after the ban, Philadelphia Eagles guard John Welbourn told *Sports Illustrated*, "The NFL basically scapegoated ephedra. The Chinese have been taking it for two thousand years. It's stupid. I worry a lot more about all the anti-inflammatories NFL teams hand out."

In late July 2003, an attorney for Korey Stringer's widow said she was suing the NFL, alleging that the league's policies led to Stringer's death from heat stroke during training camp in 2001. Stan Chesley said Kelci Stringer's suit would also name football helmet maker Riddell Sports Group, Inc., and some NFL medical advisers. There was no mention of ephedra in the lawsuit.

Chesley said the federal lawsuit would include a wrongful death claim on behalf of Stringer's widow and son, and a class-action claim on behalf of all NFL players. "What's on trial here is the rules and procedures and the culture" of the NFL, Chesley said. "Frankly, it's no coincidence that the average football player in the NFL plays for four and a half years. They use them up and spit them out."

It All Comes Back to Steve Bechler

At the time, many baseball players believed that ephedra shouldn't have been banned—possibly because many of them used it to endure a 162-game schedule, not to mention spring training and possible playoff games. Orioles outfielder Jay Gibbons said he used ephedra in both college and pro ball. In the same *PR Newswire* piece mentioned above, he said, "It's a good supplement if taken right. I've never had any problems with it. I've never had any dizziness with it. It's just like caffeine." Gibbons indicated he used a supplement containing ephedrine to help drop about fifteen pounds before the 2002 season. This past winter, he did a better job of maintaining his weight, so he didn't need to use it. Gibbons' opinion is that using ephedrine is safe as long as people are careful to follow the labels.

Gibbons's teammate, David Segui added, "There's almost a witch-hunt going on" in the aftermath of Bechler's death. "It hasn't been proven that ephedrine caused his death. There was probably some milk found in his system, too. Did that cause his death?"

Orioles catcher Brook Fordyce said Steve Bechler's death probably wouldn't deter him from using ephedra. "It has no ill effect on me that I know of, and I use it safely. So if I was tired, I probably would take one, like if we had a day game after a night game. I'm not afraid of it."

It's important to note that the *PR Newswire* article (in which Orioles owner Peter Angelos called for a ban on ephedra and which quotes several baseball players) originated with Cytodyne Technologies—which changed its name to Nutraquest, Inc.—the maker of the ephedra product that Steve Bechler consumed.

Pharmacists and the AMA Prescribe Ban

The American Society of Health-System Pharmacists (ASHP) has urged the FDA to ban the sale of dietary supplements containing ephedra. The ASHP said labeling changes proposed by the FDA will not protect the public from the dangers of the products. ASHP also encouraged the agency to work with Congress to amend the Dietary Supplement Health Education Act (DSHEA) to require that dietary supplements must at least meet the same legal requirements as nonprescription drugs. It's easy to see where ASHP's interests lie—in filling prescriptions of pharmaceutical drugs, or at least guaranteeing the purchase of OTC medications.

Big Pharma (as it's often referred to in industry and political circles) has another powerful friend, the American Medical Association (AMA), which also wants to do away with ephedra. It's no secret many physicians feel threatened by dietary supplements. They see many of the claims as "hype" and worry about patients using unproven products in lieu of traditional medical treatments. From the outset, it was the clear intent of Congress in enacting DSHEA that consumers should be provided with products, information, and education that would help promote health and prevent disease. Yet, since Congress noted in its "findings" section of the act that "consumers should be empowered to make choices about preventive health-care programs based on data from scientific studies of health benefits related to particular dietary supplements," the AMA has balked.

It's important to remember some things from an earlier chapter: who today provides much of the education for doctors? The pharmaceutical industry, of course.

Mass Media or Mass Hysteria?

Reporters faced with tight deadlines and shrinking budgets are sometimes forced to resort to the FDA and other regulatory industry press releases churned out by government agencies and other organizations for background material on complicated issues.

This certainly was true when the subject was ephedra. As a result, these products were almost always reported in the popular press as potentially unsafe. That's why it's easy to find the same statements repeated over and over and over. As you know, the more something is repeated, the more likely it will eventually be accepted as truth.

Believe it or not, sometimes these organizations get it wrong. Here's a perfect example. On February 28, 2003, a consumer advisory on ephedra was distributed by the National Center for Complementary and Alternative Medicine (NCCAM), which is part of the National Institutes of Health. The first line of the advisory reads, "Dietary supplements containing ephedra, which have been in the news recently because of the deaths of well-known athletes, may cause rare but serious health consequences."

Which "well-known athletes"? Sean Riggins, the high school player in Illinois? Steve Bechler, who wasn't sure he would even make the Orioles team? Neither of them fit the description "well-known" (unless, of course, you count the publicity they received after they died). Korey Stringer? He had an ephedra product in his locker, but there is no evidence that he took it. Are we now supposed to assume that he did take the product simply to help build more evidence for the case against ephedra?

Consider how the issue is covered in a May 1, 2003 *Sports Illustrated* article entitled, "NFL puts support behind supplement regulation laws." The article states, "The NFL banned ephedra after the death of Minnesota Vikings offensive tackle Korey Stringer during training camp in 2001. . . ." Doesn't that imply he died from ephedra? Shouldn't there be a caveat such as "although there is no evidence he ever took it"? By not including a clarifying statement, the sentence very much implies that ephedra caused Stringer's death. Even those who know better might conclude that new evidence surfaced without them knowing it.

So who are the "well-known athletes" NCCAM had in mind when it wrote its consumer advisory? I don't have a clue, but you can bet the statement is now widely accepted as fact. Once a barn door is opened. . . .

Side Effects: Ephedra vs. Pharmaceuticals

In the last chapter I discussed the findings of the seven scientists who, in August 2000, appeared at the Office of Women's Health at the Department of Health and Human Services for two days of hearings about the safety of ephedra. You heard or read about these findings didn't you? What—you didn't hear about them? No surprise there, I suppose—the hearings garnered little publicity.

There's a greater chance you read this story, which appeared in *USA Today* on July 17, 2003. Here's the headline: "As Backlash Against Ephedra Mounts, Congress Drags Feet."

There was a three-year gap between the panel's findings and the *USA Today* story. Much had to have changed in that time, right? More evidence of ephedra's dangers, a higher percentage of adverse side effects and many more deaths from its use, wouldn't you think? Well, let's see:

- Baseball player Steve Bechler died.
- High school football player Sean Riggins died.
- Korey Stringer had an ephedra product in his locker.

Now let's look at some other statistics. Over those same three years, it's estimated that:

- 300 people died as a result of using acetaminophen.
- Thousands of people died due to the misuse of aspirin (some studies place the number as high as 48,000).
- 137,000 people die each year just as a result of taking prescription medications where no prescription errors or abuse are involved.
- 300,000 died from alcohol use.*
- 1,300,000 died from cigarette use.*
- (*These are not regulated by FDA)

Now look at the data from the 2001 National Household Survey on Drug Abuse, SAMHSA, 2002 regarding Emergency Department

Trends from the Drug Abuse Warning Network. In 2000, 43 percent of those who ended up in hospital emergency rooms from drug overdoses—nearly a half million people—were there because of misusing prescription drugs. Not illicit drugs, but perfectly legal prescription drugs.

In seven cities in 2000 (Atlanta, Chicago, Los Angeles, Miami, New York, Seattle, and Washington, D.C.), 626 people died from overdose of painkillers and tranquilizers. By 2001, such deaths had increased in Miami and Chicago by 20 percent. From 1998 to 2000, the number of people entering an emergency room because of misusing hydrocodone (Vicodin) rose 48 percent, oxycodone (Oxy-Contin) 108 percent, and methadone 63 percent. The rates are intensifying: from mid-2000 to mid-2001, oxycodone misuse went up 44 percent in emergency room visits.

By comparison, the highest number of deaths attributed to ephedra is 130—and that's for the herb's roughly decade-long use as a weight-loss and fitness aid. (Although I've seen this number stated a few times, I have no idea where it originated.) But even that number is highly questionable. According to the RAND study, there were only seventeen sentinel events where death was only one outcome. And even these deaths, since they are based on AER data, could be wrong. Some experts put the number of deaths where there is no question that ephedra was the culprit at only two. Yet here's a sample of media reports reporting the number of ephedra deaths:

October 8, 2002 Associated Press
"FDA Cracks Down On Illegally Promoted Ephedra Product"
" . . . said Sen. Dick Durbin, an Illinois Democrat. He said Food and Drug Administration reports link ephedra to eighty-one deaths and 1,400 incidents of heart attack, high blood pressure and stroke."

February 26, 2003 *Sports Illustrated*
"Why the Federal Govt. Needs to Come to Terms with Ephedra"
"But Bechler didn't listen, and he joins a grim roll of nearly 90 deaths. . . ."

May 16, 2003 *State Journal-Register* (Illinois)
"Ephedra-based products have been blamed for dozens of deaths, including that of 16-year-old Lincoln Community High School football player Sean Riggins, who took it along with caffeinated soda, believing his athletic performance would be enhanced."

May 26, 2003 *San Diego Union-Tribune*
"Ephedra, blamed for nearly 120 deaths, drew national attention after officials investigating the February heatstroke death of Baltimore Orioles pitching prospect Steve Bechler linked it to a diet pill containing ephedrine, ephedra's active ingredient."

Although the number seems to climb by date, that is merely a coincidence. If there were that many new deaths, you would have heard the specifics. In fact, it would have been unavoidable.

The Media Gets It Wrong—Again

Let's look a little closer at the July 17 *USA Today* story, which by the way, has no byline: "Years after diet supplements containing ephedra surged onto store shelves without government regulation or consumer warnings, concerns about serious risks to users finally are forcing meaningful changes. On Monday, New Jersey's attorney general joined a parade of more than one hundred lawsuits against the ephedra industry."

Actually, there is government regulation—DSHEA, for one, as well as the power of the FDA to remove any product it deems dangerous. And there have been consumer warnings. His mention of "meaningful changes" is correct, especially if the author is referring to the changes in labeling. However, that doesn't quite jive with the next sentence about the lawsuits. Sorry if I seem picky, but did the lawsuits bring about the "meaningful changes"? Or did the author add that sentence simply for dramatic affect?

The next paragraph states, "The popular herbal supplement, which is linked to at least 120 deaths and 1,400 serious reactions, also is under assault from state legislatures, medical groups—and the marketplace. Last week, CVS, the nation's second-largest drugstore chain, announced it will stop selling ephedra diet products."

The article is 100 percent correct about CVS's actions. But what it fails to report is that when CVS announced it would stop selling ephedra-based products it also stated its belief that ephedra-based products are safe when used as directed. This is similar to a statement made by the largest American vitamin and dietary supplement chain, General Nutrition Centers (GNC), in May when it announced it would stop selling the herb. Here are the exact words from the GNC release dated May 2, 2003, "We believe that ephedra-based products are safe when used as directed. Nonetheless, the current business climate dictates that we move in a different direction," said Michael K. Meyers, GNC's president and CEO.

Could it be both chains are simply responding to a lessening demand for the products? Are they afraid of liability for future and past sales of ephedra? Probably so, especially considering the phrase "the current business climate dictates that we move in a different direction" in GNC's press release. It's also interesting that CVS will still gladly sell you prescription drugs, OTC pain relievers, and in most locations, cigarettes.

Later in the *USA Today* article, the author writes: "Congress continues to protect the diet supplements industry, the source of $4 million in political contributions during the past six years."

I have heard this charge many times. If I didn't know better, I'd be incensed. Four million dollars in campaign contributions over the past six years? Those scalawags! But wait—while $4 million is certainly a lot of money, according to the Center for Responsive Politics the total amount of political contributions from dietary supplement companies in the 2002 election cycle was $969,642 with the large majority of it—$847,750—coming from one company, Metabolife. During the same period, the pharmaceutical companies gave $26.9 million. Yes, you read that right—$26.9 million.

This is probably a good time to talk a little about Metabolife. On August 15, 2002, the Justice Department launched a criminal investigation of Metabolife to determine whether the herbal diet pill manufacturer lied about ephedra's safety. The next day, Metabolife, with estimated annual sales of $500 million, produced thirteen thousand consumer complaints about ephedra products. The company said that these health-related complaints were not released because they hadn't been analyzed properly. The explanation angered U.S. Food and Drug Administration officials, who had sought access to the documents since 1997. Calling it "disingenuous," then–Acting FDA Commissioner Lester Crawford declared that, "Metabolife has refused and resisted us every step of the way."

Back to the *USA Today* story, which continues, "While a House subcommittee resumes desultory hearings next week on the supplement's dangers, there's little movement toward what's really needed: government regulation of ephedra and other largely untested and unproved diet supplements."

Not so. Already pending before the U.S. Senate was the proposed legislation S.722 ("Dietary Supplement Safety Act of 2003"). Which, as I covered earlier, could be the first step toward the dismantling of the DSHEA codes, ultimately affecting how your supplements are regulated, their cost, and their availability.

The article continues, "The RAND Corp. think tank issued a review in February concluding that while several instances of death and illness are clearly linked to ephedra use, the product does not result in long-term weight-loss benefits or improvements in athletic performance." As I've already pointed out, the RAND report says nothing of the sort. Gee, I wonder who fed them this misinformation.

More Bad Reporting

Consider another story, this time appearing on MSNBC in April 2001. Entitled "Unsafe Supplements?" it is almost entirely inaccurate and misleading. I've already covered many of the issues that correspondent Robert Hager raises, so I'll only discuss other issues.

First of all, the theme of the report is that public health is being endangered by the lack of oversight in the diet supplement industry, and that new government regulation is needed. As I've said repeatedly—and will say again—the FDA already has the authority to remove dangerous products from the marketplace.

I think we need to follow the money. What health and safety worries does the NIH really have about dietary supplements if, according to government figures, it allocates a mere 1 percent of the amount expended annually for medical and health research to supplements? That's right—1 percent! If it really were concerned about establishing, through legitimate research, the safety and/or dangers of ephedra and other supplements, wouldn't it dedicate more of its funds to that endeavor?

The MSNBC story stated that the FDA is often not informed of adverse reactions. "The government doesn't hear about the vast majority of health problems associated with dietary supplements, according to an unpublished report from the inspector general of the Department of Health and Human Services."

The story talks about one particular problem—state poison control centers aren't communicating with the FDA. While this may be true, wouldn't this be the case with any substance people take, not just supplements? And wouldn't these communications channels be easily established if there was sufficient data to warrant such an action?

The MSNBC story also states that the FDA "was unable to determine the ingredients in 32 percent of the products mentioned in adverse event reports." According to the FDA's own regulation, as of March 23, 1999 dietary supplement products must include an ingredient statement and information panel titled "Supplement Facts," in which all ingredients in the product must be declared.

The MSNBC story goes on to say, "in a recent year when the FDA received 470 reports of bad reactions to dietary supplements, the nation's poison control clinics actually treated 13,000." First, just as we indicated in the discussion about AERs , it is impossible to determine if these cases can be directly attributed to dietary supplements, whether they were only a contributing factor, or if the supplements were merely present in the victims' stomachs. We also don't know whether they were due to a deliberate overdose, an accidental overdose or people not following directions on the label. But even if they do point to supplements as the culprits, this means that thirteen thousand reports of adverse reactions represent less than one-hundredth of one percent of the 150 million Americans taking supplements, or approximately one person out of 11,536.

The article then mentions the ephedra uproar. The MSNBC story states, "Research on ephedra that was commissioned by the FDA concluded that the supplement poses risks that far outweigh any benefits it might have. Results were published in the *New England Journal of Medicine*."

There are a couple problems with this. First, this *NEJM* article was not new. Second, it certainly was not clinical research. Rather, it was a study of anecdotal reports collected by the FDA. Anecdotal reports don't constitute unbiased research, nor do all experts agree with the conclusions in the *NEJM* article.

One of the EEC's panel of seven, Dr. Grover M. Hutchins, conducted his own analysis of twenty-two reports from the same FDA data in which death occurred. In a letter to the *NEJM*, Dr. Hutchins stated that the data "showed no consistent clinical or pathological features of the reported adverse events and showed that ephedrine-type alkaloids were not likely to have been causative or contributing factors in the deaths. . . . With an adequate explanation of the reported adverse events, the implication of ephedrine-type alkaloids in deaths from a wide variety of conditions that occur in the general population is no more than idle speculation."

Bruce Silverglade, from the Center for Science in the Public Interest, is also quoted in the article. He said, "Right now consumers are playing a game of Russian roulette because no one is sorting out products that work from those that don't." His statement is not entirely true.

Reputable supplement manufacturers do conduct efficacy research. Also, two agencies in the federal Department of Health and Human Services (HHS)—the Office of Dietary Supplements and the National Center for Complementary and Alternative Medicine—are funding efficacy research. Additionally, the Office of Dietary Supplements has created a database of research about dietary supplements—IBIDS—which now contains nearly half a million bibliographic records about dietary supplements from 1986 to the present.

As for product testing to find out which supplements "work," the Web site ConsumerLab.com compares products with formulations shown to be effective in clinical trials. Finally, other organizations are developing third-party testing and certification programs.

Boozer Under Attack

Next, the MSBNC story saw fit to take a swipe at the research by Dr. Carol Boozer, whom I mentioned earlier, by stating, "While the FDA has received claims of 70 deaths among ephedra users, an industry-financed study turned up no problems."

In describing Dr. Boozer's research as "industry-financed," MSNBC implies it was automatically biased and therefore, crooked. Most research on drugs is at least partially financed by the pharmaceutical companies. (I cover a number of medical conferences, so I know.)

Actually, while the FDA "study" was no study at all, but rather a review of unproven anecdotal cases, Boozer's study used the gold standard of research: a randomized, double-blind, placebo-controlled clinical trial. Isn't this what everyone wants?

While Metabolife contributed their product and some funding to Dr. Boozer's study, the funding was indirect; the money went through Science Toxicology and Technology, an independent consulting firm of physicians and toxicologists based in San Francisco that underwrote the research.

While accurately quoting Dr. Boozer as saying, "The bottom line is that in our studies we found that there were no real health consequences, significant health consequences, to individuals that were taking these products," it said she was affiliated with the New York Obesity Research Center. For the average person, this would mean nothing. The story neglects to mention that the New York Obesity Research Center is affiliated with the prestigious Columbia Medical School.

Dr. Boozer did manage to make an excellent point in the MSNBC article. Referring to the *NEJM* article mentioned above, Boozer noted that twelve million people took ephedra in 1999. She pointed out that whenever twelve million people do the same thing—such as get haircuts, drink water, take aspirin, or drive to work—some will have heart attacks, develop high blood pressure, or suffer strokes—and some will die either because of or in spite of their activities. (As you'll see later, the ephedra enemies weren't done with Dr. Boozer.)

As its final point, the MSNBC story lists three recommendations from the report given by the inspector general of the Department of Health and Human Services. One of those recommendations is that "ingredients in supplements should be standardized to guard against contamination." That's misleading. Contamination is largely caused by poor manufacturing practices—things like incomplete cleaning of machines—and not raw materials. For eight years—since DSHEA went into effect—the FDA has promised to develop "good manufacturing practice" (GMP) standards that all supplement manufacturers will be required to meet. The National Nutritional Foods Association (NNFA) already has a GMP inspection and certification program in place, complete with a seal that companies can place on their labels.

Even without a GMP, dietary supplements are already required to be both safe and pure (free of pathogenic contaminants) under the FDA's current GMP standards for foods, which supplements can be held to as a fall-back position. The FDA's new GMP standards for dietary supplements are expected to be tougher than those for foods largely because the procedures for processing supplements are more complex and in some ways more technically challenging than those for foods.

The Ultimate Witch Hunt

In July 2003, at the two-day U.S. House Subcommittee on Oversight and Investigations the tone was set early by Billy Tauzin, U.S. Representative from Louisiana and chairman of the House Energy and Commerce Committee:

> This week the gentleman from Michigan [Mr. Dingell] and I and all of the members of the Committee on Energy and Commerce had to face a horrible realization: This week we faced

the parents of Steve Bechler, the 23-year-old pitcher for the Baltimore Orioles, who died of a heart attack at that young age taking ephedra tablets, tablets which we in 1994 voted to exempt from FDA safety regulations. I have got that on my conscience now. In 1994, you and I decided, those of you who were here with me, that safety did not matter when it came to ephedra.

Mr. Speaker, as the Justice Department criminal investigations are under way and as our own Committee's investigation is under way, we learned this week that over 17,000 serious events have occurred as a result of the use of unregulated ephedra; young athletes, young people, dying, suffering strokes, heart attacks, like Steve Bechler, because we voted in 1994 to say that safety did not count when it came to ephedra.

Is it any wonder that today Tauzin is president of the ultra-powerful PhARMA lobby group?

The July 2003 hearings were vastly different in tone and substance from the August 2000 gathering at the FDA and CFSAN-sponsored meeting at the Office of Women's Health (OWH) when scientists, government officials, industry experts, and interested parties met in Washington for two days of hearings about the safety and risks of ephedrine alkaloids. The official title of the July 203 hearings was "Issues Relating to Ephedra-containing Dietary Supplements." But, they were really only interested in hearing from one side—unless they could fling mud at those defending the herb. This time, not one member of the panel put together by the Ephedra Education Council was invited, nor were any of the other doctors who spoke in support of ephedra. Were they discredited in the ensuing three years, making their testimony suspect? Outside of receiving honorariums from the Ephedra Education Council—a fact none of them tried to hide—their testimony and research is still being cited. You may be saying to yourself, "But they were paid by a pro-ephedra organization—can we really trust their statements?" That's exactly the kind of question a House Subcommittee member might ask. But as you'll see later, the last people who should criticize the receiving of funds are many of the House Subcommittee members.

Let the Hunt—Uh, Hearings—Begin

The mood of the hearings was established before they even began. As a July 23, 2003 article in the *New York Times* stated while quoting "unnamed officials," "For several years, the industry had refused to give the regulators all the data from the study, which was conducted at medical centers in New York and Boston in the late 1990s. But last February, the Food and Drug Administration made an unusual deal to gain access to the data, officials say." The study the *New York Times* is referring to is the Boozer/Daly study.

The article, "Expert Panel Finds Flaws in Diet Pill Safety Study" and written by Christopher Drew and Ford Fessenden, continues:

> The agency had to make the deal, the officials say, because it was in a bind. While drug companies are required to prove the safety of their products and must turn over safety data and consumer complaints to the FDA, the agency, under a 1994 law, has no such authority over the makers of dietary supplements like ephedra.
>
> The notion that a federal regulatory agency had to make a deal to investigate a health threat also goes a long way, critics say, to explaining how the ephedra companies have been able to keep the government at bay through nearly a decade of complaints about their products.

At first, it appears the *New York Times* raises some interesting points, that is until you hear the rest of the story. According to Dr. Boozer in a phone interview and e-mails we exchanged in early September 2003, she had told Metabolife before she conducted the first study that she planned to publish the results in a medical journal, regardless of the outcome. When she and an industry attorney struck a deal after many months of negotiation with the FDA for her data, the agreement was that the FDA would ask independent scientists to review the data. On top of this, the FDA agreed to provide her with copies of these reviews prior to the government making them public in any form. You can imagine her surprise when portions of their reviews showed up in the *Times* article before she saw them.

In the same *New York Times* article, the reporters also wrote, "Top agency officials said they agreed to the deal to counter industry concerns that the agency's scientists were biased against ephedra. Representative James C. Greenwood, a Republican from Pennsylvania and the chairman of the House subcommittee that will hold a hearing on ephedra today, said the deal made sense because the outside experts ended up showing that the study was 'seriously flawed.'"

Naturally Boozer was stunned when she read this, and two months later, still could not get the *New York Times* to correct their article. Should they? I think they should, and not just based on what Dr. Boozer says. I saw the documents provided by the FDA to the House subcommittee.

Included with the reviews is a letter stamped May 14, 2003 from Charles W. Prettyman of HHS to then–FDA Commissioner Dr. Mark McClellan. There are two interesting points in this letter. First, as we already mentioned, the FDA had agreed to share the results of the reviews with Dr. Boozer and an industry lawyer before releasing it to the public. Yet, somehow the *New York Times* obtained them first. (In fact, when Dr. Boozer testified at the July hearings she still hadn't seen the reviews. The Prettyman letter was not made public until August 8.)

Second, in his letter Mr. Prettyman wrote:

> The main points I gather from the three reviews [one still hadn't come in] are as follows:
> • The study was generally well designed and conducted.
> • The formulation may or may not represent what is being marketed.
> • The controls, subject selection, exclusion criteria, and monitoring do not represent real world use conditions.
> • The product seems to offer some short-term weight loss.
> • The product should only be used with the monitoring of a learned intermediary.
> • One expert believes the study was seriously compromised due to some mix-up in the active and placebo preparations.

Can't the *New York Times* distinguish between "expert" and "experts"? It makes a big difference. More later.

As I considered the concerns raised by the article and began reviewing the list of those scheduled to speak, I wondered why Dr. Wanda Jones, deputy assistant secretary for women's health at NIH who headed the 2000 meeting, was not asked to testify at the current hearings. She would be objective, I thought. But she wasn't invited. When I further scrutinized the presenters' names, I had a gut feeling this had the potential to be more a witch hunt than objective inquiry.

Here's how James Greenwood, Chairman of the Subcommittee on Oversight and Investigations opened the meeting:

> Good morning and welcome to the first day of hearings on issues relating to ephedra-containing dietary supplements. Baltimore Orioles pitcher Steve Bechler and high school athlete Sean Riggins probably thought they were helping themselves when they used ephedra supplements either to lose weight or enhance athletic performance. Tragically, these two young men, twenty-three years and sixteen years of age respectively, died. And coroners who investigated their cases believed ephedra played a role in their deaths. . . .

Could Mr. Greenwood have been any more blatant in his bias against ephedra? As they say, the die was cast.

The first two witnesses were Pat and Ernie Bechler, parents of Steve Bechler. They were accompanied by their attorney, Todd Macaluso. In June, the Bechlers filed a civil action charging wrongful death, product liability, negligence, fraud, and misrepresentation against Cytodyne Technologies, Inc., and Phoenix Laboratories, the manufacturers of Xenadrine RFA-1, the diet supplement their son had been taking at the time of his death. Why did they need an attorney there? Most likely to guide them in their responses in case questions were raised about a story appearing in the *Sun-Sentinel* of Fort Lauderdale in March. In the story, Mrs. Bechler said her son suffered "a couple of heatstrokes" while in high school. "He was probably sixteen, seventeen years old," Pat Bechler told the newspaper. "Both of them happened when he was playing baseball."

In an ESPN story run the same time, which also used Associated Press material, Ernie Bechler said Steve Bechler's half-brother, Ernie Jr., died at age twenty from a brain aneurysm. "He came in from playing baseball one day. He was hot, and he suddenly had a severe headache. He collapsed on the floor, and he was dead by the time the paramedics got there."

The Bechler's testimony was heart wrenching, with Mrs. Bechler tearfully asking how many others "will have to die to prove these products are not safe?" The Bechler's appearance set the tone for the entire hearing.

The next witness was Kevin Riggins, father of the late Sean Riggins and founder and director of the Sean Riggins Foundation for Substance-Free Schools in Lincoln, Illinois. Here's part of what Riggins said:

My wife and I were not familiar with this particular substance; in fact, we had no idea that Sean had been taking it. As we were to discover later through investigation and conversations with Sean's teammates, numerous teenagers, including athletes and young people trying to lose weight, were using these products. The teens could buy these pills at the corner gas stations with pocket change. The little packages, which promote weight loss, performance and energy enhancement, were being sold right next to the Twinkies and candy bars. In fact, the use of these products was so casual, none of the kids believed that they were taking a drug. With the marketing style and the ease in which they could be obtained, the teens thought nothing of it. "They sell these things in the stores, they are not illegal, so they must be OK." This was a quote from one of my son's friends. As it turns out, the vast majority of the American public believes this as well.

Mr. Riggins then went on to bash DSHEA:

As Americans, we believe that our regulatory organizations, in this case the FDA, are protecting our interests by not allowing dangerous products to be sold, especially in regards to what we put in our bodies. In the case of ephedra, we could not be more wrong. As you well know, the Dietary Supplement Health and Education Act of 1994 allows dietary supplement companies to operate with virtually no federal oversight. A company does not need a license to produce these products, nor are there any no pre-market approval requirements. There have never been any Good Manufacturing Practice guidelines developed for these companies and they have a voluntary adverse event reporting system. When a supplement poses a risk of serious injury or death, the burden of proof falls to the Government to prove cause and effect. This is the exact opposite of the rules and regulations set up for drug companies.

Mr. Riggins was followed by Mr. Michael Vasquez—along with his lawyer, Fred G. Cohen, via satellite. In a court deposition the previous August, Vasquez, a nurse and former Metabolife employee, said the company had nurses on ten telephone lines receiving calls from consumers. He testified he handled about five adverse event calls per day. In an article appearing in the August 25, 2002 edition of the *Union-Tribune of San Diego*, Vasquez said one out of five calls were about cardiovascular symptoms, and during the four months he worked at Metabolife, he said he received about ten calls from emergency room physicians seeking information about Metabolife ingredients as they tried to provide emergency treatment to patients who had taken the pills and complained of illness.

Vasquez said all calls of serious consumer injury were forwarded to a supervisor, and the reports were discussed with Metabolife's legal department at least once a week. In some cases, Metabolife footed the costs for emergency room treatments of some of its customers.

Next up was Steven Heymsfield, M.D., deputy director of the Obesity Research Center at St. Luke's-Roosevelt Hospital, where Dr. Carol Boozer worked. Here's part of his testimony:

There exist three categories of chemical agents available for weight loss treatment. The first two categories are prescription drugs and over-the-counter drugs. The Food and Drug Administration regulates these agents under carefully controlled guidelines for safety and efficacy. The process is particularly rigorous for weight loss agents.

Prescription and over-the-counter drugs are rigorously tested, using modern scientific guidelines and procedures to ensure public and individual safety. In 1994 a third category of agents emerged referred to as "dietary supplements."

Dr. Heymsfield then talked specifically about ephedra: "By avoiding medical oversight, overweight and obese consumers purchasing dietary supplements make the false assumption that dietary supplements and herbal preparations are inordinately safe and may pose no or very little risk. . . ."

Later he said,

> There exist very few careful safety and efficacy trials that meet the current standards set forth for evaluation of pharmaceutical weight-loss agents. A concern regarding the well-controlled clinical trials is that subjects were appropriately medically screened prior to entry into the trial so as to reduce the medical risks of those exposed. One such trial was carried out at our institution and only those subjects deemed medically acceptable were entered into treatment.

While Dr. Heymsfield makes some valid points, it's important to note he is speaking prior to testimony scheduled later by his colleague, Dr. Carol Boozer. Dr. Boozer's clinical studies, which I reported on in chapter 4, found ephedra to be safe. Dr. Heymsfield's testimony seems to downplay, if not refute, what she is prepared to say before she even gets to say it.

Dr. Raymond Woosley, M.D., Ph.D., vice president for Health Sciences at the Arizona Health Sciences Center, University of Arizona, was next to speak: "I have consistently recommended that the FDA take steps to have non-prescription products containing ephedrine removed from the market." Enough said.

Next was Douglas Zipes, M.D., director of the division of cardiology at the Krannert Institute of Cardiology, Indiana University School of Medicine in Indianapolis:

Laboratory analysis of these products has disclosed that there is considerable variation in the composition of herbal supplements from one manufacturer to another and often from lot to lot from the same manufacturer. Most of these herbal products have not been tested rigorously, with the accepted norm of standardized, controlled, prospective, randomized trials that we use to test medical drugs and devices. In addition to lack of efficacy for the claimed use, some of these products produce important side effects either directly or by interactions between the herbal remedies and prescription drugs and over-the-counter drugs.

Dr. Cynthia Culmo, R.Ph., a former official with the Texas Department of Health followed. She discussed how the previous year, the Texas department, spurred by reports of more than seven hundred cases of side effects and eight deaths linked to ephedra, tried on several occasions to impose regulations that would have required a prescription to purchase ephedra products. At the time, there were charges that the ephedra supplement industry mounted an intense lobbying effort, and Metabolife contributed generously to local politicians and helped bankroll lobbying efforts.

Next to testify was Dr. Marcia Crosse, Ph.D., acting director of Health Care-Public Health and Science Issues in the U.S. General Accounting Office (GAO):

> In summary, FDA has determined that dietary supplements containing ephedra pose a significant public health hazard based on the 2,277 adverse events reports it has received. The number of adverse event reports FDA has received for dietary supplements containing ephedra is fifteen times greater than the number it has received for the next most commonly reported herbal dietary supplement. While it is difficult to establish with certainty that a particular adverse event has been caused by the use of ephedra, based on the pattern of adverse event reports it has received and the scientific literature it has reviewed, FDA has concluded that ephedra poses a risk of cardiovascular and nervous system effects among consumers who are young to middle-aged.

She then reported a total of five deaths attributed to ephedra.

I've already discussed the GAO report, but one thing bears repeating—the GAO had found the AERs were insufficient evidence for the FDA to impose stricter limits on daily doses of ephedra.

Dr. Crosse also mentioned ephedra caused fifteen times more adverse effects than the next most common dietary supplement. This brings us to a study appearing in the March 18, 2003 issue of *Annals of Internal Medicine* entitled, "The Relative Safety of Ephedra Compared with Other Herbal Products." Commonly referred to as the Bent Study, since the lead author's name is Stephen Bent, M.D., the study found the risk for adverse events attributable to ephedra accounted for 64 percent of all adverse reactions to herbal products in the United States, yet these products represented only 0.82 percent of herbal product sales. The researchers concluded "ephedra use is associated with a greatly increased risk for adverse reactions compared with other herbs, and its use should be restricted."

Not everyone concurs. Comments filed independently with the FDA set forth a rigorous critique of this article. Poison experts, including Richard Kingston, Pharm.D., vice president and senior clinical toxicologist at PROSAR International Poison Center, and associate professor at the University of Minnesota, wrote that the authors of this paper committed serious errors, misrepresenting the data as well as committing methodological flaws.

Regarding factual misrepresentations, these authors reported that:

> All the incidents that were tabulated under the ephedra containing product categories represented "adjudicated" reports of adverse effects. . . . They [the authors of the Bent Study] failed to acknowledge that the vast majority of these calls undergo no process of authentication. As any poison center specialist who has ever fielded an exposure-related inquiry in a public poison center can attest, just mere fact that someone calls the poison center does not always mean that the event in question is accurately depicted or reported. In fact, these incidents are rarely verified by independent medical practitioners. More often than not, these incidents represent reports from the general public, often made anonymously, and typically accepted at face value.

This ended the first panel. So far, the "Anti-Ephedra" team had completely dominated the contest. In fact, the "Defend Ephedra" team hadn't even been allowed to make a peep.

Panel Two: Perp Walk

Any hopes of turning the tide in defense of ephedra with the second panel were dashed before the first words—or lack thereof—were uttered. Of the many companies selling ephedra products, the subcommittee issued subpoenas for executives from only three:

• Five officials from Metabolife: More than eighty-five consumer lawsuits are now pending against the company.
• One official from Cytodyne Technologies: Manufactured the product implicated in the death of Steve Bechler.
• Two officials from NVE Pharmaceuticals: Manufactured the product linked to the death of Sean Riggins.

Before the hearing, FDA and HHS officials told the *New York Times* they were trying to determine whether Metabolife's founder, Michael Ellis, lied when he told the Food and Drug Administration in 1998 that the company had never received notice of "any serious adverse health event" among users of Metabolife 356, its flagship product, which contains ephedra.

As expected, Mr. Ellis, along with a former Metabolife chief executive, David Brown, and the company's head nurse, Daniel Rodriguez, all refused to testify at the hearing, invoking their Fifth Amendment right to avoid compelled self-incrimination.

K. Lee Blalack II, a lawyer for Mr. Rodriguez, said his client declined to testify because he was cooperating with Justice Department investigators. Mr. Blalack said Mr. Rodriguez has received immunity from prosecution.

Robert Occhifinto, the president of NVE Pharmaceuticals, acknowledged that he had twice been convicted of federal crimes, including selling raw materials to a maker of illegal drugs, and that his company had never employed a doctor or chemist in creating the ingredient formulas for its products.

Dr. Carol Boozer was also a member of this panel, but they tried to sink her before she began. For one thing, they included her on the same panel as the ephedra-selling executives (whose problems we just documented). Was this a deliberate attempt at guilt by association?

Press reports prior to the hearing showed that experts hired by the FDA had found shortcomings in a study led by Dr. Boozer, saying supplement industry officials had promoted the study as suggesting that ephedra diet pills are safe.

Also prior to the hearings, the *New York Times* reported, "Documents released by Mr. Greenwood's subcommittee show that the three scientists hired to review the data all ended up criticizing the study. One of the agency's experts noted that through a mix-up, some of the participants who were supposed to receive placebos were given a mixture of ephedra and caffeine similar to what is in most of the diet pills, thus making the study 'impossible to rely on.'"

Let's go back to the letter from Mr. Prettyman of HHS, which stated, "The study was generally well designed and conducted." Adds Dr. Boozer, "The primary shortcomings cited were that the study would have been better if it were larger and longer—statements that are true about any study."

And what of the pill mixup? The article quotes one reviewer as saying that the amount of mixup between the placebo pills and ephedra pills—which was only 1.5 percent of the total—made the study impossible to rely on. "But none of the other three reviewers (including one from the FDA) mentioned this as a problem," says Dr. Boozer. "The *New York Times* article also implies that it was the reviewer who found the problem, when actually, I was the one who found the error, investigated it and reported it to both the journal editors and the FDA—prior to initiation of the reviews." Dr. Boozer also indicated this was pointed out by one of the reviewers, Dr. Richard Atkinson, and by a colleague, Dr. Allan Geliebter, in a letter to the editor of the *Times*, published on July 26.

The *Times* article continued:

Another FDA expert, Dr. Norman Kaplan, a hypertension specialist at the University of Texas Southwestern Medical

Center at Dallas, said that with only 87 participants completing the six-month study, the group was too small to assess safety. He also said the researchers had played down increases in heart rates and blood pressure among study participants, which could translate into a 20–40 percent increase in strokes and heart attacks among ephedra users.

Dr. Boozer points out that the article failed to mention that another reviewer, Dr. Atkinson, stated that these changes were "clinically insignificant." "The truth is that scientists differ in their interpretation of the clinical relevance of these changes," says Dr. Boozer.

Again, the *Times:* "In addition, the reviewers said the study would be a poor predictor of what might happen to the general public. Two reviewers noted that the study enrolled only people in near-perfect health, using a series of rigorous tests to eliminate 11 percent of the volunteers before the trial began."

To this point, Dr. Boozer responded, "It is standard practice in clinical trials to screen out individuals who are not healthy to avoid exposing such individuals to potential risks, and to avoid confounding the results."

Although she defended her studies during her testimony, Dr. Boozer concluded with the following statement:

> While efficacy of ephedra in promoting weight loss is established, it is not my position that the safety of herbal ephedra is proven for different populations or with different usage. Additional research would be required to determine effects in people who are not healthy, or who consume ephedra at levels above those studied, or for periods longer than six months, or in combination with prescription or illicit drugs. But, at present, there is no scientific data proving that consumption of ephedra/caffeine combinations for weight loss are unsafe, when consumed in accordance with appropriate warning labels. Additional research on the effects of ephedra on weight loss and in other areas, such as athletic performance, is clearly needed. I urge those who are responsible for policy to promote such research and to be guided by its findings.

Despite all the efforts to discredit her, Dr. Boozer's testimony stood out, more for her neutral and forthright position in a hearing brimming with agendas and politics.

Unfortunately, additional research and studies were not in the cards at this time. Again, according to the *New York Times*, citing "several scientists [who] criticized studies paid for by the dietary supplements industry," said "given the possible dangers, it would now be unethical to ask anyone to take ephedra as part of a clinical trial."

There are two problems with this statement. The first questions of ephedra safety were raised a decade ago. Why didn't the NIH initiate any large-scale trials in that time? The NIH is comprised of twenty-seven separate components, mainly institutes and centers. It receives funding of $23,256,571,000 in Congressional appropriations. At present there are only two small-scale studies being conducted on ephedra, by the National Center for Complementary Medicine and Alternative Health (and we already saw what they thought of ephedra with their "Consumer Alert" in chapter 5).

The second problem is that with the current massive tide of negativity against the herb, what scientist would be interested in putting together a grant proposal, especially if the attitude of "several scientists" is that it now would "be unethical to ask anyone to take ephedra as part of a clinical trial." What? Are we to believe no controversial pharmaceutical drugs are clinically tested?

Also appearing on the panel was Dr. Carlon M. Colker, M.D., chief executive officer and medical director for Peak Wellness, Inc., in Greenwich, Connecticut. At first glance, Dr. Colker looked out of place on this panel, which could be loosely defined as the pro-ephedra panel—warts and all. You had all the company execs with some clouds in their past, plus Dr. Boozer, who endured more negative pre-publicity than anyone. Yet, here was Dr. Colker proudly defending ephedra.

During his testimony Dr. Colker said, "I have personally taken a variety of ephedra-based dietary supplements for the purpose of losing weight. I found that they worked well for me, over and above any adjustments to my diet and exercise. I also use ephedra-based products in my practice."

Top Recipients of Political Donations within the Pharmaceutical-Health Products Industry

Top 20 Members of the House; Election Cycle 2002

Rank	Candidate	Amount
1	Johnson, Nancy L. (R-CT)	$211,317
*2	Dingell, John D. (D-MI)	$130,498
*3	Tauzin, Billy (R-LA)	$119,750
*4	Ferguson, Mike (R-NJ)	$113,718
*5	Burr, Richard (R-NC)	$104,210
6	Thomas, Bill (R-CA)	$103,475
*7	Bilirakis, Michael (R-FL)	$95,742
8	Hastert, Dennis (R-IL)	$94,050
9	Blunt, Roy (R-MO)	$83,066
10	Sununu, John E. (R-NH)	$82,999
11	Eshoo, Anna (D-CA)	$70,506
12	Bonilla, Henry (R-TX)	$67,845
13	Graham, Lindsey (R-SC)	$67,481
*14	Greenwood, James C. (R-PA)	$66,475
15	Morella, Connie (R-MD)	$64,989
16	Upton, Fred (R-MI)	$64,424
17	Thune, John (R-SD)	$60,625
18	Ramstad, Jim (R-MN)	$60,401
19	Holt, Rush (D-NJ)	$58,361
20	Frelinghuysen, Rodney (R-NJ)	$58,113

Methodology: The numbers on this page are based on contributions from PACs and individuals giving $200 or more. All donations took place during the 2001–2002 election cycle and were released by the Federal Election Commission on Monday, April 28, 2003. Feel free to distribute or cite this material, but please credit the Center for Responsive Politics.

Top Recipients of Political Donations within Dietary Supplement Industry; Election Cycle 2002

Rank	Candidate	Amount
1	Istook, Ernest J. (R-OK)	$37,000
2	Kennedy, Patrick J. (D-RI)	$17,000
3	Burton, Dan (R-IN)	$9,000
4	Kucinich, Dennis J. (D-OH)	$6,500
5	Pallone, Frank Jr. (D-NJ)	$2,500
6	Thune, John (R-SD)	$2,000
*6	Deutsch, Peter (D-FL)	$2,000
6	Bonilla, Henry (R-TX)	$2,000
9	Morella, Connie (R-MD)	$1,000
9	Graham, Lindsey (R-SC)	$1,000
9	McInnis, Scott (R-CO)	$1,000
9	Lantos, Tom (D-CA)	$1,000
9	Cunningham, Randy (R-CA)	$1,000
9	Solis, Hilda L. (D-CA)	$1,000
9	Phelps, David (D-IL)	$1,000
16	DeFazio, Peter (D-OR)	$500
16	Kolbe, Jim (R-AZ)	$500
18	Wu, David (D-OR)	$250

Dr. Colker's credentials seem impeccable: he is an attending physician at Beth Israel Medical Center in New York, as well as Greenwich Hospital in Connecticut. He was appointed by the State of Connecticut to the posts of assistant medical examiner and probate court physician. He is also a fellow in the American College of Nutrition, and a member of the American College of Physicians and the American College of Sports Medicine, among many other professional medical organizations. There's one little problem with his resume—he accepted money from Cytodyne to perform a clinical evaluation of their ephedra product Xenadrine RFA-1. Another attempt at guilt by association? Is that what the panel designers were after? We're not sure, and no one will say.

Still, Dr. Colker was firmly in the pro-ephedra camp. Not only that, he made recommendations the industry and government should be more interested in noting if public health is their overriding concern. Here's what Dr. Colker said: "While ephedra-based dietary supplements, including Xenadrine RFA-1, are appropriate for some people, there are populations for whom I think ephedra-based dietary supplements are not appropriate." Specifically, Dr. Colker mentioned people with contraindicated conditions—particularly without being monitored by their physician. He also said he believes there is significant abuse potential among youth and athletes. "Young people tend to fall into the scary mindset that 'more is better,'" said Dr. Colker. "Regulations should be designed accordingly to prevent sales to minors. Similarly, in general, athletes have a significant abuse potential in that some are willing to go to extremes to get an edge."

Panel Three was more of the same. While the Major League Baseball Players Association defended ephedra, the rest of the testimonies were provided by sports organizations that already have banned ephedra, as well as Major League Baseball.

If you were keeping score the final tally was:

Anti-Ephedra	23
Defended Ephedra	2
Draw (Dr. Boozer)	1

Oh, there was another potential point for the "Defended Ephedra" team that was ultimately withheld. This was the letter from forensic pathologist Dr. Michael Baden, former New York City chief medical examiner, who stated his opinion that the ephedra product taken by Orioles pitcher Steve Bechler very likely did not contribute to his death. The letter was never read during the proceedings.

Also, not called were Bechler's teammates, one who said when Bechler reported to spring training out of shape that he was pushed extremely hard in the workouts. Twice, Orioles' manager Mike Hargrove pulled Bechler out of workouts and even considered a "special conditioning" program for the pitcher.

Another person not called was the aforementioned Dr. Colker, who stated after Bechler died, "I don't see how ephedra could have contributed. This was clearly a case of heatstroke. Taking ephedra as directed does not lead to heatstroke."

Two other speakers did testify at the hearings: FDA Commissioner Mark B. McClellan, M.D., and J. Howard Beales, III, director of the Bureau of Consumer Protection of the Federal Trade Commission. Dr. McClellan said once the agency finishes evaluating scientific data, probably later this summer, "we will take action." At the time, whether that meant a ban on sales or new restrictions on the labels and marketing, was unclear. According to the *New York Times* account, "McClellan said the agency needs to make sure the evidence it is reviewing, such as studies on the herb and health complaints submitted to companies that use it in their products, could support a ban under the law. The 1994 statute requires the FDA to prove that a dietary supplement is harmful rather than having the manufacturer prove that it is safe, as with drugs."

It's very obvious that those who watched the hearings or read any accounts of them would come away with one unmistakable impression—ephedra is bad, bad, bad. But hey, I'm certain that was the desired outcome.

Chicken or Egg?

I finished up the hearing with the McClellan quote from the *New York Times* for a reason. It was only the last of many references during witnesses' testimony comparing drugs to dietary supplements; in particular, how unfair—and unsafe—the regulatory system is. It actually began with the *New York Times* article prior to the hearings, when the authors wrote, "While drug companies are required to prove the safety of their products and must turn over safety data and consumer complaints to the FDA, the agency, under a 1994 law, has no such authority over the makers of dietary supplements like ephedra." I'm not going to challenge these assertions until the next chapter, because I think there's something as important you should also know.

Remember this chapter's opening quote from Congressman Billy Tauzin? Perhaps the most telling aspect of his comments is when and where he made them. He didn't say this during the ephedra hearings, but rather at the time of the vote in the House on drug importations a few days later. Was Mr. Tauzin so moved by the testimony he heard, or was he trying to soften up the members of the House for a possible vote against ephedra and DSHEA?

It's impossible to tell whether companies, individuals, or industries contribute funds to certain politicians because they already support their causes, or to nudge them to the contributor's way of thinking. Probably a better question is, does it really matter? Even if a member of Congress supports one particular piece of legislation favorable to an industry—for argument's sake, let's say the pharmaceutical industry—isn't that member of Congress likely to continue to support the industry's future positions as long as the dollars keep pouring in?

Let's look more closely at some aspects of Congress' relationships with the pharmaceutical and supplement industries First, here are the members of the Subcommittee on Oversight and Investigations, which was the key subcommittee for the July 2003 hearings "Issues Relating to Ephedra-containing Dietary Supplements."

Subcommittee Members
- James C. Greenwood, Pennsylvania, Chairman
- Michael Bilirakis, Florida
- Cliff Stearns, Florida
- Richard Burr, North Carolina
- Charles F. Bass, New Hampshire
- Greg Walden, Oregon, Vice Chairman
- Mike Ferguson, New Jersey
- Mike Rogers, Michigan
- W. J. "Billy" Tauzin, Louisiana (ex officio)
- Peter Deutsch, Florida, Ranking Member
- Diana DeGette, Colorado

- Jim Davis, Florida
- Jan Schakowsky, Illinois
- Henry A. Waxman, California
- Bobby L. Rush, Illinois
- John D. Dingell, Michigan (ex officio)

On the following pages are two lists: one shows the top recipients of pharmaceutical campaign contributions, and the other shows the top recipients of supplement industry contributions, with subcommittee members indicated with an asterisk (*). Five of the top seven members of the House of Representatives receiving campaign contributions from the pharmaceutical industry are on this subcommittee. One member of the subcommittee—Peter Deutsch—received contributions from dietary supplement companies.

Money talks, and you can definitely tell whose money is doing the talking here. Only one member of the House Subcommittee received money from the dietary supplement industry (and it was a measly $2,000), while six of the subcommittee members received funds from the pharmaceutical industry, with those contributions ranging from approximately $66,000 to $130,000. Simply put, the supplement industry contributions amount to nothing more than chump change when compared to the drug dollars.

You might wonder why I went off on a tangent earlier and talked about the House of Representatives' vote on "Drug Importation" in August 2003, which received wide bipartisan support. According to the Center for Responsive Politics, campaign contribution figures show that lawmakers who sided with pharmaceutical interests (voting "no" on the bill) received an average of nearly three times the contributions from drug firms as those who took the alternate position (voting "yes"). Members who voted against the bill received an average of $39,813 in individual and PAC contributions from pharmaceutical manufacturers between 1989 and 2002. Members who voted for the bill received an average of $13,917 from the industry during that time.

The July 24, 2003 House vote on drug reimportation was unusual in that it did not break down along strict party lines, as many votes do. But the vote was not unusual in at least one major respect: campaign contributions were a solid indicator of the outcome.

The bill, which would ease the way for low-cost prescription drugs sold abroad to be "reimported" to the United States, passed by a vote of 243–186. Eighty-seven Republicans joined 155 Democrats and one Independent to support the bill in what represented a startling rebuke of the pharmaceutical industry, one of the most influential interests in Washington. Not surprisingly, the industry lobbied hard in opposing the bill.

Supporters of the bill say it would help to lower the cost of prescription drugs that are available at far cheaper prices abroad than they sell for domestically. The measure's opponents argue that reimported drugs could pose safety risks to consumers and hamper the innovation of new drugs.

It's interesting, if not helpful, to note how the Subcommittee on Oversight and Investigations—the subcommittee that conducted the July 2003 hearings regarding ephedra—voted on the bill. All six members on the above top-twenty list of contributions—Dingell, Tauzin, Ferguson, Burr, Bilirakis and Greenwood—voted "no" (in support of the pharmaceutical industry). Here's how the rest of the subcommittee members voted (the "yes" votes are noted with an asterisk):

House Member	Vote	2001–2002 Contributions	1989–2002 Contributions
Stearns (FL)	N	$25,813	$81,613
DeGette (CO)	N	$12,503	$20,003
Waxman (CA)	N	$10,000	$87,850
Davis (FL)	N	$5,500	$10,567
Rogers (MI)	N	$7,000	$17,500
*Deutsch (FL)	Y	$5,000	$40,200
Rush (IL)	N	$3,500	$5,500
Walden (OR)	N	$3,500	$8,700
*Bass (NH)	Y	$500	$1,750
*Schakowsky (IL)	Y	$0	$0

Are these subcommittee members, who will largely be responsible for the fate of ephedra—and possibly DSHEA—"in bed" with the pharmaceutical industry? While it's difficult to prove definitively, the numbers certainly support the notion.

For the sake of argument, let's say that those who voted against the bill really could have had legitimate concerns with the bill, and thus voted "no." Well, let's look at what one of these representatives—Billy Tauzin from Louisiana—had to say about the issue:

> Mr. Speaker, I join my colleague, the ranking member of our committee, the gentleman from Michigan [Mr. Dingell], in opposing this bill because it is dangerous.
>
> And with this bill tonight, its authors I know are well-intentioned, angry at the price of drugs in America, angry at Canada because they impose price controls that take advantage of our citizens, angry at those trade laws that let it happen, they are asking us tonight to do exactly what we did in 1994—to vote for a bill that says safety does not matter when it comes to drugs, that safety does not really count; that we are going to repeal tonight, if they get their way, the language that is in the law that says that FDA must certify the safety of any drugs that are imported into this country; to take away the language that says FDA must do those things appropriate to ensure that the drug supply in this country is never compromised; that bogus, counterfeit, diluted, old, rotten drugs are not permitted into this country.
>
> I voted wrong in 1994. I am not going to vote wrong tonight. I will never vote to compromise safety again in the use of drugs or products for our young people and our old people and our citizens.
>
> Tonight we will learn about those rotten drugs that are coming into this country from Canada, yes, and from a lot of other countries, transhipped through Canada. We will have the smoking gun for tonight to show what is about to happen if we open the door to that awful problem.

It's kind of funny to see what lengths this guy will go to take shots at DSHEA and the supplement industry.

And what does PhRMA, the super-pharmaceutical lobby group, have to say on the issue? Here's a statement made by Alan F. Holmer, president of PhRMA:

> To best benefit patients, Congress should focus on enacting Medicare drug coverage legislation and not on legislation dangerous to patients. The Gutknecht importation bill would jeopardize the safety of our nation's medicine supply and import foreign governments' price controls.
>
> However, we are pleased that a broadly bipartisan group of 53 Senators last night reiterated their strong opposition to changing current safety protection for patients. They urged the chairmen of the House-Senate Conference Committee to maintain the strong safety requirements pertaining to importation of drugs.

Hmmm, a lot of this language sounds awfully familiar, wouldn't you agree?

Suddenly Silent

When the ban on ephedra went into effect, not a peep was heard from the Congressmen who chastised the FDA for their shoddy evidence in 1997 when the GAO report came out, remember?

"I am concerned about the apparent lack of scientific data behind the FDA's actions," said House Science Committee Chairman F. James Sensenbrenner, Jr. "For the FDA—one of the most important regulatory agencies in government—to use such poor science for a dietary supplement raises warning flags for the other products the agency regulates."

Also this, "According to the GAO report, FDA missed the mark in their proposed regulation," said Congressman Ralph Hall. "Documentation of FDA's work was inadequate, they failed to record key steps in their analysis, they neglected to review the AERs for reliability, they arbitrarily inflated the benefits of their regulation and all of this fed into their proposed rule." Hall added, "I would suggest that FDA withdraw the proposed rule, do their job right and see whether we can't come up with a rule that everyone can support grounded in real science and reliable data."

After the ephedra ban we heard nothing from these people even though the FDA's case was essentially the same. What happened? Who got to them?

12

Is DSHEA Doomed?

As with any controversy, there are plenty of rumors. There's no question that important facets of DSHEA—such as Good Manufacturing Practices (GMPs)—have never been implemented and enforced. Some Washington insiders say FDA staffers have admitted, off the record, that they have not been forthcoming with regulations such as Good Manufacturing Practices (GMPs)—as DSHEA required the FDA to do eight years ago—because they wanted to create an issue that would result in rewriting, if not eliminating DSHEA.

This begs the question: was (and is) ephedra really the monster it was made out to be? Did it indeed kill large numbers of people, including athletes, or result in innumerable cases of heart attack, stroke, and other dangerous side effects?

Consider this prepared testimony given by Douglas Zipes, M.D., Professor of Medicine Pharmacology and Toxicology at Indiana University School of Medicine in Indianapolis at the U.S. House Subcommittee on Oversight and Investigations Hearing in July 2003, "Issues Relating to Ephedra-Containing Dietary Supplements. "In my opinion, the Dietary Supplement Health and Education Act (DSHEA) passed in 1994 has not provided a satisfactory framework to protect the public health by allowing dietary supplements to be marketed without prior approval of efficacy or safety by the FDA. Though DSHEA limits certain health claims for dietary supplements, these products are marketed in such a way that consumers believe they are effective to cure or treat many of the conditions that afflict the population, including obesity."

At this point you might be asking yourself why the dietary supplement industry is characterized by so many as an out-of-control, undependable trade run by a scurrilous lot of incompetents and crooks. Well, those are especially strong words so let me rephrase the question—why are so many people out to hinder, if not destroy, the dietary supplement industry?

Consider this possibility: the ephedra controversy is simply a wedge issue—a ploy put forth by the pharmaceutical industry and others—designed to crack the door to DSHEA, enact tighter supplement controls, and ultimately destroy the dietary supplement industry. Before you want to fit me for a tin-foil hat or ask who I thought was on the grassy knoll, at least consider the possibility.

Maybe a lesson from ancient Greek mythology can provide a helpful illustration. According to the well-known legend celebrated in the *Iliad* and the *Odyssey* of Homer, the Trojan horse was a huge, hollow wooden structure constructed by the Greeks to gain entrance into the city of Troy during the Trojan War in the twelfth or thirteenth century B.C. In traditional accounts, Paris, son of the Trojan king, ran off with Helen, wife of Menelaus of Sparta, whose brother Agamemnon then led a Greek expedition against Troy. The ensuing war lasted ten years, finally ending when the Greeks pretended to be defeated and sailed to the nearby island of Tenedos to hide. Before doing so, they left behind a large wooden horse with a raiding party of armed warriors cleverly concealed inside. Sinon, a Greek who feigned desertion, convinced the Trojans that the horse was an offering to Athena that would make Troy impregnable.

Despite warnings of a devious plot, the Trojan horse was wheeled inside the city gates by the Trojans, who did not realize that Greek soldiers were hidden inside. That night, while the Trojans celebrated their victory, the Greeks snuck out of the wooden horse, opened the gates to their comrades—who had returned from Tenedos undiscovered—and succeeded in conquering Troy.

This brings us once again to the idea that perhaps the entire uproar was not about ephedra only. Could it instead be a sort of Trojan horse, employed by the drug industry and others to gain access to the fort surrounding DSHEA? If this is a plot with designs that extend beyond public safety, then shame on the perpetrators in hiding. I'm sure everyone agrees the public deserves safe and effective dietary supplement products. However, they also ought to have straightforward, balanced, and responsible reporting by both the media and government on the safety and benefits of these products.

Getting Around the Act

The Food, Drug, and Cosmetic Act defines "drug" as any article (except devices) "intended for use in the diagnosis, cure, mitigation, treatment, or prevention of disease" and "articles (other than food) intended to affect the structure or function of the body." These words permit the FDA to stop the marketing of products with unsubstantiated "drug" claims on their labels.

Here's one viewpoint. According to the Institute of Food Technologists' "IFT's Summary," published in the July 1999 issue of *Food Technology*, this act broadened the definition of supplements to include ingredients not recognized as traditional nutrients, such as botanicals and hormones.

"Prior to DSHEA, these ingredients could have been challenged by the FDA as unapproved food additives, [but they are now] exempt from additive regulations applicable to conventional foods," note summary authors Mary Ellen Camire, Ph.D., University of Maine, and Mark A. Kantor, Ph.D., University of Maryland.

Although supplement manufacturers should ensure that their products are safe and be able to provide information to support any labeling claims, the FDA bears the burden of showing that a supplement is unsafe or mislabeled before it can restrict or ban the product's use, say Camire and Kantor. "The passage of DSHEA has created an economic and regulatory environment favorable to the expanded marketing, sales, and distribution of dietary supplements," they note. "Opportunities for consumers to purchase supplements in a free market economy are vastly increased, but [false] expectations remain that government agencies provide [consumer] protection from unsafe or mislabeled products. One of the future challenges with respect to supplements will be to reconcile these apparently opposing forces."

Money Talks

It should be obvious by now that there are those in and out of the HHS and FDA who have objected to DSHEA since its inception as just a bad law, and who have used ephedra as the poster child of their objections. Of course, the cynic in me believes it has to do more with what is so often the root of much disagreement today—that's right, money. For example, one company making ephedra-caffeine products reportedly grossed $946 million yearly during its peak. If you consider the growth of the supplement industry into a $4-billion-a-year industry since DSHEA passed in 1994, well, it's not hard to believe that there are parties outside the industry that desire a piece of the pie—especially those who already own their own chain of bakeries.

Although not many people are anxious to speak on the record about whom they think is really pushing for a ban on ephedra and overhauling DSHEA, at least one man is. "The pharmaceutical industries have huge political lobbies," said Dr. Richard Kreider, Ph.D., of Baylor University. Dr. Kreider, who is also president of the American Society of Exercise Physiologists, also pointed out that Dr. Frank Greenway, one of the EEC Seven and an internationally recognized expert in bariatric medicine from the Pennington Biomedical Research Center, reported that ephedra worked as well and was more cost effective than several diet drugs, which must have at least some pharmaceutical companies nervous. "The pharmaceutical lobby also has an interest to see supplements that may work as well as some (other) drugs be restricted."

Could Dr. Kreider be right? This is a good time to take a closer look.

Worst-Case Scenario

When attacking DSHEA and the supplement industry, critics usually cite variations of one of two themes:

1. At best, supplements don't do anything but waste people's money. And at worst, they can harm—or even kill—you.
2. Government regulators are powerless to regulate supplements under DSHEA.

To show how this first issue works—apart from ephedra—let's look at a study appearing in the April 10, 2002 issue of the *Journal of the American Medical Association*. In that issue, *JAMA* published the results of the NIH's first large-scale trial on St. John's wort (*Hypericum perforatum*) and depression. You might remember the news accounts generated from the study, which didn't vary much from a headline appearing on a press release from the National Institute of Mental Health (NIHM): "Study Shows St. John's Wort Ineffective for Major Depression of Moderate Severity."

There are a few things of interest here. First, on the bottle of St. John's wort (SJW) I take, it says it is for "mood enhancement," not necessarily moderate depression. I find when I'm under stress, it helps take the edge off and my focus improves.

But here's the most interesting finding of the study. It found that neither SJW nor the prescription drug Zoloft (sertraline) were more effective than placebo in this particular trial. Media coverage fixed solely on SJW, erroneously reporting that "St. John's wort doesn't work," yet they did not even mention Zoloft's ineffectiveness. Just to be sure, here is what the authors stated in the abstract of their study: "Interventions patients were randomly assigned to receive *H. perforatum*, placebo, or sertraline (as an active comparator) for eight weeks. Based on clinical response, the daily dose of *H. perforatum* could range from 900 to 1,500 milligrams and that of sertraline from 50 to 100 milligrams. Responders at week eight could continue blinded treatment for another eighteen weeks. "Results on the two primary outcome measures, neither sertraline [Zoloft] nor *H. perforatum* was significantly different from placebo."

And what did the NIMH say about the study? "The multi-site trial, involving 340 participants, also compared the FDA-approved antidepressant drug sertraline (Zoloft) to placebo as a way to measure how sensitive the trial was to detecting antidepressant effects."

It continued, "The trial . . . was launched in response to the growing use of St. John's wort in the United States and a need for more definitive data on its use for different types of depression. Although several smaller European studies have suggested that St. John's wort is useful in treating mild to moderately severe depression, experts who reviewed those studies concluded that they had limitations and more rigorous trials were needed before firm conclusions could be drawn."

You then have to traverse five dense paragraphs about SJW and depression before you reach this (emphasis is mine): "The overall response to sertraline on the primary measures *was not superior to that of placebo, an outcome which is not uncommon in trials of approved antidepressants. In fact, this apparent lack of efficacy occurs in up to 35 percent of trials of antidepressants.*"

Did I miss something? Why didn't the article writers investigate more closely why Zoloft, which is marketed for depression and which costs far more than St. John's wort, didn't perform better? I think the real story here is that if this study is any indicator of truth, it demonstrates that a drug, with sales of over $2 billion and prescribed to millions of Americans for severe forms of depression, may be no more effective than placebo. Zoloft costs around $100 for thirty pills, St. John's wort ranges between a few to several dollars for a month's supply, and a placebo costs virtually nothing! Again, shouldn't the news report have at least mentioned this?

Then, in February 2005 another study on St. Johns wort appeared that should have garnered headlines—especially with all the news about antidepressants—but this time, didn't. This time, *Reuters Health* reported a high-grade extract of St. John's wort proved to be more effective at treating moderate to severe depression than at least one commonly prescribed antidepressant drug, Paxil. According to the article, researchers compared the treatment of more than 250 patients between eighteen and seventy years of age for six weeks. At the end of the study, fully half of the patients in the St. John's wort extract group reported improvement in their depression, while only a third of those in the Paxil group reported any benefits at all. Perhaps just as important, the side effects experienced by the St John's wort group were much fewer and farther between than in the drug group.

But St. Johns wort isn't the only herb (besides ephedra, of course) that's been under attack.

Kava Controversy

Kava is one of the world's most popular herbs, or at least it was. Significant sales declines were seen in many herbs: Information Resources, Inc., reports that sales of kava plummeted by 68.7 percent in 2004.

Kava has been used for medicinal and ceremonial purposes in the South Pacific for at least two thousand years and is one of the top selling herbs in Europe and the U.S. It is typically used for anxiety, depression, and insomnia. Studies have indicated that kava roots contain fiber, proteins, potassium, and compounds known as kavalactones.

In European studies, kava has been shown to reduce nervousness as well as other symptoms of anxiety such as heart palpitations, chest pains, headache, dizziness, and stomach upset while not hampering mental function. In studies compared with oxazepam—a drug similar to Valium—kava was better tolerated and was shown to improve mental function in contrast to the drug which was shown to inhibit mental function.

On May 17, 2002 CNN News bleated throughout the day, "The Food and Drug Administration warns that the popular herb kava may cause liver damage!" Other media outlets also picked up the story. According to the FDA's consumer advisory, this alert was based on twenty-five reports of "adverse events" linking possible liver damage with kava use in Europe, where it has been a hugely popular alternative medicine for several years. In the United States, the FDA had received a report of a previously healthy female requiring a liver transplant, as well as several other reports of suspicious liver-related injuries.

Could it be kava was taking away too much of the market from the prescription medications used for the same purpose? Could it be that moneyed interests might be trying to discredit kava's safety for financial reasons? Could it be in the cases of liver damage, that other drugs were being taken at the same time and that kava might not have been the culprit, but only the scapegoat?

After the original AERs surfaced, a scientific review was commissioned by a coalition of industry groups, including NNFA, the American Herbal Products Association (AHPA), the Council for Responsible Nutrition (CRN), and the Utah Natural Products Alliance. Donald Waller, Ph.D., the board-certified toxicologist and professor at the University of Illinois in Chicago who conducted the review, concluded there was "no clear evidence that the liver damage reported in the United States and Europe was caused by the consumption of kava." However, Waller warned that the public should be made aware there can be adverse events with concomitant use of kava and prescription drugs, excessive alcohol consumption, and preexisting liver disease.

Aside from potential health risks associated with kava, it has been scientifically demonstrated to reduce anxiety. In fact, the Psychopharmacology Research Group published results of a pilot study demonstrating 120 milligrams of kava relieved stress and alleviated insomnia.

Also, studies conducted at Duke University show kava is safe and as effective as prescription drugs for treating stress and anxiety. "Kava has several advantages over conventional pharmacological treatments for anxiety—in clinical settings, kava has been associated with better tolerant capability and lack of physiological dependence and withdrawal," wrote Drs. Connor, Davidson, and Churchill. They found kava was as safe as placebo by comparing withdrawal symptoms, heart rate, blood pressure, and sexual function. The conclusion was that kava could be safely and effectively used to treat anxiety disorders. In addition, an analysis of seven clinical trials published in the *Journal of Clinical Psychopharmacology* supported the beneficial effects of kava to relieve the symptoms of anxiety. No cases of liver toxicity were revealed.

To investigate the liver problems reported in Europe, the American Herbal Products Association commissioned a toxicology report on kava based on the available adverse reports. The researchers found that in 18 cases out of the 30 cases, patients were taking prescription or over-the-counter drugs with known or potential liver toxicity along with kava preparations. The remaining cases were people using these potent extracts for long periods of time. According to Donald P. Waller, Ph.D., a professor of pharmacology and toxicology, "kava, when taken in appropriate dosages for reasonable periods of time, has no scientifically established potential for causing liver damage." Basically, the odds of having kava "hepatotoxicity" are one in four million.

I'm not trying to put lipstick on a pig here. There are some side effects from long-term use of kava. For example, kava has caused a scaly skin rash but only after long-term heavy usage. Also, as a member of the pepper family, kava can be excessively warming and cause conditions described in Chinese medicine as being due to liver heat. These include headache, pressure behind the eyes, hot flashes, and disturbed sleep. The overriding facts are that it's effective against depression and liver problems are minimal. Yet, if you remember Senator Durbin's bill and other bills in the House, minimal problems, like the first report of a "scaly rash," would allow the FDA to yank it off the shelves after the first complaint if they wanted. Meanwhile antidepressants that cause suicidal thoughts and other serious problems are just fine in the eyes of the FDA. Just slap a warning label on 'em.

Shell Games

You would think with the popular arthritis drugs Vioxx, Bextra, and Celebrex under fire because of health risks including death that there would be an all-out effort to find replacements. Instead, we're deluged with ads for alternative pain relievers. Well, there is a substitute, glucosamine sulfate, which is often combined with chondroitin. These natural substances have been shown to significantly reduce or even reverse the effects of arthritis.

Glucosamine is an important component of the body's basic structure that make up body tissues, including tendons and ligaments, cartilage, synovial fluid, mucus membranes, several structures in the eye, blood vessels, and heart valves.

Glucosamine sulfate contributes to the cushioning nature of the joint fluids and surrounding tissues. For instance, it helps to make the synovial fluid in joints and vertebrae thick and elastic. When this fluid becomes thin and watery, due to insufficient glucosamine production, the cushioning lessens and the bones and the cartilage scrape against each other inside the joint space, causing damage. Weakened bursa sacs in the joints can also cause tendons to rub against the hard edges of bones, increasing the chance that the cartilage will erode and cause problems with movement and flexibility.

Unlike the others, glucosamine is not an analgesic or an anti-inflammatory agent, but rather appears to halt the disease process. Improvements occur more slowly with glucosamine sulfate than with over-the-counter NSAIDs, but eventually glucosamine proves more effective.

In one study that compared glucosamine sulfate to ibuprofen, pain scores decreased faster in the first two weeks in the ibuprofen group. However, by the fourth week of the study, the group receiving the glucosamine sulfate was doing significantly better than the ibuprofen group. In another study, thirty patients with osteoarthritis were divided into two groups. Half of the patients received glucosamine sulfate, while the control group received a traditional arthritis drug formula. Both groups showed improvement in the early stages of the study, but by the end of the study, the group using the arthritis drug reverted almost to pretreatment levels, whereas the total symptom score of the glucosamine sulfate group improved dramatically.

But this is not what you read in the press. Instead you read reports of side effects that are totally blown out of proportion. Most of the side effects described in the clinical trials involving oral glucosamine salts are stomach or gastrointestinal disturbances, which most often are short term. One case report describes an allergic reaction to glucosamine sulfate in a seventy-six-year-old woman with hypertension and osteoarthritis. While the reaction could be related to glucosamine's shellfish origin, this was not explored.

Another concern with glucosamine supplementation is impaired insulin action. Numerous animal studies have shown glucosamine injections produce acute insulin resistance, which should be of concern but only for diabetics.

Echinacea Debunked

I talked about this earlier, but it bears repeating. In July 2005, the Office of Complementary Medicine trumpeted a study they sponsored that appeared in the *New England Journal of Medicine* showing echinacea, the second most popular selling herb, wasn't effective in preventing or treating the common cold. In other words, there was "no benefit" in taking echinacea.

Wow! Besides fighting the common cold, echinacea has been considered an effective therapeutic agent against not only colds but upper respiratory infections and sinusitis as well. It's also believed that it reduces the severity of symptoms such as runny nose and sore throat and reduces the duration of illness, and can fight staph and strep infections as well.

Earlier animal and human studies showed the herb improved the ability of white blood cells to attack foreign microorganisms and toxins in the bloodstream. Research also suggested that echinacea's activity in the blood may have value in the defense of tumor cells.

Then this one study appears and at least two dozen newspapers trip over each other to report that the herb doesn't work. If you read or viewed any of these news reports you'd be perfectly justified in thinking you'd be wasting your money if you ever took the stuff again. But before you chuck your echinacea, there are a couple of things you should know.

I reviewed seventeen of the many articles appearing the next day about the study; only the *New York Times* reported the actual dosages the subjects took. What's interesting is both the abstract at the *NEJM* site and the press release from the NIH's Office of Complementary Medicine didn't reveal the dosage study participants took, so it's impossible for the average person to gauge the effectiveness of the herb versus what they might use themselves. Could it be they didn't want us to know?

Here, take a look at the "Methods" Section of the Abstract of the study in the July 28, 2005 edition of the *NEJM*:

"An Evaluation of *Echinacea angustifolia* in Experimental Rhinovirus Infections"
Ronald B. Turner, M.D., Rudolf Bauer, Ph.D., Karin Woelkart, Thomas Hulsey, D.Sc., and J. David Gangemi, Ph.D.

Methods: Three preparations of echinacea, with distinct phytochemical profiles, were produced by extraction from E. angustifolia roots with supercritical carbon dioxide, 60 percent ethanol, or 20 percent ethanol. A total of 437 volunteers were randomly assigned to receive either prophylaxis (beginning seven days before the virus challenge) or treatment (beginning at the time of the challenge) either with one of these preparations or with placebo. The results for 399 volunteers who were challenged with rhinovirus type 39 and observed in a sequestered setting for five days were included in the data analysis.

It doesn't say what the dosages were, does it? You might think that that's not unusual, but it is.

Here are two other abstracts from the *NEJM* that appeared at about the same time. (I selected these randomly, I assure you.)

This one is from the July 14, 2005 issue of the *NEJM*:

"Erlotinib in Previously Treated Non–Small-Cell Lung Cancer"
Methods: Patients with stage IIIB or IV non–small-cell lung cancer, with performance status from 0 to 3, were eligible if they had received one or two prior chemotherapy regimens. The patients were stratified according to center, performance status,

response to prior chemotherapy, number of prior regimens, and prior platinum-based therapy and were randomly assigned in a 2:1 ratio to receive oral erlotinib, at a dose of 150 mg daily, or placebo.

This second one is from the August 11, 2005 issue of the *NEJM*:

"One Year of Alendronate after One Year of Parathyroid Hormone (1–84) for Osteoporosis"

Methods: In the data reported here, women who had received parathyroid hormone (1–84) monotherapy (100 µg daily) in year 1 were randomly reassigned to one additional year with either placebo (60 subjects) or alendronate (59 subjects). Subjects who had received combination therapy in year 1 received alendronate in year 2; those who had received alendronate monotherapy in year 1 continued with alendronate in year 2. Bone mineral density at the spine and hip was assessed with the use of dual-energy X-ray absorptiometry and quantitative computed tomography (CT).

See? Both studies indicate the dosages administered to the subjects. Why didn't the echinacea study do the same? Is it important? You bet it is.

Mark Blumenthal, founder and executive director of the nonprofit American Botanical Council said in a released statement it would have been optimal if this trial had tested the echinacea preparations at more frequent and/or higher doses. "Dosage is one of the most important aspects in assessing any therapeutic agent. Many clinicians who recommend echinacea for treatment of upper respiratory tract infections related to colds and flu normally utilize a frequency of use and/or a total daily dose that is higher than the one used in this trial."

What would happen in you only took a third of any recommended dosage of anything? Would it be as effective? Of course not. The "suggested" German dosage they used is also suspicious. These happen to be the standard dosages recommended—and that scares people—that could be adopted if Codex goes into effect. I'll cover this in greater detail in a later chapter. I just wanted to give you a heads-up.

I decided to do a little digging. It turns out the lead investigator of the echinacea study, and the one quoted most often in news accounts is Ronald B. Turner, M.D., professor of pediatrics at the University Of Virginia School of Medicine in Charlottesville, Virginia. While Dr. Turner's credentials are impressive, and he's considered an expert in the field, there's one aspect of his career he didn't disclose, and the press hasn't investigated. I think it could be a potentially serious conflict of interest.

At a roundtable discussion at the 2002 American Thoracic Society Meeting about viral respiratory infections at the ATS, Dr. Turner was compelled to reveal—these are ATS's words not mine—"A significant relationship with industry." Turns out Dr. Turner's "significant relationship" was with a company named ViroPharma that developed a drug named Pleconaril, a compound targeting the primary viral cause of the common cold.

This is an interesting drug. From 1997 to 2002 there were nearly a thousand news stories on Pleconaril in newspapers and on television. In an article in the *British Medical Journal,* reporters wore out their thesaurus' trying to come up with superlative terms for the drug such as "cure," "miracle," "wonder drug," "super drug," and "a medical first." It was described as "good news for physicians and their patients," "potentially huge," and as a treatment that "may drastically help relieve your misery." It was compared with the search for the Holy Grail and with humankind's landing on the moon. Most of the stories reported that the drug appeared to cause few side effects, none serious. In January 2000 the Associated Press wire service ran a story quoting one ViroPharma-funded investigator saying, "This *is* the cure for the common cold."

In a December 2001, the *Los Angeles Times* ran a story entitled "The Cold Virus Meets Its Match." The article quoted Dr. Turner pontificating about Pleconaril and another drug under investigation that, "Both of these drugs are very potent antiviral agents that work against a broad spectrum of different rhinoviruses." Wow! He should know, even though even in that article Dr. Turner didn't admit he was involved in the clinical trials for Pleconaril.

A few months later, the FDA issued a "not approvable" letter for an oral tablet formulation of Pleconaril for treatment of the common cold in adults. The FDA cited clinical data showing subjects taking Pleconaril reduced the span of cold symptoms by only a day. As for those "few side effects, none serious," it seems the drug upset the menstrual cycle in many women and to their dismay, a few women on birth control pills testing the drug became pregnant. Oops! I guess Dr. Turner missed that pesky little side effect. Oh well, back to the drawing board.

In the same *BMJ* article, Dr. Turner blamed the media for the hype. He called the news coverage a disservice to the public, contributing to the public's science illiteracy. "People can't distinguish between valid results and charlatanism," he told the *BMJ*. "You pick up the paper one day and read that cholesterol causes heart attacks and you pick it up the next day and read that it doesn't. It becomes easy for people to feel that scientists don't know what they're doing."

OK, Dr. Turner. Thanks for clearing that up.

Three years after the oral formulation failed to receive approval, ViroPharma licensed rights to develop and commercialize intranasal Pleconaril in the United States and Canada from Sanofi-Synthelabo. Then, late in 2004, ViroPharma entered into an option agreement to license ViroPharma's intranasal formulation of Pleconaril to Schering-Plough for the treatment of the common cold in the United States and Canada. The latest reports say it could be on the market in 2006.

So let's recap. An oral formulation of a drug fails, so the company develops an intranasal formulation. One of their researchers— without revealing he has had ties to the company—then tests a low-dosage version of a popular herbal competitor as the drug being developed by the company he had or has "a significant relationship" with, and declares the competitor's product doesn't work.

Uh-uh. I don't buy it.

Double Whammy

Soon after the echinacea study appeared, another study slammed two popular herbs, kava-kava (again) and valerian root, a non habit-forming herb that relieves anxiety and nervous irritability. It is also used as a sedative and sleep aid.

In a study appearing in the July 2005 issue of *Medicine*, Dr. Bradly P. Jacobs from the University of California-San Francisco performed an "Internet trial" to evaluate the effectiveness of kava and valerian. Potential subjects who reported anxiety and insomnia were recruited through e-mail and Web sites. The final study included 391 participants from forty-five states.

By mail, one group of patients received kava plus an inactive valerian placebo and one group received valerian plus kava placebo; a third group received double placebos. After four weeks of treatment, subjects used a secure Web site to complete follow-up questionnaires.

The researchers say the herbal extracts were no more effective than placebo in reducing the symptoms they were intended to treat. Anxiety scores decreased by 25 percent for patients taking placebo, compared to about 21 percent with either kava or valerian.

The effects on insomnia were also similar—in all three groups, insomnia scores and time to falling asleep decreased by about 50 percent. The results were comparable across patient subgroups, such as those with higher vs. lower depression scores.

Here is one important point brought out in the study: The researchers say the study was performed "before recent safety warnings concerning liver damage related to kava. However, none of the patients taking kava reported any liver-related side effects."

Of course they didn't. I already talked about the kava–liver damage link. Here they're perpetuating the myth once again.

Then there's the "smell test" I brought up with the echinacea study. That is, what were the dosages? Here are the pertinent parts of the abstract appearing in the journal *Medicine*:

"An Internet-Based Randomized, Placebo-Controlled Trial of Kava and Valerian for Anxiety and Insomnia."

Medicine. 84(4):197-207, July 2005.

Jacobs, Bradly P., M.D, M.P.H.; Bent, Stephen, M.D.; Tice, Jeffrey A., M.D.; Blackwell, Terri, M.A.; Cummings, Steven R. M.D., FACP

"We randomly assigned 391 eligible participants to 1 of the following 3 groups, and mailed 28 days' supply: kava with valerian placebo (n = 121), valerian with kava placebo (n = 135), or double placebo (n = 135). The primary outcome measures were changes from baseline in anxiety (STAI-State questionnaire) and insomnia (Insomnia Severity Index [ISI]) compared with placebo."

Again, as with the echinacea study no dosage amounts are listed. We don't know what they took.

But there's one other interesting element here. One of the author's names is Stephen Bent. Does that name ring a bell? He was a co-author of a study I mentioned in chapter 11, commonly referred to as the Bent Study, since the lead author's name is Stephen Bent, M.D. If you recall, the study found the risk for adverse events attributable to ephedra accounted for 64 percent of all adverse reactions to herbal products in the United States, yet these products represented only 0.82 percent of herbal product sales. Poison experts, including Richard Kingston, Pharm.D., vice president and senior clinical toxicologist at PROSAR International Poison Center, and associate professor at the University of Minnesota, wrote that the authors of this paper committed serious errors, misrepresenting the data as well as committing methodological flaws.

E Is for Exasperated

At the American Heart Association meeting in New Orleans in November 2004, researchers presented a study claiming there is an increased risk of death for those consuming vitamin E at amounts greater than 400 IU/day. The study, which appeared in the *Annals of*

Internal Medicine, also made the front page of *USA Today* and numerous other national media outlets.

I have been taking 800 IU/day of natural vitamin E for many years. I was a bit startled to say the least and immediately cut my dose in half. Then I looked a little closer. I realized the study was not a controlled trial to determine if supplementation with vitamin E increased the risk of death. Rather it was a meta-analysis of other previously published studies from 1993–2004 in which vitamin E was supplemented at doses ranging form 16.5–2,000 IU/day. The authors used nineteen studies in their analysis, with the subjects in nine of the studies taking supplements of vitamin E only. The subjects involved in the studies in the analysis had a pre-existing condition, or were at a significantly increased risk of developing the disease that was being investigated in the respective study, which could have impacted the findings.

In a press release issued by the Dietary Supplement Information Bureau, Dr. C. Wayne Callaway, an expert in internal medicine, endocrinology, metabolism, and clinical nutrition, and former head of the lipid and nutrition programs at the Mayo Clinic, disputed the findings. "It is important to point out that those participating in the study suffered from a range of degenerative diseases, with varying levels of severity," said Dr. Callaway in an article. "To focus on a relatively small increase in vitamin E in some patients who also had heart failure ignores other risk factors."

I looked at the different factors Dr. Callaway cited. It turns out the patients of the study were at least fifty-five years old with vascular disease or diabetes mellitus, and at least one other significant cardiovascular risk factor. Of 7,030 patients enrolled, 916 were deceased at the beginning of the extension, 1,382 refused participation, 3,994 continued to take the study intervention, and 738 agreed to follow-up. Study participants received a daily dose of natural-source vitamin E (400 IU) or matching placebo over a median of 7.0 years.

Also, subjects in the study were typically taking five different medications in addition to vitamin E—including beta-blockers, anti-platelet agents, statins, diuretics, calcium-channel blockers, and ACE inhibitors—yet the increase in heart failure (from 12.1 percent in the placebo group to 13.5 percent in the vitamin E group) was attributed exclusively to vitamin E, with no adjustment for pharma-cotherapy. Total vitamin E blood levels may appear to be normal but the person is still at risk because of the small, dense lipoprotein par-ticles—another factor that appears not to have been addressed by the study in question.

"Numerous scientific studies have attested to vitamin E's great health benefits and safety," said David Seckman, executive direc-tor and CEO of the National Nutritional Foods Association (NNFA). "Not only for cardiovascular health, but also for immune function, DNA repair and to help protect the body against the effects of free radicals. Vitamin E continues to be a safe and effec-tive part of a healthy diet, and the suggested findings are incom-plete and misleading."

After investigating the study on my own, I started taking 800 IU of vitamin E again.

Swimming Against the Tide

The NIH often touts its National Center for Complementary and Alternative Medicine (NCCAM) and Office of Dietary Supple-ments as clearinghouses and research centers for alternative medi-cine, including dietary supplements, (if you discount the misleading article NCCAM featured about athletes dying from ephedra, of course). Well, with friends like these . . .

I showed you what the other NIH office, the National Institute of Mental Health (NIHM) did with St. John's wort. Maybe NCCAM would do better and the ephedra article was an aberration. Man, was I disappointed. I went to their site and searched for kava. This is the first item that appeared:

"Kava Linked to Liver Damage"

Of the other seventeen items listed, not one discussed any of the other clinical trials. They did a little better with glucosamine. To their credit they are in the midst of a major clinical trial, the "Glucosamine/Chondroitin Arthritis Intervention Trial (GAIT)."

Upcoming Legislation

Here are a few of the bills pending that could damage access to dietary supplements. I'll warn you, though. Even if these should wither or be withdrawn, you can be sure they'll be replaced by other onerous bills:

• Senator Richard Durbin from Illinois has submitted an amendment to prohibit the sale of any supplements containing a stimulant on a military installation or in a commissary or exchange store. Tucked away in the "National Defense Authorization Act for Fiscal Year 2006" (S.1042), it would also establish Adverse Event Reporting by supplement manufacturers.

• Senator Durbin has also reintroduced SB729, which would create a new federal food safety agency. Congresswoman Rosa DeLauro has introduced a similar bill in the House (HR 1507). Some industry observers who have analyzed the bill say it could cause DSHEA to be repealed and reclassify and regulate dietary supplements as drugs.

• The Dietary Supplement Access and Awareness Act (HR 3156) would require an Adverse Reaction Reporting System for botanicals that could permit the FDA to ban any non-vitamin dietary supplement without evidence that the substance caused harm. This could allow the Secretary of Health and Human Services to ban a product if he had "determined that risks outweighed benefits." Besides burdening the manufacturers with additional reporting requirements as I've said before, isn't this the government's job? Frankly, if there's a problem with a substance, I don't want the company that stands to profit to tell me, I want my "objective, unbiased" regulatory agency to warn me.

Here are more reasonable alternatives:

• Introduced as a substitute amendment for Senator Durbin's bill by Senators Tom Harkin from Iowa and Orrin Hatch from Utah, is an amendment that would help ensure that DSHEA finally be fully implemented, funded and enforced. It also directs the FDA to develop an appropriate system for the reporting of serious adverse reactions to dietary supplements.

• There is another bill, HR 2352, the Consumers' Access to Health Information Act, which would allow accurate labeling claims on the "curative, mitigation, treatment, and prevention effects" of foods and dietary supplements on disease and health-related conditions while not causing products to be treated as a drug by the FDA. The bill would ensure that the FDA does not suppress accurate health claims.

No preliminary results are available yet.

Then there's vitamin E. Of the eighty-two links listed, guess which one is listed first? Here's a recap:

March 18, 2005

What are the results of the HOPE-TOO Study?

"A report published in the March 16, 2005 issue of the *Journal of the American Medical Association* finds no clear evidence that men and women who had vascular disease or diabetes and who took 400 IU of vitamin E daily for 7 years reduced their risk of cancer compared to others with these conditions who took a placebo. The study was not large enough to determine if vitamin E could prevent specific cancers."

Is the Pattern Clear Yet?

Let's go back to the list of the top-selling drugs in the United States that I presented in chapter 2:

1. Lipitor, $6.8 billion, cholesterol, Pfizer, Inc.

2. Zocor, $4.4 billion, cholesterol, Merck & Co.

3. Prevacid, $4.0 billion, heartburn, TAP Pharmaceutical Products, Inc.

4. Procrit, $3.3 billion, anemia, Johnson & Johnson
5. Zyprexa, $3.2 billion, mental illness, Eli Lilly & Co.
6. Epogen, $3.1 billion, anemia, Amgen Inc.
7. Nexium, $3.1 billion, heartburn, Merck & Co.
8. Zoloft, $2.9 billion, depression, Pfizer, Inc.
9. Celebrex, $2.6 billion, arthritis, Pfizer, Inc.
10. Neurontin, $2.4 billion, epilepsy, Pfizer, Inc.
11. Advair Diskus, $2.3 billion, asthma, GlaxoSmithKline PLC
12. Plavix, $2.2 billion, blood clots, Bristol-Myers Squibb Co.
13. Norvasc, $2.2 billion, high blood pressure, Pfizer, Inc.
14. Effexor XR, $2.1 billion, depression, Wyeth
15. Pravachol, $2.0 billion, cholesterol, Bristol-Myers Squibb Co.
16. Risperdal, $2.0 billion, mental illness, Johnson & Johnson
17. OxyContin, $1.9 billion, pain, Perdue Pharma
18. Fosamax, $1.8 billion, osteoporosis, Merck & Co.
19. Protonix, $1.8 billion, gastrointestinal reflux disease, Wyeth
20. Vioxx, $1.8 billion, arthritis, Merck & Co.

Vitamin E is a threat to numbers 1, 2, 13, and 15. Kava and St. John's wort could impact numbers 5, 8, 14, and 16. Glucosamine acceptance could supplant numbers 9 and 20. That's ten of the top 20 selling drugs representing many billions of dollars in sales each year.

With the amount of money we give to NIH and its offices, shouldn't there be a greater effort to investigate whether dietary supplements offer a better and cheaper alternative to expensive drugs? Is the "billions and billions of dollars in sales" the real deterrent for them to do so?

In the introduction to this book I mentioned an e-mail I sent to an editor of a popular health magazine asking what she thought about the vitamin E study I just talked about. If you recall, she sent me the following reply: "There is some consensus that the vitamin E study was a planned 'negative' study—actually one among several others due out in the next few months—to create a 'soft landing' for Codex. Many people in the industry think that the Codex international guidelines is a back door being used by the pharmaceutical industry to control/regulate the natural products industry in the U.S."

Her mention of Codex set off alarms in my head, as it should in yours. You see—besides the desire by some to dismantle DSHEA there's something even more odious in our midst.

13

The Hidden Threat of Codex

Early this year I received an e-mail that stated, "You're out of vitamins C and E. You go to your natural food store, but you can't find the kind you want on the shelf. You ask a clerk to find them for you. She says you can't get your vitamin E as mixed tocopherols (the best natural form) anymore, and asks if you like your vitamin C in the 100- or 200-milligram size. The 1,000-milligram size, you say.

"Where have you been?" she asks. "The types and sizes of vitamins you just asked for have been declared illegal by the Dispute Settlement Body of the World Trade Organization!"

Near the bottom it states, "As a member of the World Trade Organization, the United States does commit to act in accordance with the rules of the multilateral body. The United States is legally obligated to ensure national laws do not conflict with World Trade Organization rules."

The contents of the e-mail were from an article written by Jonathan V. Wright, M.D., medical director and founder of the Tahoma Clinic in Renton, Washington. What Dr. Wright wrote about had to do with an international movement to forcing the U.S. to conform to international guidelines and standards. As investigative journalist Peter Byrne states in his article "The Fate of Vitamins," "A low-profile organization created by the United Nations is about to ban global trade of many essential nutrients—and there may be nothing you can do to stop it."

Many people think the ephedra issue is part of a larger plan to not only undermine DSHEA, but also to join a worldwide movement that would essentially destroy the dietary supplement industry. Seem too much like a "conspiracy theory" sort of statement? Maybe, but consider this. There exists an organization, called the Codex Alimentarius (which is Latin for "Food Code"), a United Nations commission that is also part of the World Health Organization (WHO). The goal of the Codex Alimentarius Commission is to set international standards for anything consumed by humans. For dietary supplement products, the intent is to establish an international guideline stating that no supplements can be sold for preventive or therapeutic purposes.

No problem there you might think, such a guideline already exists under DSHEA. That's purely wishful thinking, but you're not alone. Many health organizations believe that and Codex proponents are more than happy to perpetuate that dream-like scenario. What many others believe is that the Codex commission came under the influence of the pharmaceutical lobby and instead of focusing on food safety, it is using its power to promote worldwide restrictions on vitamins. At the same time, our U.S. Codex delegation made matters worse. For instance, in 1996 at a meeting in Bonn, Dr. Elizabeth Yetley of the FDA illegally seconded a motion to shift deliberations on herbs out of Codex, where, consistent with U.S. law, at least, they were considered foods to a secret panel at WHO that considers herbs as drugs, making them only available by "prescription."

But here is where it gets even scarier. Some say the Codex Alimentarius Commission also wants to limit over-the-counter sales of dietary supplements to very low potencies based on the German Risk Assessment Institute (BfR) maximum permitted levels. These approved levels—determined by official jargon know as "science-based risk assessment" which, frankly, is more appropriate for chemicals than dietary supplements. It's expected these levels will be well below the therapeutic range—in some cases even lower than the U.S. Recommended Dietary Allowance (RDA) levels, possibly as low as 15 percent. (If the "German Risk Assessment" sounds vaguely familiar, you have read about it before. They were the source for the low levels of echinacea in the clinical trial I talked about earlier in this book. Do you see the pattern emerging yet?)

Safe upper limits (SUL)—which typically are much higher than RDAs and many consumers approach for maximum benefit—will have no bearing on the dosages allowed. Any product that contains higher levels of vitamins, minerals, or other ingredients than the allowed amount—such as your daily multivitamin or the bottle of vitamin C on the grocery store shelf—would theoretically become pharmaceuticals. In other words, you would probably need a prescription to get a daily multivitamin. Who would be behind this? Take a wild guess. Those fighting Codex say it's simply a plot to enrich multinational food and chemical corporations under the guise of promoting human health, all with the blessing of the FDA and USDA. Once again, it's the old risk versus benefit equation. Codex is all about "risk" and bases their limits on minimal and questionable criteria.

Although you may not have heard of the Codex controversy (don't feel bad if you haven't, you're in the vast majority of Americans), it is not a new issue. Here's what well-known dietary consultant and author Gary Null wrote about the Codex Alimentarius Commission back in the September 1999 issue of *Penthouse* magazine:

> In recent years . . . big medicine, the pharmaceutical establishment, and their allies in big government all joined forces to protect their own interests. These threatened groups engage in fear-mongering before Congress to get legislation that would sic state medical boards on alternative therapies, let dietitians control the dispensing of nutritional advice, and keep the public from having freedom of choice by turning as many nutrients as possible into prescription drugs. This is what the future will bring unless we take action.

He continues, "Not far into the twenty-first century you may be saying so-long to your St. John's wort, goodbye to your Ginkgo biloba. These and many other supplements may become things of the past, at least as reasonably priced over-the-counter items."

Paranoia? Perhaps. But as a friend once told me, "Just because you're paranoid doesn't mean people aren't out to get you."

Some say Codex isn't a threat at all. Others, meanwhile, are orchestrating letter-writing campaigns charging, among other things, that many of the dietary supplement trade groups are being infiltrated by the big pharmaceutical companies and are hell-bent to destroy the industry. Could that be true?

Codex and the United States

The United States is one of the 165 member countries of the Codex Alimentarius Commission, an international food standards program created by the Food and Agriculture Organization (FAO) and the WHO. The Codex commission is mostly composed of corporate officials from the agribusiness, pharmaceutical, and chemical industries, and government officials that "regulate" those industries. The U.S. delegation has many familiar names.

As I've stated, one of the purposes of the Codex commission is to "harmonize" international food trade. If Null and others are right, here are a few of the implications:

• WHO would get to classify all dietary supplements as drugs.
• The Codex commission would limit over-the-counter sales of dietary supplements while reclassifying others as pharmaceuticals, available only through a pharmacist.
• Under World Trade Organization (WTO) rules, Codex guidelines override the regulations of individual countries.
• Member countries (including the U.S.) that refuse to accept and enforce the WTO directives are subject to severe trade sanctions.

And here's something else to ponder. The person who opened the door for U.S. participation in Codex recently resurfaced as a senior nutrition research scientist in the Office of Dietary Supplements (ODS) at NIH. ODS is supposed to be an objective research and disseminating arm of NIH regarding alternative medicine. At times I've noticed them getting facts wrong either by an honest mistake or, perhaps deliberately. Steve Bechler's death is one example; the echinacea study is another. Coupled with the reports that some of the dietary supplement associations have been infiltrated by executives from pharmaceutical companies, it makes you wonder, could this all be part of the Codex plot?

As Jenny Thompson from the Health Sciences Institute writes, "Incredible, isn't it? Our freedom to make our own healthcare choices may simply be taken away by an international commission. But at this point, the imposition of the Codex guidelines isn't necessarily a done deal. And although the situation is not promising, it's still not too late to help prevent it from happening."

John C. Hammell, president of the International Advocates for Health Freedom (IAHF) Hammell will never win a Mr. Congeniality award, but I doubt he cares. Hammell talks and writes about the issue of dietary substances with great passion and he takes no prisoners. He has fought for the rights of consumers for years, and proudly states that he played a key role in pushing for DSHEA in the early 1990s. Hammell knows his stuff, but often ruffles feathers until others dig in their heels, and in some cases, I suspect, disagree with him just on principle.

Hammell also claims that the pharmaceutical companies have infiltrated the dietary supplement industry and are working from inside to destroy it. The organization he singles out for particular harsh criticism is IADSA (International Alliance of Dietary Supplement Trade Associations), which IADSA says was created to "defend the interests of the dietary supplement industry" as a UN NGO participant at Codex. Hammell writes:

Appearances can be deceiving. It is IAHF's opinion that Pfizer did not become the world's number-one pharmaceutical company by accident—they got there by being very shrewd businessmen, and that includes having a very solid grasp of politics—and how to manipulate perceptions. It is IAHF's opinion that Pfizer has a vested interest in suppressing the dietary supplement industry worldwide.

It is IAHF's opinion that Pfizer's game plan is to have their employee, Randy Dennin, make contributions via Pfizer subsidiary Capsugel to numerous dietary supplement industry causes and functions (e.g., American Association for Health Freedom, Citizens for Health, NPI Center, etc.); and to join numerous vitamin industry trade associations, (e.g., NNFA, AHPA, CRN, IADSA) in order to create an *appearance* of loyalty to the dietary supplement industry.

Mr. Dennin is, in fact, chairman of IADSA. Since its creation in 1998, IADSA has developed into an alliance of more than fifty dietary supplement associations spread over six continents. There are at present more than 9,500 companies now part of IADSA member associations. Hammell also takes NNFA to task because of their relationship with Dennin and has demanded they scrutinize their bylaws and kick Capsugel out of the organization because of "conflict of interest."

Is there any merit to Hammell's many accusations?

Actions Speak Louder

On July 4, 2005, the UN's Codex Alimentarius Commission ratified a framework to create a global trade guideline for vitamins and minerals. The most controversial section of the "Codex Guidelines for Vitamin and Mineral Food Supplements" dictates the establishment of upper limits for the amount of a nutrient that will be allowed in a supplement product.

While business interests are celebrating a regulation that these upper limits will be based on science, consumer health advocacy groups are fearful that it's defective science that will be used, resulting in inappropriately low ceilings; that the "safety standards" imposed by the commission, in essence, treat vitamins as potentially dangerous drugs, imposing "Maximum Safe Permitted Levels" of potency that would make them practically useless.

Hammell says that in November 2005, Codex will move to fill in the blanks on allowable potency levels. "The methodology being employed by the World Health Organization to fill in these blanks is scientifically biased given that it is only examining supposed 'risks' of vitamins," writes Hammell, "while completely ignoring benefits."

Contrast that statement with a press releases issued by IADSA in July days after the decision of the Codex Alimentarius Commission to adopt the Guidelines for Vitamin and Mineral Food Supplements: "The Codex decision was hailed by IADSA Chairman, Randy Dennin, as 'a significant step on the path to better regulation worldwide.' The development of the Codex Guidelines for Vitamin and Mineral Food Supplements, under the auspices of the World Health Organization and the United Nations' Food and Agriculture Organization, has been a priority for IADSA since its creation in 1998."

The National Nutritional Foods Association (NNFA) agrees with IADSA's viewpoint. In a press release, David Seckman, NNFA's executive director and CEO, said:

> Protecting our members' rights to sell dietary supplements goes hand-in-hand with ensuring they receive accurate information about government policies that affect their businesses. Although we have regularly communicated the facts to our members about Codex and other international activities, with all the misinformation that has been circulating, we think it will be helpful to have accurate information collected in one convenient place.

Seckman added that if DSHEA—the Dietary Supplement Health and Education Act of 1994—were to actually be imperiled, whether from an international or domestic threat, it would be NNFA's first priority to take any necessary steps to ensure the law is preserved.

NNFA says it has lobbied for the adoption of DSHEA-style laws or regulations in the international arena. "NNFA has been and will continue to be very active with the Codex commission by attending meetings and filing comments that press for Codex's adoption of DSHEA and other provisions of U.S. law, such as the ability to use structure/function and health claims."

NNFA points out industry champions in Congress don't believe neither Codex nor CAFTA will affect how dietary supplements are regulated in the United States. They point to a talk given by Senator Tom Harkin from Iowa, one of DSHEA's co-sponsors during

NNFA's recent annual meeting. Senator Harkin acknowledged that "there are rumors out there" about CAFTA, but "American consumers' access to supplements is governed by U.S. law." Harkin also noted that, "Any new law applying to supplements will have to go through the United States Senate. And I assure you that Senator Hatch and I will not let any international guidelines define what supplements can be made available here in the U.S. market." Also, in a recent letter to his congressional colleagues, Representative Chris Cannon from Utah warned his fellow representatives to "not fall prey to the false allegations that the implementation of CAFTA will limit access to dietary supplements." Cannon added that "CAFTA will in no way affect the sales of dietary supplements."

The Council for Responsible Nutrition (CRN) has taken a similar stand. They say the Codex guideline for vitamin and mineral supplements will benefit both manufacturers and consumers and that those who opposed the decision have looked for ways to misinterpret its implications.

CRN says the latest effort involves the numerous references being made to the Central American Free Trade Agreement (CAFTA). They say critics of the decision by Codex to adopt the long-needed guideline on vitamins and minerals cite the adoption of CAFTA as an imminent danger to consumer access to dietary supplements. "Nothing could be farther from the truth," CRN said in a press release. "CAFTA contains no reference to dietary supplements, and in fact contains no language at all that is different from language contained in the North American Free Trade Agreement (NAFTA), the Free Trade Agreement of the Americas (FTAA), the World Trade Organization (WTO) and General Agreement on Tariffs and Trade (GATT) or any other of the seminal international trade agreements that have been concluded over the course of the past several decades."

Ah, therein lies the rub, say Codex and CAFTA critics. They say the devil is in the details and even supporters of Codex and CAFTA don't fully understand the implications. With the Codex Guidelines for Vitamin and Mineral Food Supplements now officially available to be enforced by the WTO, health freedom advocacy groups point out that some terms in CAFTA would strengthen the movement to force the U.S. to weaken DSHEA.

At this point, you may be thinking this is a chapter about the opinions of John Hammell versus everyone else. It's not. He has plenty of allies, including the American Holistic Health Association, Citizens for Health, the Coalition for Health Freedom, and numerous health and consumer advocates. Another organization that disagrees with the IADSA assessment is the Alliance for Natural Health (ANH), a pan-European association of manufacturers, distributors, and consumers. As ANH's executive director recently stated, "It appears that the Codex guidelines for food supplements include faulty procedures that contradict Codex's own rules, as pointed out by the U.S.-based National Health Federation, itself a Codex participant. We have also demonstrated that the risk assessment system being considered by Codex is scientifically flawed."

Patrick McGrath, associate director of Citizens for Health, said CAFTA could "weaken protection of dietary supplement consumer choices" through the establishment of a CAFTA committee that would consult with the Codex Alimentarius Commission.

Hammell says ANH, along with all other critics of WHO's biased methodology, were barred from participation in a "Nutrient Risk Assessment Workshop" presided over by an FDA employee, Dr. Christine Lewis Taylor, "an unelected bureaucrat with a known bias against the Dietary Supplement Health & Education Act of 1994 and against consumer access to vitamins and minerals within the therapeutic range." Hammell says that given the well-demonstrated bias and flawed scientific methodology being employed, it is highly probable that Codex will fill in the blanks for allowed potencies of vitamins and minerals to potencies that are well below the therapeutic range—even lower than RDAs in some instances.

Hammell remains undaunted. "Immediate action is required to stop a finalized Codex vitamin standard from being rammed through on November 1, 2004 at the Codex meeting of the Committee on Nutrition and Foods for Special Dietary Uses."

Trading on Our Health

As the debate over the Central America Free Trade Agreement (CAFTA) raged during the summer, there was concern on the part of many that as part of the agreement dietary supplements would be affected. In an e-mail message, Hammell pointed out that Section 6 of CAFTA requires the United States to form a Sanitary Phyto-sanitary Measures Committee for the purpose of insuring that we harmonize our laws under the terms of the SPS Agreement in the WTO. Also, that Article 3 of the WTO's SPS Agreement requires us to harmonize our food safety laws, which includes DSHEA, to Codex standards. Hammell points out that even though this is a trade agreement with a small part of Latin America, it gives Codex the authority to set the standards for food safety, including vitamins and minerals.

What are SPS measures? That's a good question. The U.S. Department of Agriculture's Foreign Agricultural Service (FAS) defines SPS measures as "any measure, procedure, requirement, or regulation, taken by governments to protect human, animal, or plant life or health from the risks arising from the spread of pests, diseases, disease-causing organisms, or from additives, toxins, or contami-nants found in food, beverages, or feedstuffs." FAS points out that virtually all countries, including the United States, supported the development of new and strengthened SPS rules in the Uruguay Round in 1995. Before the Uruguay Round, trade rules for SPS measures were so vague that countries could protect domestic pro-ducers from international competition by establishing import restrictions justified only by the country's assertion that the meas-ure existed for "health reasons." These restrictions were of partic-ular significance for U.S. agriculture, as countries could cite unfounded risks of a pest or disease as reason to keep out U.S. exports. With the Uruguay Round's removal of other agricultural market access barriers, rules for disciplining the use of SPS measures became even more important.

CRN says the CAFTA and SPS argument is nonsense. They say the only quality unique to CAFTA was it was recently under negotiation, and therefore in the news. "Cynically, Codex critics have effectively taken old wine and placed it in new bottles in an effort to tie the completely unrelated adoption of a vitamin and mineral supplement guideline at Codex with a trade agreement that, while headline news, is nothing more than another agreement in a series of agreements negotiated over several decades. The real target of the critics is the global trading system."

As the CAFTA debate raged on—sadly only among the most ardent people with strong feelings both pro and con—the average American tuned out. The measure passed the Senate and squeaked through the House by only one or two votes (depending on who you talk to) after a late-night vote and considerable arm-twisting. While the victors pontificated on the wonderment of free trade elevating our neighbors to the south and creating jobs here at home (yeah, right—consumers in El Salvador making pennies per hour are lining up to buy our SUVs and computers as we speak). What many didn't notice is CAFTA awarded pharmaceutical companies with measures that protect and extend their monopoly rights in Central America.

At Glacier-Like Speed

Hammell says his critics and defenders of Codex either have their head in the sand or are being purposefully mislead—or are misleading people themselves. He claims the movement to overturn DSHEA and adopt international standards for dietary supplements is a long-range plan implemented by glacier-like steps so as not to attract attention, having learned their lesson after consumers got wise and pushed for the passage of DSHEA in 1994. "They have convened high-level think tanks with the best and brightest PR and legal minds in the world to create flow charts of just how to methodically subvert the will of the American people who voted with their feet against FDA tyranny in 1994 via the biggest outpouring of letters and phone calls ever sent to the U.S. Congress in the *history* of Congress."

With no GMPs for dietary supplements in place, the fear is that more stringent requirements will be forced on dietary supplements.

To do so, critics say, they'll draw on some of the most damaging evidence they can find. *If* you don't believe that, you need only glance across the Atlantic Ocean.

The U.K. Experience

In April 2005, many health advocates cheered a victory, however minor and however temporary. Here's what happened: In August 2005, dietary supplements in the European Union were scheduled to be regulated by the Food Supplement Directive approved by the European Parliament and the Council of the European Union in June 2002. The directive calls for regulating vitamins and minerals by establishing a "positive list," which presently only includes thirteen vitamin forms and fifteen mineral forms. If a nutrient is not on the list it would be considered "banned" from being sold in the EU.

Trade groups, led by the Alliance for Natural Health, had lobbied to overturn the legislation, claiming it would ban thousands of vitamin and mineral supplements. The ANH—which has fought the measure—said the approved substances are broken down by chemical composition, with synthetic compounds favored over natural forms. That means that not on the list are several forms of vitamin C, natural forms of folic acid, certain antioxidants, and a range of minerals, including boron, vanadium, silicon, mixed tocopherols, tocotrienols, sulphur, chelated/plant-derived forms and natural forms of vitamin E and selenium. Based on the positive list, the EU directive effectively banned 300 of the 420 forms of vitamins and minerals present in 5,000 products currently on the U.K. market.

Trade groups, including the Alliance for Natural Health, the National Association of Health Stores, and the Health Food Manufacturers Association, lobbied to overturn the legislation, claiming it would ban thousands of vitamin and mineral supplements. Then the ANH filed a lawsuit.

In response to the ANH suit, Advocate General Geelhoed of the European Court of Justice in Luxembourg recommended invalidating the EU directive, but he upheld the concept of using a positive list to shape international markets, and he urged EU officials to correct what amounts to technical glitches in the wording of the directive, so that the positive list can be effectuated this summer.

In August, however, the European Union's high court upheld proposed restrictions on the sale of food supplements. The European Court of Justice said the EU law was "appropriate for securing the free movement of food supplements and ensuring the protection of human health."

Back in the U.S.A.

Here's how it could affect us in the United States. The positive list will prohibit the importation of excluded substances and products into European Community markets. Also, we can expect the list to be incorporated into the Codex guidelines for vitamins and minerals. Why? Because Codex is mandated to look to "accepted international standards" to determine which substances are allowed and not allowed and at what doses. Many observers believe that Codex will adopt the EU directive's positive list as its own standard, since there is no other internationally accepted standard.

Adding a substance to the list can be tricky and expensive. In order for a nutrient substance to be added to the positive list, a comprehensive risk-assessment study must be performed, with favorable results submitted to the Office of the EU Communities by July 12, 2005. Even then, it can only remain on the positive list until 2009. These expensive scientific studies can only be undertaken by governments or corporations with deep pockets. In sum, the EU directive will likely destroy any European health supplement business that produces or sells commonly accepted vitamin and mineral products.

Also, as for upper limit doses, the Codex commission is looking to adopt the specifications of a study conducted by the FAO/WHO and others, including the Alliance for Natural Health. The study will set upper limit supplement dosage levels in the near future, and those standards, which will be based upon risk-assessment values—not health benefits—will be incorporated into the Codex Alimentarius regulations.

That's not all. In 2004, the Institute of Medicine (IOM), a quasi–governmental body based in Washington, D.C., that performs scientific studies on spec from government and private companies under contract with the FDA, issued a report called "The Proposed Framework for Evaluation of Dietary Supplements." The report shifts IOM's previous focus upon health benefits to focus on scientific risk assessment. As in the Codex guidelines, and the EU directive, IOM's report calls for safety issues to be considered as if there are no health benefits attached to the use of a vitamin or mineral. It also recommends a method of setting maximum doses that could distinguish low levels for typical usage from prescriptive use, where only medical professionals will be authorized to prescribe supplements above certain dosages. The IOM report recommends putting the burden of supplying safety data upon industry, *not* the government. *If* you recall, that's just what Senator Durbin and the bills in the U.S. House propose to do. (Is it getting even clearer yet?)

This could cripple many small health-focused businesses. As Suzan Walter, president of the American Holistic Health Association, says, "Have you noticed the growing number of situations where dietary supplement companies are being required to submit costly documentation to prove that a vitamin or mineral is safe, even when there is extensive research already demonstrating its safety and effectiveness?"

Walter says the negative economic impact of what is currently happening in Europe and Canada is changing the landscape of the entire industry. She asks some important questions. Are we seeing a scenario where small companies will either have to sell out to larger supplement companies or fold? Where many of the larger companies are being bought out by pharmaceutical companies? Do current events support the strength of the supplement companies or the pharmaceutical companies?

Some organizations seem to be going along since they believe it will affect their ability to export to other countries. It seems that the American Herbal Products Association has bought into the propaganda, that Codex standards won't supersede DSHEA or affect U.S. supplement sales even though their impact on international sales is less clear. An AHPA representative said in a statement that the Codex standards could "be used under World Trade Organization agreements to force countries to allow the importation and sale of products that conform to the guidelines." Or, it could do the opposite, dry up existing markets because of stringent requirements. A more realistic assessment is Codex will seriously impact the export business of U.S.-based supplement companies and could eventually result in similar product restrictions being implemented here.

Since Codex is mandated to look to "accepted international standards" to determine which substances are allowed and not allowed and at which doses, American supplement manufacturers and distributors will be locked out of the European regional markets, and the local markets of any country that adopts the Codex standards in order to benefit from trade with Europe.

The FDA and some CRN members pooh-pooh the alarmists. They say compliance with Codex is "voluntary." Further, according to a U.S. Department of Agriculture official, the United States has never changed its laws or regulations to conform to any standards or guidelines adopted at Codex. He noted further that the United States does not, as a matter of practice, officially accept, accept in part, accept free distribution, or accept standards or guidelines adopted by the Codex commission. Therefore, it doesn't appear that any changes to U.S. law or regulations would likely occur as a result of any adoption by the Commission of the vitamin and food supplement guidelines.

That may be, but non-compliance would result in trade sanctions or expulsion from the WTO. I doubt the multi-nations and corporate lobbyists will allow such things to happen, because since the creation of the World Trade Organization and its internal operating agreements, every member nation knows that its laws and regulations can become the object of a WTO ruling and the object of political pressure to harmonize.

Who Represents Our Interests at the Codex Meetings?

The Department of Agriculture and the Food and Drug Administration represent the official U.S. position. From the corporate side, official Codex participants include Amway Corp., Wyeth Pharmaceutical Co., DSM Nutritional Products, Mead Johnson Nutritionals, Bristol-Myers Squibb Co., Nestle USA, Herbalife International, and the trade group Council for Responsible Nutrition (CRN). CRN's membership includes Archer Daniels Midland Co., Cargill Health & Food Technologies, Bayer Corp., Wyeth Consumer Health, Weider Nutrition International Inc., Shaklee Corp., Nutraceutical Corp., Herbalife International of America, Kemin Foods, General Nutrition Centers, Inc., Cadbury Adams USA LLC, DSM Nutritional Products, Eastman Chemical Company, Mingtai Chemical LLC, and Monsanto Life Sciences Company.

Some of the corporate participants have multiple interests at the meetings, since they have representatives from various divisions representing their diverse interests, such as pharmaceuticals, chemicals, and supplements.

Is Codex a Threat or Just Some Alarmist Hand Wringing?

I think syndicated radio host Robert Scott Bell says it best:

> You have a multi-billion-dollar cartel whose survival depends upon the continuity and escalation of disease across the globe. On the other side, there is a multi-million-dollar industry dominated by a bunch of naïve do-gooders attempting to promote self-responsibility and disease prevention. Use the power and force of government to discredit and curtail the growth of the natural products industry. If that does not work, buy up the companies that make up the bulk of its sales, co-opt them, and control them. If that does not work, plan for the nuclear option and use international treaties to destroy the

national sovereignty of all nations so that you can harmonize all laws to be pro-drug and anti-supplement in the name of *free trade*. Codex is the nuclear option "fail safe" for the inevitable failure of Big Pharma to win the hearts and minds of Americans in the war against true health, freedom and independence.

And Robert Scott Bell is a Libertarian!

The idea that the United States would ever succumb to international law like Codex seems unfathomable, and yet we see it happening in other industrialized countries. Both NNFA and CRI have pledged to uphold DSHEA. They must be held to that promise. Shrugging their shoulders after the fact will not be acceptable.

14

Conclusion:
It's Up to Us

There is a basic marketing axiom that says if you repeat a statement often enough, people will accept it as truth. And it's even more believable if you can get someone else to say it. It works with advertising—think Viagra, Cialis, Crestor, Prilosec, etc.—and it works with media reports that perpetuate inaccurate statements such as, "The FDA has no control over dietary supplements."

So if you hear that a supplement is dangerous—or even better, if you can get the media to say it is dangerous—many, many people will simply believe it. The same can be said for DSHEA. If people continuously read and hear that dietary supplements are unregulated and/or dangerous and that the FDA's hands are tied, making it unable to exert any authority on the industry putting public's health at risk, the message resonates even more.

I have to admit, I'm very frustrated. I fully intended to end this book on a positive note and a call to action to preserve our access to effective and safe dietary supplements. But then I picked up the *Atlanta Journal and Constitution*'s sports section. There was an article about Baltimore Oriole player Rafael Palmeiro's suspension for testing positive for steroid use. The article stated, "The Food and Drug Administration doesn't regulate dietary supplements. No government agency does."

Once I picked myself up off the floor, and got beyond the irony that the late Steve Bechler *also* played for the Orioles, I also read this: "Weakening the plausibility of Palmeiro's claims are reports the Orioles slugger tested positive for stanozolol, a powerful anabolic steroid not available in dietary supplements. Still, there's an outside chance that a supplement you buy at your local health food store contains a trace amount of a banned steroid, which could generate a positive test."

He continued, "There are documented cases of steroids contaminating supposedly non-steroidal supplements, and athletes often claim to be the latest victim. Two of the nine big-league players suspended for steroid use have blamed supplements, and Palmeiro has hinted that a contaminated supplement could have led to his positive test."

By using the term "dietary supplements," anyone reading the article might question whether the multivitamin they take is laced with steroids. Frankly, I don't know what he's referring to. What I do know is his claim that "steroids contaminating supposedly non-steroidal supplements" doesn't even pass the logic test. Does he suppose that companies manufacturing dietary supplements just happen to have some "powerful anabolic steroids" lying around that somehow managed to contaminate a totally unrelated substance?

I decided to send an e-mail and blast the writer, but realized it was doubtful I'd receive a response since he couldn't defend what he wrote. I decided instead to test his level of understanding of DSHEA, so instead I wrote:

Dear Mr. Knobler:
In your August 3 article "Steroid Case Plays Two Ways,'"near the end you stated, "The Food and Drug Administration doesn't regulate dietary supplements. No government agency does."
Are you sure that's true?
Sincerely,
Mike Fillon

He wrote back:
"The truth of what I wrote depends on how you interpret the

word 'regulate.' I should have written 'strictly regulate.' While the FDA technically has regulatory authority, it does not regulate supplements in the same way that it regulates foods and drugs."

He then cut and pasted the following gobbledygook:

"Under the Dietary Supplement Health and Education Act of 1994, the dietary supplement manufacturer is responsible for ensuring that a dietary supplement is safe before it is marketed, the FDA says. The FDA thus provides no checks or guarantees that supplements contain what they say they contain, which was the context of the article. The FTC regulates product advertising, but it also does not go so far as to check or guarantee a supplement's contents.

"Thanks for reading my article and our paper."

In this book I've repeatedly shot down the misinformation he reported. It's obvious the days of a reporter asking, "I wonder if that's true?" are over. If you slap together a couple of quotes in an article with no probing or independent digging to see if someone is guilty of a verbal snow job, that's OK in today's media. Plus when it comes to drugs, food, and dietary supplements, they seem content to repeat whatever the pharma-sponsored FDA tells them. Maybe one saving grace is that only 11 percent of the U.S. population bothers to read newspapers anymore. Then again, maybe this type of reporting is a reason why readership is so low.

Every week I receive the FDA reports on recalls of items within their jurisdiction. FDA inspectors find more contamination problems and ingredient shortages with food items and drugs than with dietary supplements. This despite the FDA dragging its feet for ten years to establish Good Manufacturing Practices (GMP).

The *AJC* article makes it sound like the dietary supplement industry is populated by mad scientists mixing test tubes in the back of a rusted pickup truck. If anything, responsible dietary supplement manufacturers have erred on the side of caution and overcompensated for the lack of GMPs. Of course there are fly-by-night companies making outlandish health claims about their products, but the FDA, the FTC, and other agencies have the power to stop them. Don't believe them when they say they don't or can't.

What Happened?

Over the past thirty years, the pharmaceutical industry has infiltrated and wrestled away control of every aspect of medicine from the laboratory to the FDA advisory panels along with medical journals and doctors' continuing medical education courses. Do you or your doctor actually know if cholesterol-lowering statin drugs *really* prevent us from suffering a heart attack, as the studies claim, or cause muscles to break down and destroy kidneys? Is this another case of the risk versus benefit shell game without a pea under any of the shells?

Bayh-Dole has also led to cozy relationships between the academics upon whom we depend for unbiased medical information and drug companies whose main goal is profitability. Today, it is not uncommon for clinicians at medical schools to add to their incomes $1,000-a-day consulting contracts with pharmaceutical companies, patent royalties, licensing fees, and big-payoff stock options. In 1984, drug companies contributed $26 million to university research budgets. By 2000, the amount skyrocketed to $2.3 billion.

At least eight studies have shown that industry-sponsored research that gets published tends to produce pro-industry conclusions, according to a review by Yale University researchers that appeared last year in *JAMA*. By reanalyzing data from eight separate studies of the effect of conflict of interest on 1,140 published scientific papers, the researchers found that papers based on industry-sponsored research are significantly more likely to reflect favorably on a sponsoring company's drug or device than research that is supported by a non-profit entity or the federal government.

Sometimes there isn't much that journal editors can do to separate good science from that which has been massaged to a corporate sponsor's specs. Increasing numbers of studies that get published are actually written by PR firms, "medical communications" specialists, who then go out and recruit an academic willing to put his name on the paper, for a fee.

Which brings us back to your vitamins, minerals, and herbs.

The Truth About DSHEA

The FDA already has the power to regulate any dietary supplement under DSHEA. If the FDA claims that ephedra or any other dietary supplement is unsafe, or violates any of the following conditions, it can remove it.

A dietary supplement that is "adulterated" or "misbranded," or that bears an unauthorized drug claim is subject to seizure, condemnation, and destruction. DSHEA included additional safety requirements regarding the introduction of new dietary ingredients. The law clarified that dietary supplement ingredients marketed prior to October 15, 1994 do not require pre-market approval. However, manufacturers marketing a new dietary supplement ingredient after this date must submit safety information on the new dietary ingredient to the FDA.

Also, DSHEA provides the Secretary of Health and Human Services with the authority to remove any dietary supplement or dietary supplement ingredient that poses an "imminent hazard." If the HHS Secretary makes this decision, the government must conduct an administrative review of the case and the product cannot be sold to the public. In addition, the FTC also has the ability to remove products and punish companies guilty of fraudulent advertising and promotion.

The FDA can remove products from the market for the following reasons:

• *Misleading Labeling/Failure to Warn:* According to the FDA, many makers of dietary supplements are selling products containing significantly less—or much more—of the key ingredients than stated on the label, according to a study published in the *American Journal of Health-System Pharmacy*. Sometimes, consumers have no way of telling how much they are ingesting with each tablet. If that's the case, the FDA has to power to remove these products. But they also need to finalize the GMPs.

• *Poses a Significant and Unreasonable Risk:* The FDA does not have to prove that a product actually harmed anyone, but simply that it presents a "significant or unreasonable risk" of illness or injury. Does the scientific evidence on the safety and efficacy of ephedra's consumption show that it poses a significant or unreasonable risk? Not the studies I've seen.

On the other hand, there are people who die every year from violent allergic reactions to common foods such as peanuts and shellfish. So should we ban peanuts and shellfish? Of course not. And that's because relatively few people are adversely affected (and since I live in Georgia I know peanut farmers would storm Washington, D.C.!).

• *Contains Poisonous or Deleterious Substances:* The FDA does not have to prove that a dietary supplement contains a substance that will injure, but simply that it may render injury under the recommended or suggested conditions indicated on a product's label. Studies show that ephedra dietary supplements, when used according to industry standards are safe for most people. Perfect for everyone? By no means.

• *Is Unfit for Food:* Although dietary supplements are not considered a "food," the FDA has authority to stop the marketing of any dietary supplement that the agency believes is not fit for human consumption. There is no evidence whatsoever that any legitimate supplements are unfit for human consumption.

• *Makes Drug Claims:* If a dietary supplement's label indicates that the product can diagnose, cure, mitigate, treat or prevent a disease, then it is clearly being represented as a "drug" and is no longer considered a dietary supplement. Responsible manufacturers have labels, warnings, and directions for use for their products and do not represent their products as drugs.

• *Lacks Truthful and Informative Labeling:* By law, all dietary supplement products must contain extensive informative labeling, including detailed information about the nutrients in the product, such as name and quantity of all ingredients in the product and the name and place of business of the company, for example. Industry supports enforcement efforts of this provision. Recently the Secretary of Health and Human Services announced enforcement efforts to remove products that were marketed to minors and for illicit purposes. The dietary supplement industry has consistently urged the FDA to use its enforcement powers to remove such products from the marketplace.

There are other protections as well. The FTC monitors false advertising and also has the power to shut down fraudulent operations. Magazines, newspapers, and broadcast outlets also have a code of ethics against false or misleading advertising. Are these enforced? Of course not. I'm sure plenty of us have been suckered into buying a device that comes with the guarantee of being able to see through walls—or a magic pill that can solve a myriad of health problems. But the simple truth is that the power to ban these items exists.

So, the FDA, the Department of Health and Human Services, and the FTC all have broad powers to remove any product that is an "imminent hazard," "deleterious," "a significant risk," and so on.

This begs the question: Why did they ban ephedra? We have a right to know. According to Metabolife company records supplied to HHS, over the last five years more than 4.5 billion tablets and 50 million bottles of Metabolife 356 have been sold. The company also claimed it recorded 14,700 "incident reports," with about 78 of the reports appearing to be serious incidents, including hospitalizations and one reported death. According to some experts who have reviewed them, this level of adverse incidents is consistent with the occurrence of these conditions in the general population. That means that people taking 4.5 billion placebo or sugar pills would create just as many "incident reports."

There's also a risk of misinterpretation of data or overreaction to misread data. When Metabolife released its record of AERs, various media accounts stated that all 14,700 "incident reports" were "serious"—clearly a gross exaggeration. Where did they get this information from? They didn't make it up.

But that is probably beside the point. Many experts, including the GAO and the FDA, now say AERs are not a valid scientific basis upon which to develop regulatory policy on the safety of a substance. But, when the average consumer reads these numbers as fact, the information resonates.

It's Our Call

I've stressed one basic premise throughout this book. That is, it's better to be healthy than sick, but it's our choice. In this country we have the freedom to succeed grandly, or screw up royally.

Unfortunately, too many of us have opted for the latter. As I look around, I see half our population overweight and obese. I see people at risk for diseases such as diabetes, heart disease, and cancer and doing nothing about it except to trot off to the drugstore followed by a trip to the cookie and soft drink aisle in their favorite supermarket. Here's the sad fact: Regardless of how many people read this book, there will be hundreds of thousands of our fellow citizens who will choose to watch TV instead. During every hour they watch, they'll probably see ads for salt-, sugar- and fat-laden fast-food meals; ads for other food and drinks with all the nutrition squeezed out of them and replaced by questionable substances such as aspartame and high-fructose corn syrup.

I have no doubt that in that hour they will see multiple ads for heartburn, cholesterol, and erectile dysfunction. What they *won't* see are ads for vitamin E or coQ10, and it's highly unlikely they'll see a spot promoting exercise. Unfortunately, we as human beings don't react until it's too late.

When I think like this—with aid from articles like the one I just cited in the *AJC*—I get frustrated. But then I realize it's still worth it. Maybe you'll tell someone and they'll tell someone else. We won't reach everyone but maybe enough people will take an interest that we can make a difference.

Granted, there are many forces aligned against us. The message constantly hammered home is, "eat this, drink that, and don't worry; we have drugs for when you overindulge or get sick. Why exercise when you can plop down on the couch, hit the remote, chug our beer and watch others frolic on the beach? We offer you the easy solution plus an excuse and an escape. Isn't that what you *really* want?" The dietary supplement industry has thrown a monkey wrench into this grinding-away mindset.

If you recall, in the introduction to this book I wrote, "As you read, it's important for you to keep asking yourself one question after I present evidence. That question is: Who benefits? Hopefully, when you finish you'll know what to do about it."

So, if you are determined to push forward and optimize your heath, let's review who's pushing back and what you can do about it.

Not-So-Friendly Adversaries

The Media

If you're reading this book, it's likely you read or at least skim one newspaper per day. If so, by now you should be able to spot lazy, slanted, and misleading reporting. Hopefully, you'll notice when "medical studies" don't include dosage amounts, and you'll sit up on the rare occasions it's reported that the pharmaceutical industry pulls another fast one affecting our safety. Contact the newspaper if you spot something that you think is wrong. If it is, tell them you expect a correction.

Pharmaceutical companies pay big bucks to advertise—and let's not kid ourselves—the pharmaceutical industry helps dictate what gets reported. It's only after news of hidden dangers and missing evidence—you know, the unavoidable—that you're likely to see these types of shenanigans reported.

When you read ads in magazines or on TV for drugs, don't focus on the attractive models. Instead read the creeping text, listen to the swift-talking voice-overs, and read the fine print. That's when you'll notice things like statin drugs don't decrease the risk of heart trouble.

Likewise, if you see an infomercial or other ad for a dietary supplement that makes bogus claims, complain to the magazine, TV, or radio station along with the FDA and FTC. It doesn't take long to compose and send an e-mail or make a phone call.

The Medical Profession

I would never tell you to *not* take a drug your doctor prescribes, but you are entitled to have your questions answered to your satisfaction. I hope if your doctor reaches for his prescription pad, you'll ask him or her what the prescription is for, why it's being prescribed, and how long you're expected to take the drug. Remember to ask about alternatives.

But remember, doctors have a closet-full of free samples. Research studies show that when doctors are given samples of drugs by pharmaceutical representatives, they are more likely to prescribe those drugs instead of over-the-counter or generic alternatives, not to mention supplements or behavior modification. The influence that free samples has over physicians seems to violate professional guidelines covering physician contacts with the drug companies.

Also, as I've mentioned, most continuing medical education classes are sponsored by the drug companies and many of the medical studies your doctor's read have been authored by doctors with a financial stake in the sponsoring drug company or have been paid by them. Bottom line? Drug companies spend over $10,000 every year for every doctor in the United States. That's roughly $15 billion a year. You can call the pharmaceutical companies a lot of things but stupid isn't one of them. They spend so much because they know it's a great investment that will convert to ringing cash registers at drug stores.

Many doctors are reluctant to change even if they try to brush off the low-hanging fruit from the drug companies. I remember a story Dr. John Abramson tells in his book, *Overdosed America*. When he presented evidence that the studies on statin drugs showed that while they did reduce cholesterol they didn't reduce heart attacks, a colleague whom he knew well said, "I don't believe it." Abramson tried again by explaining the evidence differently. Again the other doctor said, "I don't believe it."

I guess the moral of this story is that we human beings are reluctant to change our opinions even when irrefutable evidence is presented. We prefer the status quo and are more comfortable with information that validates what we already believe to information that challenges our beliefs.

As I pointed out earlier, when the evidence can no longer be ignored and threatens our beliefs we suffer a cold-sweat moment. I had one when it became irrefutable that the FDA's evidence against ephedra was fabricated at best. I then flipped and noticed many more instances of questionable and deceptive tactics. I could no longer say, "I don't believe it."

Our Elected Officials

We put them in office, we pay their salaries, but despite some token lip-service, many politicians are available only to the highest bidders. Unless you're a big party donor or a high-powered lobbyist, "that ain't you."

Earlier in the book I mentioned that members of Congress have tried, and are trying, to either overturn DSHEA or wound it badly enough that it withers and dies. Serving as their accomplice is former Louisiana Congressman Billy Tauzin, who—funny how these things work out—is now president of PhRMA, the ultra-powerful drug lobby group.

Here are a few of the bills pending that could damage our access to dietary supplements. I mentioned these bills in an earlier chapter, but they bear repeating. I'll warn you, though. Even if these should wither or be withdrawn, you can be sure they'll be replaced by other onerous bills:

• Senator Richard Durbin from Illinois has submitted an amendment to prohibit the sale of any supplements containing a stimulant to be sold on a military installation or in a commissary or exchange store. Tucked away in the "National Defense Authorization Act for Fiscal Year 2006" (S.1042) it would also establish adverse event reporting by supplement manufacturers.

• Sen. Durbin has also reintroduced SB729, which would create a new federal food safety agency. Congresswoman Rosa DeLauro has introduced a similar bill in the House (HR 1507). Some industry observers who have analyzed this bill report that it could cause DSHEA to be repealed and dietary supplements would be reclassified and regulated as drugs.

• The Dietary Supplement Access and Awareness Act (HR 3156) would require an adverse reaction reporting system for botanicals that could permit the FDA to ban any non-vitamin dietary supplement without evidence that the substance caused harm. This could allow the Secretary of Health and Human Services to ban a product if he had "determined that risks outweighed benefits." Besides burdening the manufacturers with additional reporting requirements as I've said before, isn't this the government's job? Frankly, if there's a problem with a substance I don't want the company who stands to profit to tell me, I want my "objective, unbiased" regulatory agency to warn me.

Here are more reasonable alternatives:

• Introduced as a substitute amendment for Senator Durbin's bill by Senators Tom Harkin from Iowa and Orrin Hatch from Utah, is an amendment that would help ensure that DSHEA finally be fully implemented, funded, and enforced. It also directs the FDA to develop an appropriate system for the reporting of serious adverse reactions to dietary supplements.

• There is another bill, HR 2352, the Consumers' Access to Health Information Act, which would allow accurate labeling claims on the "curative, mitigation, treatment, and prevention effects" of foods and dietary supplements on disease and health-related conditions while not causing products to be treated as a drug by the FDA. The bill would ensure that the FDA does not suppress accurate health claims.

If our elected officials make a public stand, and reverse course without explanation, we must hold them accountable. The same holds true if they don't take a public stand at all. Make them. Don't be afraid to hold their feet to the fire.

Check their voting records on issue that are important to you. It doesn't take a majority of voters to make a big stink.

The Regulators

Under the umbrella of Health and Human Services the two agencies that have the biggest impact on our ability to use dietary supplements are the FDA and the Office of Complementary Medicine (OCM), although, as with the slam against St. John's wort I reported, others can get involved too.

I've spent a good deal of time hammering away at the FDA, so I won't rehash all of their mischievous antics here. The OCM is a different story. As I mentioned, in the case of the echinacea study, I think they tried to pull a fast one. They dismissed the usefulness of the herb out of hand without telling us a small dosage was used, and without revealing the pharmaceutical ties of the lead researcher.

There is a role for OCM, if only they'd fulfill it. Let's take the case of echinacea. Dr. Benjamin Kligler, assistant professor in the Department of Family Medicine at Albert Einstein College of Medicine in New York has studied the herb.

He says that, while echinacea is widely promoted for its ability to "boost" the immune system, there isn't sufficient data to support that claim. He says that a number of in vitro and animal studies have shown that echinacea appears to increase immune function, and this might be a bit technical for you, by "increasing levels of interferon and may increase phagocytosis, cellular respiratory activity, and lymphocyte activation through release of tumor necrosis factors."

Interferon is a protein produced by human cells that when invaded by viruses are released into the bloodstream or intercellular fluid to induce healthy cells to manufacture an enzyme that counters the infection. Phagocytosis is the process of ingesting and destroying a virus or other foreign matter by phagocytes. Lymphocytes are a type of infection-fighting white blood cell are vital to an effective immune system that "patrol" the body. Tumor necrosis factors are the proteins produced by white blood cells that act as chemical messengers between cells (cytokines) that help regulate the immune response and hematopoiesis (blood cell formation).

Dr. Kligler says the active components believed to be responsible for this immune-stimulating effect are the high-molecular-weight polysaccharides such as heteroxylan and arabinoglactan. "However," he writes, "because the active component has not been identified, commercial echinacea products are not typically standardized to any particular component."

It seems rather than supporting studies of questionable dosages against placebos, wouldn't OCM's budget be better spent investigating the hows and whys of echinacea? To put the optimal formulation on the market to help us? It makes one wonder what master they're really serving.

I believe this is what NIH, specifically OCM, should be doing with all herbs and other supplements: figure out how they work and why.

I recently spoke with Tod Cooperman, M.D., founder of ConsumerLab.com. In 1999, ConsumerLab began independently testing vitamins, minerals, and herbs to determine their purity and whether they contained what the label stated. He said one of the difficulties is determining what many of the components in some herbs do and how they work. He says there should be studies to determine what the right phytochemical compositions included in a product should be, but no one in HHS, NIH or the FDA is doing this.

Dr. Cooperman also sounds an all-too-familiar alarm. "The FDA already has requirements that a product contain 100 percent of what it claims, but we find that not all products do. The FDA doesn't have the personnel to enforce their own laws. That's the biggest issue the government faces, they don't have the manpower of financial resources and they don't expect to get it in order to enforce their rules."

The Pharmaceutical Industry

In July 2005, the Center for Public Integrity (CPI), a Washington-based watchdog group, reported that U.S. drug companies spent more than $800 million over the past seven years in campaign donations and lobbying that have produced favorable laws and tens of billions of dollars in extra profits.

CPI says the industry's influence campaign has also led to a more friendly regulatory policy at the FDA. Among the tactics cited in the report are lobbying to quash laws that could change drug prices and affect profits, including stopping importation of medicines from countries that cap prescription drug prices.

The industry spent nearly $128 million in 2003 alone lobbying the government. This has resulted in Congress passing, and President George W. Bush signing, the Medicare Modernization Act of 2003, a law that created a taxpayer-funded prescription-drug benefit for senior citizens. PhRMA—whose membership includes sixteen of the industry's twenty largest companies and their subsidiaries—spent $74 million since 1998, nearly double the estimated $38.8 billion in 2004 it says it spent discovering and developing new medicines.

CPI also found that U.S. manufacturers of drugs and cosmetics hired about 3,000 lobbyists, more than a third of them former federal officials, to advance their interests before the House of Representatives, the Senate, the FDA, the Department of Health and Human Services, the Office of the U.S. Trade Representative, and other executive branch offices.

Congress tops the list of targets for industry lobbying, with contacts at the House or Senate listed on about 5,500 lobby disclosure reports. A third of all lobbyists employed by the industry are former federal government employees. Fifteen are former senators, and more than sixty are former members of the U.S. House of Representatives.

It's amazing what these companies get away with. Drug companies routinely delay or prevent the publication of data that show their drugs are ineffective. The majority of studies found that such popular antidepressants as Prozac and Zoloft are no better than placebos, for instance, never saw print in medical journals, a fact that is coming to light only now that the FDA has been forced to reexamine those drugs.

Ourselves

And whose fault is this sorry state of affairs? Frankly, it's ours, at least in part. We've let the FDA take money from the pharma companies under the guise that it will speed up the development of life-saving drugs. We've let the pharma companies infiltrate the medical profession to the extent that their continued education is underwritten by them and marketing reps consult on patient care and treatment. We sit idly by while our elected representatives take junkets and other goodies from lobbyists, then they mention their "morality" or "family values," and we put them right back on the congressional automatic teller machine line.

I can understand if you get defensive when I say it's our fault since we elect people to take care of these things for us. The sad fact is that by the time many of them arrive in Washington they've also been compromised by special interests. They become more beholden to lobbyists camped outside their door than the voter at home busy walking his dog and mowing his lawn.

It's a Battlefield

Our lawmakers and regulators are constantly weighing how much freedom or limitations to impose on those of us who look to health remedies not always found in our doctor's office. How they respond to these various interests will determine the future of American medicine—whether it's a true free-market system in which the best therapies can rise on their merits, or a climate in which only the most strictly regulated and tightly controlled treatments can be used.

On one side stand the vitamin and supplement makers, nutritionists, acupuncturists, chiropractors, and other medical practitioners. It is estimated that one-third of Americans already use some form of alternative treatments.

Opposite them are the pharmaceutical companies, the American Medical Association, the pharmacy industry, HMOs, and insurance companies and their assorted lobbyists.

In general, the alternative side offers lower-price solutions and the inherent advantage of warding off disease, not just treating symptoms. The other side has deeper pockets. It's up to us to decide who wins or if there should be a truce.

Don't get me wrong; there are some positive signs. While the movements toward integrative and holistic medicine in the United States stretch back to the nineteenth century they have become more mainstream in the last few years. The difference between "integrative" and "holistic" medicine lies in the practitioners' approach to the patient. "Holistic" is the approach that the practitioner uses in working with the patient, while integrative is the combination of multiple treatment modalities from the complementary and alternative medicine realm. "The ideal approach," says Karen Lawson, M.D., president of the American Holistic Medical Association, and director of Integrative Clinical Services at the University of Minnesota's Center for Spirituality and Healing, "is both integrative in methodology and holistic in attitude."

The new options of complementary therapies, or integrative and holistic medicine are now available in 25 percent of metropolitan hospitals, in a wide range of outpatient clinical settings, and in almost a quarter of conventional medical schools and academic health centers in the United States. Individuals are being given new choices of therapeutic modalities and philosophies of care. Today, the interdisciplinary health-care team is expanding to include bodyworkers, herbalists, naturopathic doctors, practitioners of traditional Chinese medicine, homeopaths, nutritionists, mind/body teachers, chiropractors, spiritual directors, and many others.

Dr. Lawson says with this shift comes a change of relationship between providers and patients, into a patient/client-centered care model, empowering the individual to choose their team, make their own informed decisions, and steer the direction of their own healing process. "With all the new possibilities for seeking health and healing, the potential for both individual and community growth and well-being can increase, perhaps exponentially, but only through the willingness to take on the personal responsibility for our own lifestyle choices," says Dr. Lawson. "This is not a path of care for those uninterested in investing time and effort into making changes in their own lives."

It is my hope that this book will enlighten consumers about the commercial and political interests influencing efforts to change current law regarding the sale and advertisement of dietary supplements. Additionally, I hope that lawmakers will realize that the best way to determine the safety and efficacy of dietary supplements is to conduct research, and therefore increase funding, to support this work. This means that that they must realize that additional funding is necessary to help the FDA and FTC enforce existing law on behalf of the American public.

The truth is, we hold the highest office available in a republic, that of citizen. As Iowa Senator Chuck Grassley so aptly stated during the recent Vioxx controversy, "There should be only one chair at the table and that is for the American people."

Our best hope for our health is our own vigilance.

Bibliography

Publications

AHPA, CHPA, NNFA, UNPA, Citizens Petition to FDA on Ephedra Labeling, Oct. 25, 2000.

AHPA, CHPA, NNFA, UNPA, Letter to Joe A. Levitt, Oct. 23, 2000.

AHPA, CHPA, CRN, NNFA, UNPA, Letter to Paul M. Coates, Oct 23, 2000.

Alsheikh-Ali Alawi A. M.D., Marietta S. Ambrose M.D., Jeffrey T. Kuvin M.D., and Richard H. Karas M.D., Ph.D. "The Safety of Rosuvastatin as Used in Common Clinical Practice. A Postmarketing Analysis," *Circulation*, May 23, 2005.

Armstrong, W. Jeffrey, P. Johnson, and S. Duhme, "The Effect of Commercial Thermogenic Weight Loss Supplement On Body Composition And Energy Expenditure In Obese Adults," *Journal of Exercise Physiology*, 4(2): 28–34, 2001.

Avorn, J., M. Chen, and R. Hartley, "Scientific versus commercial sources of influence on the prescribing behavior of physicians," *American Journal of Medicine*, 73: 4–8, 1982.

Bell, C., J.M. Kowalchuk, D.H. Paterson, B.W. Scheuermann, and D.A. Cunningham, "The effects of caffeine on the kinetics of O_2 uptake, CO_2 production and expiratory ventilation in humans during the on-transient of moderate and heavy intensity exercise," *Experimental Physiology*, 84(4): 761–74, 1999.

Bent, S., T.N. Tiedt, M.C. Odden, and M.G. Shlipak, "The Relative Safety of Ephedra Compared with Other Herbal Products," *Annals of Internal Medicine*, 138, 2003.

Benton, D. et al., "Vitamin supplementation for one year improves mood," *Neuropsychobiology*, 32(2): 98–105, 1995.

Bero, L.A., and D. Rennie, "Influences on the quality of published drug studies," *Int J Technol Assess Health Care*, 12(2): 209–37, 1996.

Blumenthal, D., E.G. Campbell, M.S. Anderson, N. Causino, and K.S. Louis, "Withholding Research Results in Academic Life Science: Evidence from a National Survey of Faculty," *Journal of the American Medical Association (JAMA)*, 277: 1224–8, 1997.

Blumenthal, James A., Andrew Sherwood, Michael A. Babyak, Lana L. Watkins, Robert Waugh, Anastasia Georgiades, Simon L. Bacon, Junichiro Hayano, R. Edward Coleman, Alan Hinderliter, "Effects of Exercise and Stress Management Training on Markers of Cardiovascular Risk in Patients With Ischemic Heart Disease: A Randomized Controlled Trial," *JAMA*, 293: 1626–34, 2005.

Boodman, Sandra G., "Statins' Nerve Problems," *Washington Post*, September 3, 2002.

Boozer, C.N., P.A. Daly, P. Homel, J.L. Solomon, D. Blanchard, J.A. Nasser, R. Strauss, and T. Meredith, "Herbal ephedra/caffeine for weight loss: a six-month randomized safety and efficacy trial," *The International Journal of Obesity*, 26: 593–604, 2002.

Boozer, C.N., J.A. Nasser, S.B. Heymsfield, V. Wang, G. Chen, and J.L. Solomon, "An Herbal Supplement Containing Ma Huang-Guaraná for Weight Loss: a Randomized, Double-blind Trial," *Int J Obes Relat Metab Disord*, 25(3): 316–24, 2001.

Boushey, Carol J. Ph.D., *Journal of the American Medical*

"Clinical Trials: Questions and Answers," National Cancer Institute, January 14, 2004.

Caudill, T.S., M.S. Johnson, E.C. Rich, and W.P. McKinney, "Physicians, pharmaceutical sales representatives, and the cost of prescribing," *Arch of Fam Med*, 5: 201–206, 1996.

Chalmers, I. "Underreporting research is scientific misconduct," *JAMA*, 263: 1405–08. 1990.

Cho, M.K., R. Shohara, A. Schissel, and D. Rennie, "Policies on faculty conflicts of interest at U.S. universities," *JAMA*, 284: 2203–08, 2000.

"Cholesterol—And Beyond: Statin Drugs Have Cut Heart Disease. Now They Show Promise Against Alzheimer's, Multiple Sclerosis and Osteoporosis," *Newsweek*, July 14. 2003.

Circulation, 97: 1027–28, 1029–36, March 24, 1998.

Clemons, J.M., and S.L. Crosby. "Cardiopulmonary and subjective effects of a 60 mg dose of pseudoephedrine on graded treadmill exercise," *Journal of Sports Medicine and Physical Fitness*, 33(4): 405–12, 1993.

Cook, H. "Practical guide to medical education," *Pharmaceutical Marketing*, 2001.

Cox, Teri, Commentary in *Pharma Executive*, September 2002.

Daly, P.A., D.R. Krieger, A.G. Dulloo, J.B. Young, and L. Landsberg, "Ephedrine, Caffeine and Aspirin: Safety and Efficacy for Treatment of Human Obesity," *International Journal of Obesity*, 17(Supp. 1): S73–S78, 1993.

Davidson, Jonathan. et al., "Effect of Hypericum Perforatum (St John's Wort) in Major Depressive Disorder," *JAMA*, 287: 1807–14, 2002.

Davidson, R.A., "Source of Funding and Outcome of Clinical Trials," *Journal of General Internal Medicine*, 1: 155–8, 1986.

Davis, R., "Health Education on the Six o'clock News: Motivating Television Coverage of News in Medicine," *JAMA*, 259(7): 1036–38, 1988.

Davis, Ron, "Dangers of Dietary Supplement Ephedra, Statement for the Record of the American Medical Association to the Subcommittee on Oversight of Government Management, Restructuring and the District of Columbia Committee on Government Affairs," United States Senate, October 8, 2002.

Davis, C., and E. Saltos, "Dietary Recommendations and How They Have Changed Over Time." In Elizabeth Frazao, *America's Eating Habits: Changes and Consequences*, Washington, D.C.: U.S. Department of Agriculture, Food and Rural Economics Division, *Agriculture Information Bulletin No. 750*, pp. 33–50, 1999.

"Dietary Supplement Industry Calls on FDA to Adopt National Standards on Ephedra," Ephedra Education Council, Oct. 26, 2000.

"Dietary Supplements for Weight Loss: Limited Federal Oversight Has Focused More on Marketing than on Safety" (Testimony: 07/31/2002, GAO-02-985T).

"Dietary Supplements: Uncertainties in Analyses Underlying FDA's Proposed Rule on Ephedrine Alkaloids," Letter Report: 07/02/1999, GAO/ HEHS/GGD.

DiMasi, Joseph, et al., "The Cost of Innovation in the Pharmaceutical Industry," *Journal of Health Economics.* 10: 107–42, 1991.

"Drug Marketing," *New England Journal of Medicine (NEJM)*, 346: 498–505, 524–531, 2002.

"Echinacea Not Effective for the Common Cold." *Journal Watch (General)* 2005.

"Effect of Hypericum Perforatum (St John's wort) in Major Depressive Disorder: A Randomized Controlled Trial," Hypericum Depression Trial Study Group, *JAMA*, 287: 1807–14, 2002.

Elias, M., "Antidepressant barely better than placebo," *USA Today*, July 7, 2002.

Emerson, Bo, "Chewin' the Fat: Whose Fault Is Obesity?" *Atlanta Journal and Constitution*, July 5, 2003.

Federal Register, Vol. 68, No. 49, March 13, 2003.

Federal Register, Vol. 49, p. 838–39, Sept. 23, 1997.

Fessenden, Ford, "Studies of Dietary Supplements Come Under Growing Scrutiny." *New York Times*, June 23, 2003.

Flanagin, A., L.A. Carey, P.B. Fontanarosa, et al., "Prevalence of Articles with Honorary Authors and Ghost Authors in Peer-reviewed Medical Journals," *JAMA*, 280: 222–24, 1998.

Food and Drug Administration, 62 Fed. Reg. 30678, June 4, 1997.

Freemantle, N., I.M. Anderson, and P. Young, "Predictive Value of Pharmacological Activity for the Relative Efficacy of Antidepressant Drugs: Meta-regression Analysis," *British Journal of Psychiatry*, 177: 292–302, 2002.

Friedberg, M., B. Saffran, T.J. Stinson, W. Nelson, and C.L. Bennett, "Evaluation of Conflict of Interest in Economic Analyses of New Drugs Used in Oncology," *JAMA*, 282: 1453–57, 1999.

Gaster B., Holroyd J., "St. John's wort for Depression," *Arch Int Med.* 160(2): 152–56, 2000.

General Accounting Office, "Dietary Supplements: Uncertainties in Analyses Underlying FDA's Proposed Rule on Ephedrine Alkaloids," (GAO/HEHS/GGD-99-90), Washington, D.C., General Accounting Office, July 2, 1999.

Getz, K.A., "AMCs Rekindling Clinical Research Partnerships with Industry," *Centerwatch*, 1999.

Gibbons, R.V., Landry, F.J., Blouch, D.L., et al., "A Comparison of Physicians' and Patients' Attitudes Toward Pharmaceutical Industry Gifts," *JGIM*, 13: 151–54, 1998.

"GPs to stop prescribing antidepressants blamed for suicidal feelings in under-18s," *The Guardian* (UK), September 28, 2005.

Greene, J., M. Marsden, R. Sanchez, et al., "National Household Survey on Drug Abuse—main findings 1998." Rockville: Dept. of Health and Human Services, Substance Abuse and Mental Health Administration, Office of Applied Statistics, Report No.: H-11, 2000.

Greenway, F.L., "The Safety and Efficacy of Pharmaceutical and Herbal Caffeine and Ephedrine Use as a Weight Loss Agent," *Obesity Review*, 2(3): 199–211, 2001.

Gugliotta, G., "FDA Backs off Former Weight Loss Policy," *Washington Post*, Feb. 29, 2000.

"Guidelines for Communicating Emerging Science on Nutrition, Food Safety and Health," *Journal of the National Cancer Institute*, 90(3): 194–99, 1998.

Haller, C.A., P. Jacob, and N.L. Benowitz, "Pharmacology of Ephedra Alkaloids and Caffeine After Single-Dose Dietary Supplement Use," *Clinical Pharmacology and Therapeutics*, 71(6): 421–31, 2002.

Hasslberger, Sepp, "Codex Alimentarius To Approve 'Vitamin Guidelines'," *Health Supreme*, June 10, 2005.

_____, "Medical system is leading cause of death and injury in U.S.," *Health Supreme*, October 29, 2003.

_____, "Codex and the *Titanic*'s Deck Chairs," *Health Supreme*, December 4, 2003.

"The Hazards of Vitamin E" (Editorial), *New York Times*, Nov. 14, 2004.

Heart Protection Study Collaborative Group, *The Lancet*, 360: 7–22, 2002.

Hensley, Scott, "The Statin Dilemma: How Sluggish Sales Hurt Merck, Pfizer," *The Wall Street Journal*, July 25, 2003.

High-fructose Corn Sweeteners (HFCS), *American Journal of Clinical Nutrition*, 72, 1128–34, November 2000.

High-fructose Corn Sweeteners (HFCS), *Journal of Nutrition*, 130: 3077–84, December 2000.

"How Accurate is the FDA's Monitoring of Supplements Like Ephedra?" Committee on Government Reform, House of Representatives, May 1999.

"How the Media Left the Evidence Out in the Cold," *British Medical Journal*, 326: 1403–04, 21 June 2003.

Ismail, M. Asif, "Drug Lobby Second to None. How the Pharmaceutical Industry Gets Its Way in Washington," Center for Pubic Integrity, July 7, 2005.

Jacobson, N.S., L.J. Roberts, S.B. Berns, and J.B. McGlinchey, "Methods Defining and Determining the Clinical Significance of Treatment Effects: Description, Application, and Alternatives," *Journal of Consulting & Clinical Psychology,*: 67: 300–07, 1999.

Jones, G., "Interpretation of Postmortem Drug Levels," *Drug Abuse Handbook*, CRC Press: 970–87, 1998.

Jones, W.K. "Safety of Dietary Supplements Containing Ephedrine Alkaloids," Office of Women's Health Report on Public Hearing, August 8–9, 2000.

Kaitin, Kenneth I. and Elaine M. Healy, "The New Drug Approvals of 1998, 1997 and 1996: Emerging Drug Development Trends in the User Fee Era," Tufts Center for the Study of Drug Development, *PAREXEL's Pharmaceutical R&D Statistical Sourcebook*, p. 117, January 2000.

Kanfer, I., R. Dowse, V. Vuma, "Pharmacokinetics of Oral Decongestants." *Pharmacotherapy*, 13(6 Pt 2): 116S–128S,143S–146S, 1993.

Kassirer, J.P., "Financial Indigestion," *JAMA*, 284: 2156–57, 2000.

Kaufman, D.W., J.P. Kelly, L. Rosenberg, T.E. Anderson, and A.A. Mitchell, "Recent Patterns of Medication Use in the Ambulatory Adult Population of the United States: The Slone Survey," *JAMA*, 287(3): 337–44, 2002.

Kaufman, L., "Prime-time Nutrition," *Journal of Communication*, 30(3): 37–45, 1990.

Kernan, W.N., C.M. Viscoli, L.M. Brass, J.P. Broderick, T. Brott, et al., "Phenylpropanolamine and the Risk of Hemorrhagic Stroke," *NEJM*, 343(25): 1826–32, 2000.

Khan, A., H.A. Warner., and W.A. Brown, "Symptom Reduction and Suicide Risk in Patients Treated with Placebo in Antidepressant Clinical Trials: An Analysis of the Food and Drug Administration Database," *Archives of General Psychiatry*, 57: 311–17, 2000.

Kissin, W., T. Garfield, and J. Ball, "Drug Abuse Warning Network." Annual Medical Examiner Data, Bethesda: Dept. of Health and Human Services, Substance Abuse and Mental Health Administration, Office of Applied Statistics, Report No.: D-13, 2000.

Kissin, W., T. Garfield, and J. Ball, "Mid-year 1999 Preliminary Emergency Department Data from the Drug Abuse Warning Network." D-14. Bethesda: Dept. of Health and Human Services, Substance Abuse and Mental Health Administration, Office of Applied Statistics, 2000.

Korn, D., "Conflicts of Interest in Biomedical Research," *JAMA*, 284: 2234–37, 2000.

Kunin, C.M., "Clinical Investigators and the Pharmaceutical Industry," *Annals of Internal Medicine*, 89 (Suppl): 842–45, 1978.

Laise, Eleanor, "The Lipitor Dilemma," *Smart Money: The Wall Street Journal Magazine of Personal Business*, November 2003.

Lehrman, Nathaniel S., "The Bureaucratic Destruction of Patients' Faith in Their Doctors: Public Psychiatry's Negative Lessons for General Medicine," *Bulletin of the New York Academy of Medicine*, Vol. 71, No. 2; 194–217, Winter 1994.

Lenzer, Jeanne, "Drug Secrets: What the FDA isn't telling," *Slate*, September 27, 2005.

Levy, D., "Ghostwriters: a Hidden Resource for Drug Makers," *USA Today*, September 25, 1996.

Lexchin, J., "What Information Do Physicians Receive from Pharmaceutical Representatives?" *Canadian Family Physicians*, 43:941–945, 1997.

Tanner, Lindsey, "AMA Refuses to Back a Ban on Drug Ads," Associated Press, June 21, 2005.

Lutz, Katherine, "Can a Popular Antidepressant Cause Teenage Suicide?" *Boston Globe*, August 5, 2003.

Marsa, Linda, "The Cold Virus Meets Its Match," *Los Angeles Times*, December 17, 2001.

McNamara, Stephen H., and Wes A. Siegner, "FDA Has Substantial and Sufficient Authority to Regulate Dietary Supplements," Food and Drug Law Institute, 57: 15–24, 2002.

Morgenstern, L.B., C.M. Viscoli, W.N. Kernan, L.M. Brass, J.P. Broderick, E. Feldmann, et al., "Use of Ephedra-Containing Products and Risk for Hemorrhagic Stroke," *Neurology*, 60(1): 132–35, 2003.

Morton, R.H. "Effects of Caffeine, Ephedrine and their Combinations on Time to Exhaustion During High-intensity Exercise," *European Journal of Applied Physiology*, 79(4): 379–81, 1999.

Nelkin, D. "An Uneasy Relationship: The Tensions Between Medicine and the Media," *The Lancet*, 347(9015): 1600–03, 1996.

"New Antipsychotic Drugs Worrying, New Study Shows," *Globe and Mail*, September 13, 2005.

"Off the Charts: Pay, Profits, and Spending by Drug Companies," *Families USA*, Pub No. 01-104.

"The Other Drug War: Big Pharma's 625 Washington Lobbyists," *Public Citizen*, July 2001.

"The Pharmaceutical Industry Into Its Second Century: From Serendipity to Strategy," Boston Consulting Group, pp. 51–56, January 1999.

"Pharmaceutical R&D: Costs, Risks and Rewards," Office of Technology Assessment, U.S. Congress, 1993.

O'Neil, John, "Treatments: Statins and Diabetes: New Advice," *New York Times*, April 20, 2004.

Oral Testimony of the Consumer Healthcare Products Association, to the White House Commission on Complementary and Alternative Medicine Policy, Minnesota Town Hall Meeting, March 16, 2001.

Peterson, M, "What's Black and White and Sells Medicine?" *New York Times*, August 27, 2000.

"Prescription Drugs and Mass Media Advertising," The National Institute for Health Care Management Foundation, 2001.

"Prescription Drug Expenditures in 2000: The Upward Trend Continues," The National Institute for Health Care Management Foundation, May 2001.

"The Relation Between Voluntary Notification and Material Risk in Dietary Supplement Safety," *FDA Docket, 2000*, 00N–1200(41).

Rennie, D., and A. Flanagin, "Authorship! Authorship! Guests, Ghosts, Grafters, and the Two-sided Coin," *JAMA*, 271:469–71, 1994.

"Report of the Advisory Review Panel on OTC Cold, Cough, Allergy, Bronchodilator, and Antiasthmatic Products," *Federal Register*, 41:38403, 1976.

Ricks, Delthia, Roni Rabin, "Drug panelists' links under fire, *Newsday*, July 19, 2004.

Rizvi K., et al., "Do lipid-lowering drugs cause erectile dysfunction? A systematic review," *Family Practice*, 19: 95–98, Feb 2002.

Rochon, P.A., J.H. Gurwitz, R.W. Simms, et al., "A study of manufacturer-supported trials of nonsteroidal anti-inflammatory drugs in the treatment of arthritis," *Arch Intern Med.*, 154: 157–63, 1994.

"Safety Assessment and Determination of a Tolerable Upper Limit for Ephedra," *CANTOX Report on Ephedra*, CANTOX Health Sciences International, 2000.

Samenuk, D., M.S. Link, M.K. Homoud, R. Contreras, T.C. Theohardes, P.J. Wang, N.A. Estes, "Adverse Cardiovascular Events Temporally Associated with Ma Huang, an Herbal Source of Ephedrine." *Mayo Clinic Proceedings*: 77(1): 12–6, 2002.

Schoenhals, Kim, "Need a Lift? Natural Remedies for Improving Mood," *Nutrilearn.com*, Virgo Publishing, July 20, 2005.

Sensenbrenner, F. James, "GAO Report Questions Science Behind FDA's Action on Ephedrine Alkaloids," Committee on Science, August 4, 1999.

Siegner, Wes A. "New laws are not needed," *USA Today*, July 16, 2003.

Siig, Melissa, "Life After Lipitor: Is Pfizer product a quick fix or dangerous drug? Residents experience adverse reactions," *Tahoe World*, January 29, 2004.

Shekelle, P.G., M.L. Hardy, M. Maglione, and S.C. Morton, "Ephedra and Ephedrine for Weight Loss and Athletic Performance Enhancement: Clinical Efficacy and Side Effects." *Agency for Healthcare Research and Quality*, 2002.

Sternberg, Steve, Julie Appleby, "Researchers Deal Crestor Another Blow," *USA Today*, May 24, 2005.

Suissa, S., P. Ernst, J.F. Boivin, R.I. Horwitz, B. Habbick, D. Cockroft, et al., "A Cohort Analysis of Excess Mortality in Asthma and the Use of Inhaled Beta-agonists," *Am J Respir Crit Care Med.*, 149:604, 1994.

Swain, R.A., D.M. Harsha, J. Baenziger, R.M. Saywell Jr. "Do Pseudoephedrine or Phenylpropanolamine Improve Maximum Oxygen Uptake and Time to Exhaustion?" *Clin J Sport Med.*, 7(3): 168–73, 1997.

Taylor, H., and R. Leitman, eds. "Widespread Ignorance of Regulation and Labeling of Vitamins, Minerals and Food Supplements, According to a National Harris Interactive Survey," *Harris Interactive Health Care News*, 2(23): 1–5, 2002.

"Top-selling drug (Seroxat/Paxil) linked to increased suicide risk," *London Times*, August 22, 2005.

Turner, Ronald B., et al., "Echinacea," *NEJM*, 353: 341–48, July 28, 2005.

Turner, Ronald, B., M.D., Margaret T. Wecker, Gerhardt Pohl, Theodore J. Witek, Eugene McNally, Roger St. George, Birgit Winther, Frederick G. Hayden, "Efficacy of Tremacamra, a Soluble Intercellular Adhesion Molecule 1, for Experimental Rhinovirus Infection: A Randomized Clinical Trial," *Journal of the American Medical Association (JAMA)*, 281: 1797–04, May 19, 1999.

"Tylenol Deaths," *Journal of Pediatrics*, 132, 1998.

Vahedi, K., V. Domigo, P. Amarenco, and M.G. Bousser, "Ischaemic stroke in a sportsman who consumed Ma Huang extract and creatine monohydrate for body building," *Journal of Neurol Neurosurg Psychiatry*, 68(1): 112–13, 2000.

Vansal, S.S., and D.R. Feller, "Direct Effects of Ephedrine Isomers on Human Beta-adrenergic Receptor Subtypes," *Biochemical Pharmacology*, 58(5): 807–10, 1999.

"Vitamin E Roundup," Council for Responsible Nutrition (CRN), Mar 2005.

Walker, A. "The Relation between Voluntary Notification and Material Risk in Dietary Supplement Safety." *FDA Docket, 2000*, 00N–1200.

Wazana, A. "Physicians and the Pharmaceutical Industry: Is a gift ever just a gift?" *JAMA*, 283, No. 3, 2000.

Wheatley, D., "Kava and Valerian in the Treatment of Stress-induced Insomnia," *Phytotherapy Research*, 15: 549–51, 2001.

Whitaker, Robert, "Anatomy of an Epidemic: Psychiatric Drugs and the Astonishing Rise of Mental Illness in America," *Ethical Human Psychology and Psychiatry*, Volume 7, Number I: 23–35, Spring 2005.

White, L.M., S.F. Gardner, B.J. Gurley, M.A. Marx, P.L. Wang, and M. Estes, "Pharmacokinetics and cardiovascular effects of ma-huang (*Ephedra sinica*) in normotensive adults," *J Clin Pharmacol*, 37(2): 116–22, 1997.

Willman, David, "How a New Policy Led to Seven Deadly Drugs," *Los Angeles Times*, December 20, 2000.

Winslow, Ron, "The Birth of a Blockbuster: Lipitor's Route out of the Lab," *Wall Street Journal*, January 24, 2000.

Woelk, H., "Comparison of St. John's wort and imipramine for treating depression: randomized controlled trial," *BMJ*, 321(7260): 536–39, 2000.

Wolfe, Sidney M., "Ephedra: Scientific Evidence Versus Money/Politics," *Science*, April 19, 2003.

Wolfe, S.M. "Why do American drug companies spend more than $12 billion a year pushing drugs? Is it education or promotion?," *J of Gen Int Med*, 11: 637–39, 1996.

Wood, A.J.J., C.M. Stein, and R. Woosley, "Making medicines safer—the need for an independent drug safety board," *N Engl J Med.*, 339: 1851–54, 1998.

Books

Abramson, John, M.D., *Overdosed America*. New York: HarperCollins, 2004.

Angell, Marcia, M.D., *The Truth About the Drug Companies*. New York: Random House, 2004.

Bian, Tonda R., *The Drug Lords: America's Pharmaceutical Cartel*, No Barriers Publishing, 1997.

Chang, H.M. and P.P.H. But, *Pharmacology and Applications of Chinese Materia Medica*, World Scientific, 1986.

Cohen, Jay, *Over Dose: The Case Against the Drug Companies: Prescription Drugs, Side Effects, and Your Health*. New York: Penguin, 2001.

Fried, Stephen M., *Bitter Pills: Inside the Hazardous World of Legal Drugs*. New York: Bantam Doubleday Dell, 1998.

Greider, Katharine, *The Big Fix: How the Pharmaceutical Industry Rips Off American Consumers*. New York: Public Affairs, 2003.

Hawthorne, Fran, *Inside the FDA*. New York: John Wiley & Sons, 2005.

_____, *The Merck Druggernaut: The Inside Story of a Pharmaceutical Giant*. New York: John Wiley & Sons, 2003.

Higgs, Robert (ed.), Ronald W. Hansen, Paul H. Rubin, *Hazardous to Our Health? FDA Regulation of Health Care Products*, Independent Institute, 1995.

Hilts, Philip J., *Protecting America's Health: The FDA, Business, and One Hundred Years of Regulation*, New York: A.A. Knopf, 2003.

Huang, K.C,, *The Pharmacology of Chinese Herbs*, CRC Press, 1993.

Kassirer, Jerome P., M.D., *On the Take: How Medicine's Complicity with Big Business Can Endanger Your Health*, New York: Oxford University Press, 2005.

Marsa, Linda, *Prescription for Profits: How the Pharmaceutical Industry Bankrolled the Unholy Marriage Between Science and Business*, New York: Scribner's, 1999.

Miller, Henry I., John J. Cohrssen, and Terry L. Anderson, *To America's Health: A Proposal to Reform the Food and Drug Administration*, Hoover Institution Press Publication, 2000.

Moore, Thomas J., *Deadly Medicine: Why Tens of Thousands of Heart Patients Died in America's Worst Drug Disaster*. New York: Simon & Schuster, 1995.

Mundy, Alicia, *Dispensing With the Truth: The Victims, the Drug Companies, and the Dramatic Story Behind the Battle over Fen-Phen*. New York: St. Martin's Press, 2001.

Papas, Andreas M., and Jean Carper, *The Vitamin E Factor: The Miraculous Antioxidant for the Prevention and Treatment of Heart Disease, Cancer, and Aging.* New York: HarperCollins, 1999.

Ravnskov, Uffe, M.D., Ph.D., *The Cholesterol Myths: Exposing the Fallacy that Saturated Fat and Cholesterol Cause Heart Disease.* Winona Lake, IN: New Trends Publishing, 2000.

Stauber, John, and Sheldon Rampton, *Trust Us We're Experts: How Industry Manipulates Science and Gambles with Your Future*, Los Angeles: J.P. Tarcher, 2002.

Tang, W. and G. Eisenbrand, *Chinese Drugs of Plant Origin.* New York: Springer-Verlag, 1992.

Web sites

Alliance for Natural Health: www.alliance-natural-health.org

American Botanical Council: www.herbalgram.org

American Council on Science and Health (ACSH): www.acsh.org

American Holistic Health Association: www.ahha.org

American Obesity Association: www.obesity.org

Robert Scott Bell, "Jump Start Your Health": www.rsbell.com

Centers for Disease Control and Prevention: www.cdc.gov

Center For Consumer Freedom (CCF): www.ccf.org

Center for Media and Democracy (PR Watch): www.prwatch.org

Center for Public Integrity: www.publicintegrity.org/dtaweb/home.asp

Center for Science in the Public Interest (CSPI): www.cspinet.org

Consumer Labs: www.consumerlab.com

Council for Responsible Nutrition: www.crnusa.org

Ephedra Education Council: www.ephedrafacts.com

FDA News: www.fda.gov/opacom/hpwhats.html

FDA conflicts of interest Web site: www.lasikinfocenter.net/Webpages/FDA%20Conflicts%20of%20Interest%20Webpage.htm

FDA Review.Org—A Project of the Independent Institute: www.fdareview.org/glossary.shtml#elixir

Food and Nutrition Board (FNB) of the National Academy of Sciences: www.iom.edu/IOM/IOMHome.nsf/Pages/About+FNB

Food Policy Institute at the Consumer Federation of America: www.consumerfed.org

Harvard School of Public Health Nutrition Source: www.hsph.harvard.edu/nutritionsource

International Advocates for Health Freedom: www.iahf.com

International Food Information Council Foundation (IFIC): www.ific.org/food

Steven Milloy: www.junkscience.com

National Advisory Council for Complementary and Alternative Medicine (NAC-CAM): www.nccam.nih.gov

National Food Processors Association: www.nfpa-food.org

National Institutes of Health: www.nih.gov

News Target: www.newstarget.com

Office of Dietary Supplements, National Institutes of Health:
    www.dietary-supplements.info.nih.gov

PharmaVoice: www.pharmalinx.com

Pharmaceutical Research and Manufacturers of America: www.phrma.org

Physicians Committee for Responsible Medicine: www.pcrm.org

Public Citizen: www.citizen.org

QuackWatch: www.quackwatch.com

RAND Report:
    www.fda.gov/OHRMS/DOCKETS/98fr/95n-0304-bkg0003-ref-07-01-
    index.htm

RxPolicy: PhRMA Watch: www.rxpolicy.com/phrma.html

University of California-Berkeley Wellness Letter: www.berkeleywellness.com

Index

Hastert, Dennis 285
Hatch, Orrin 24, 326, 314, 348
HDL cholesterol 33
Health food retailers 70
Health Sciences Institute 14, 323
HealthDay Reporter, 204
health-food industry 20
HealthPartners Research Foundation 148
heart disease 12, 31, 33–39, 41, 45–46, 48–53, 55, 68, 76, 80, 82, 86–87, 102–104, 106–108, 110–113, 120–121, 123–124, 179, 212, 214, 225, 231–232, 344, 356–357, 367
Heart Protection Study 103, 121, 360
heartburn 28, 34, 39, 42–43, 45, 58–59, 78, 94, 150–151, 185, 315–316, 344
heatstroke 221, 227, 265, 288
Helicobacter pylori 44
Hemingway, Mariel 23
hepatitis 129
Herb Research Foundation 85
Herbalife International 334
herbs 13, 24, 28, 32, 52, 59, 64–65, 109, 222, 224–225, 250, 280, 301, 310, 320, 340, 350, 367
hereditary blood disorders 141
heroin 92
Hershey Foods 188

Heymsfield, Steven, M.D. 277
high-fructose corn sweeteners (HFCS) 106–107
high-protein diet 36
Hippisley-Cox, Julia 173–174
histamine 42
Holguin, Fernando M.D. 47
Holmer, Alan F. 292
Holt, Rush 285
homocysteine 49, 78, 111–112
hormone replacement therapy 86–87
hormones 25, 86–87, 102, 111, 297
horny goat weed 53
Horowitz,, B. Zane, M.D. 40
horse chestnut 53
Horton, Richard 174
Hospital for Sick Children 141, 143
House Subcommittee on Oversight and Investigations 11, 271, 295
Huber, Gary 242
Hughes, Howard 19
Hulsey, Thomas C., D.Sc. 306
human guinea pig 70, 127, 129, 131, 133, 135, 137, 139, 141, 143, 145, 147, 149, 151, 153
Hutchins, Grover M., M.D. 239, 269
hydrochloric acid 43
hydrocodone 264
Hyman, Phelps & McNamara, P.C. 21
hyperlipidemia 81

hyperosmolar coma 146
hyperreflexia 164
hypertension 31, 41, 49, 73, 78, 80, 104, 111, 113, 189–190, 206–211, 214, 225, 229, 282, 305, 356
hypochlorhydria 44
hypohydration 228
hypomania 164
hypothermia 237

IBM 8
ibuprofen 45, 100, 111, 174, 233, 304
Illinois Retail Merchants Association 258
IMS Health 33, 51, 184, 190
Indiana Bible College 155–156
Indianapolis Police Department 160
Indianapolis Star 157, 160, 162, 164
inflammation 36–38, 44–45, 53, 102, 106, 124
infomercials 26, 68, 81, 132, 184
insomnia 53, 157, 230, 244, 252, 301–302, 310–311, 365
Institute of Food Technologists 25, 297
Institute of Medicine (IOM) 149, 332
institutional review board (IRB) 89
insulin 63, 107, 111, 305
interferon 349
International Advocates for Health Freedom (IAHF) 323–324, 369

Tagamet 151
Tahoma Clinic 319
TAP Pharmaceutical
  Products, Inc. 34, 152,
  315
Targeted Genetics Corp.
  138
Tauzin, Billy 11, 271,
  288–289, 292, 347
teenagers 55, 159, 276
Texas Department of
  Health 279
thalassemia 141
*The Truth About the
  Drug Companies* 55,
  185, 366
Thomas, Bill 285
Thompson, Jenny 14,
  323
Thomson Corp. 128
thrombosis 133–134,
  144
Thune, John 285–286
Tice, Jeffrey A., M.D.,
  311
tobacco 113, 187–188,
  222, 257
tofu 48
tomatoes 46, 48
Topol, Eric 125
Tostitos Light 83
tranquilizers 264
Trans World Airways
  19
tranylcypromine 225
Traub, Michael, N.D.
  132
Travis, Randy 23
Treacy, John 98
tremor 164, 252
triglycerides 36, 39, 107
trimethylglycine 59, 78
Trippe, Juan 23
Trojan horse 296–297
Trudeau, Kevin 68
Tums 42

tuna 48, 196
turmeric 46
Turner, Ronald B., M.D.
  306, 308
Tylenol 61, 157, 365

Ucyclyd Pharma 152
ulcers 42, 44, 53
unfunded mandates 25
University of
  Washington Study 73
Upjohn 188
Upton, Fred 285
urinary incontinence
  158
U.S. Court of Appeals
  for the First Circuit 21
U.S. Department of
  Agriculture (USDA) 1,
  85, 328, 333, 358
U.S. House 19–20,
  196–197, 271, 295,
  332, 351
U.S. National Library of
  Medicine 93
U.S. Postal Service 26
U.S. Public Interest
  Research Group 116
USA Today 96–98, 104,
  152, 263, 265–267,
  312, 358, 362, 364
Utah Natural Products
  Alliance 243, 302

valdecoxib 174
valerian 53, 310–311,
  365
Vasquez, Michael 277
Vaughan, Bill 118
vegetables 46, 48–49, 79
Viagra 81, 337
Vicodin 264
Vioxx 10, 34, 51, 79, 81,
  99–100, 115–116, 127,
  154, 172–179, 181,
  203, 303, 316, 354

ViroPharma 308–309
vitamin B12 43, 111
vitamin B6 111
vitamin C 47, 319, 321,
  330
vitamin E 6, 11–12, 30,
  47, 59, 78, 110, 190,
  311–313, 315–316,
  319, 330, 344, 360,
  365, 367
vitamins 13, 20, 23–24,
  28, 30, 36, 45, 47–49,
  59, 64, 70, 78, 102, 109,
  319–321, 324–328,
  330–331, 340, 350, 364
Vytorin 103

Walden, Greg 289
Wall Street Journal 165,
  178, 183, 189, 360,
  362, 366
Waller, Donald P.,
  Ph.D. 303
Wal-Mart 54
Walton, Ralph G., M.D.
  83
Warner Lambert 105
watchdogs 7, 89
Waxman, Henry A.
  289
WebMD 2, 4
weight loss 4–5, 42, 52,
  82, 184, 202–203, 220,
  224, 232, 235,
  241–244, 249–251,
  274, 276–277, 283,
  355–356, 358–359, 364
Weiss, Avrum Geurin,
  Ph.D. 165
Welbourn, John 259
Whelan, Elizabeth M.
  186
Whelton, Seamus 49
whistle-blowing 145
whole grains 46, 48, 79
Wilson, James 138

About the Author

Mike Fillon has written about health and medical topics for more than fifteen years. For *Popular Mechanics*, he has written over four hundred articles on a broad variety of medical, technological, and scientific subjects. Recently he wrote six cover stories, including two articles for two of the top-selling issues in the magazine's hundred-year history. Fillon has written more than five hundred consumer-oriented news and feature stories for WebMD, CBS HealthWatch, Doctor's Guide, MSNBC, and the *Reader's Digest* Web sites. He has written both short and feature-length pieces for more than two dozen other publications, including *Health Week, NCN News, Information Week, Arthritis Today, Great Life, Let's Live,* and *Science Digest.* He has also written for the American Cancer Society, Emory University, and the Centers for Disease Control and Prevention. Additionally, he has been interviewed on numerous radio shows and has appeared on the *Weekend Today Show* and *American Morning with Paula Zahn.*

Fillon has recently published three successful health books: *Real RDAs for Real People, Ephedra Fact & Fiction,* and *The Good Digestion Guide,* as well as the booklets *Conquering Caffeine Dependence* and *Conquering Food Triggers.* He also had two books published in 1999: *Natural Prostate Healers* and *Young Superstars of Tennis.* He has contributed a number of chapters for the *Reader's Digest* book *Looking After Your Body.*

Fillon has a master of science degree from the State University of New York Maritime College. He is a member of the American Medical Writer's Association and the National Association of Science Writers.

A native New Yorker, Fillon and his family live in Atlanta.